# Developing Occupation-Centered Programs for the Community

SECOND EDITION

**Linda S. Fazio**, Ph.D., OTR/L, FAOTA

*Professor of Clinical Occupational Therapy*
*Division of Occupational Science and Occupational Therapy*
*University of Southern California*
*Los Angeles, California*

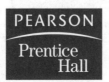

PEARSON

Prentice
Hall

Upper Saddle River, New Jersey

**Library of Congress Cataloging-in-Publication Data**

Fazio, Linda S.
  Developing occupation-centered programs for the community: a workbook for students and professionals/Linda S. Fazio. —2nd ed.
     p. cm.
  Includes bibliographical references and index.
  ISBN-13: 978-0-13-170808-2
  ISBN-10: 0-13-170808-2
  1. Occupational therapy services—Planning.   2. Community mental health services—Planning.
  [DNLM: 1. Occupational Therapy—organization & administration.   2. Community Health
Services—organization & administration.   3. Program Development—methods.   WB 555 F287d
2008]   I. Title.


  RC487.F39 2008
  362.2'2—dc22

                                                                                            2007009367

**Publisher:** Julie Levin Alexander
**Publisher's Assistant:** Regina Bruno
**Executive Editor:** Mark Cohen
**Editorial Assistant:** Nicole Ragonese
**Managing Production Editor:** Patrick Walsh
**Production Management:** Stratford/TexTech
**Production Editor:** Kathy Glidden
**Manufacturing Manager:** Ilene Sanford
**Manufacturing Buyer:** Pat Brown

**Senior Design Coordinator:** Maria Guglielmo
**Director of Marketing:** Karen Allman
**Senior Marketing Manager:** Harper Coles
**Marketing Specialist:** Michael Sirinides
**Marketing Assistant:** Wayne Celia
**Cover Design:** Maria Vicareo
**Cover Illustration:** Getty Images
**Printer/Binder:** Edwards Brothers
**Cover Printer:** Phoenix Color Corporation

Pearson Education LTD.
Pearson Education Australia PTY, Limited
Pearson Education Singapore, Pte. Ltd
Pearson Education North Asia Ltd
Pearson Education Canada, Ltd.
Pearson Educación de Mexico, S.A. de C.V.
Pearson Education—Japan
Pearson Education Malaysia, Pte. Ltd
Pearson Education Inc., Upper Saddle River, New Jersey

Pearson Prentice Hall™ is a trademark of Pearson Education, Inc.
Pearson® is a registered trademark of Pearson plc.
Prentice Hall® is a registered trademark of Pearson Education, Inc.

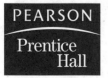

                                                              10 9 8 7 6 5 4
                                          ISBN-10: 0-13-170808-2
                                          ISBN-13: 978-0-13-170808-2

*To my daughters, April and Holly, who are always at the
center of my community, sharing in many of
my occupations, and untiring in their contributions
to the meaning in my life.*

# Contents

| PART I | BUILDING A FOUNDATION   1 |
|--------|---------------------------|

**PART III**          **DEVELOPING THE PROGRAM: PREPARATION AND IMPLEMENTATION PHASE     161**

**PART IV**                                    **REVIEW AND EVALUATION PHASE   263**

# *Preface*

Developing Occupation-Centered Programs for the Community is a practical guide to mark the way for the return of occupational therapy to community practice. Some practitioners, of course, have never left. Rather, they have remained at the center of their patients'/clients' communities throughout their practice, and their models for intervention have always been inclusive of the context and dynamics of community.

For others who may have aligned themselves with the medical/institutional models for treatment returning to community practice may be a reawakening or at least a reminder of the power of the human spirit to forge ahead and to seek out opportunity. We can inspire our communities through skill building and coaching via occupation. We can recognize the intricacy involved in the simplicity of meaning and help our clients to achieve it. We can guide those who embrace wellness and autonomy in achieving that status regardless of the presence of illness or differing abilities. We can advocate for a strong and optimistic future for our clients and for our profession. We can create and build positive communities as well as contribute to existing ones in the interest of equality and social justice.

For the occupational therapy practitioner of one, five, or twenty-five years, the world of practice may have been enlightening, satisfying, disappointing, or all of these things, but it has seldom been without challenge. Practice today and in the future represents yet another challenge—or better, an opportunity.

Beyond the entry-level skills that must be exceptional to practice in the community, the practitioner must have creativity, ingenuity, and resourcefulness. In addition, he or she must have the accompanying commitment to the rights of everyone to have the opportunity, knowledge, and skills to lead a self-assessed and productive life with dignity and quality.

There has never been a time when choosing the community as our context for practice is more appropriate or more needed. And for the student, it is a place to begin. As Margaret Mead has said:

> Never doubt that a small group of thoughtful committed citizens can change the world. Indeed it's the only thing that ever has.
>
> Lecture, University of Wisconsin-Milwaukee (1973)

When I first heard these words during graduate school, they inspired me. Although I had "given up" on occupational therapy for a time, her words encouraged me to return—and to return with a vengeance. I knew that occupational therapy could change the world, even if for only one patient. Later I discovered that neither occupational therapy nor one patient could change the world. In fact, it was occupation and the impact of occupation-centered interventions within the context of community that held this power to bring about change.

I have shared this belief with students for some time and have, with their help, devised ways to bridge their admission into community practice. It is my expectation that this book will guide you in the introductory process of developing occupation-centered community programming. It will help you begin. The spirit and energy that is required to create change is up to you.

I am reminded of a story told by the potter Paul Soldner as he demonstrated his techniques during a student workshop in Colorado during the 1960s. As a student he had observed a photo of a clay pot in an artist's journal. He was enamored with the form and the stature of the pot and tried for years to raise a similar example from his potter's wheel. Finally successful, he raised the pot of his dreams, just like the photo, to a striking four feet in height. It was some time before he discovered that the pot in the photo, his dream for years, was only four inches high. This is what I would like you to do with my community programming examples—take them from four inches to four feet!

The glue that holds the world together is community—in place, in spirit, and in meaning.

*Linda S. Fazio*

# Acknowledgments

The programming described in this text represents the ideas and work of many over a number of years. Most of the examples do not exist as they are described but, in fact, have been collapsed and redesigned into "best practice" scenarios. Not all of them have been tried, and some of the ones that have did not always happen in the way they are presented; you are benefitting from the experiences of many. Nothing happens just right the first time and sometimes not even the second or third times.

Although they have been modified, many of the programming examples were very much influenced by the work of colleagues and students. I have been privileged to enjoy the company of students for most of my professional life. My students have been instrumental in teaching me that the world is not flat; perhaps it cannot even be described in any terms with which we have become comfortable because the world changes with our perceptions. To most students, occupational therapy is a very small window on reality based on a few observations that are most likely made in the hospital or institutional setting. To others, occupational therapy is a fairly unknown commodity and is little more than a blank canvas of opportunity upon which one is preparing to paint a future. I am always amazed by the creativity of students and their hard work and most of all by their untiring "goodness" and trust in the buoyancy of the human spirit. If practice is changed, they will be the ones to do it.

I would like to thank all of my colleagues, first at Texas Woman's University and now at the University of Southern California and Mount St. Mary's College. They have contributed to my thoughts and ideas, some reflected in this book and some not.

I specifically would like to thank Florence A. Clark, Chair of the Division of Occupational Science and Occupational Therapy at the University of Southern California, through her leadership an environment has been created that is rich with ideas and opportunities—an environment that fosters creativity, excitement, and exploration.

I would also like to thank Lynn Whitley, Education Program Coordinator for the Sea Grant Program at the University of Southern California, who so generously shared information and cooperation as we worked together in the development of the Sea Grant/Parent-Child Education Program. In addition, I would like to thank Dyanne Van Peter, Research and Development Coordinator for the Social Science Research Institute and Project Coordinator of the Parent-Child Education Program, who provided many of the photographs.

I most certainly wish to thank my students both at the University of Southern California and in the former Occupational Therapy Assistant Program at Mount St. Mary's College in Los Angeles. Specifically, I would like to thank the following former students for their ideas and work that are represented in this book: Karly Ackermann, Aileen Agcaoili, Leslie Ann Ambrosius, Allison Anodide, Madeleine Arel-Davis, Amy Beneck, Bridget Brown, Lisa Broze, Yvonne Bueno, Christine Carlson, Della Chaffe, Kristy Chow, Lauren Cosgrove, Jennifer Cukingnan, Jan Daimaru, Tegan DaRe, Heather Pyle-De Renne, Aimee Levine-Dickman, Mary Dockter, Shawn Donovan, Hilary Dorinson, Jennifer Doyle, Holly Eck, Julie Faldmo, Lisa Feldman, Sharon Fritz, April Furlong, Ilene Fuson, Dina Gagliano, Denise Goddeyne, Mary Graddon, Karen Green, Melissa Gutierrez, April Haller, Mark Harrison, Angelina Herridge, Junie Hong, Minako Hongo, Joanie Hooper, Lindsay Hughes, Theodore Johnson, Kazumi Kasuya, Harpreet Khandpur, Lydia Kim, Kelly Koelbel, John Kriege, Teri Ladwig, Kelly Lenti, Tricia Lo, Maria Lopez, Kealii Lum, Diana Martin, Tracey Martin, Yoko Masuda, Laura Matsumoto, Carol McAlister, Patricia Harmon-Mills, Marsha Mitchell, Amy Muhlenpoh-Armstrong, Stacy Neill, Brigette Nisly, Suzanna Oses, Amy Peacock-McClennan, Terry Peralta, Shawn Phipps, Michelle Plasch, Shellie Reeder, Jennifer Reimer, Carly Rogers, Sheila Ruiz, Deborah Ryan, Nora Serelis-Garunketis, Rekha Shastry, Randy Siegel, Carrie Spalding, Stephanie Staley, Elly Steese, Teresa Sullivan, Kristin Sutliff, Maria Tan, George Toth-Fejel, Joelle Tran, Sarah Turner, Dyanne Van Peter, Jacy Ver Maas-Lee, Audra Wagner, Ava Wang, Karen Wong, Marcia Wang, Tina Wong, Leslie Wooten, Erin Wyman, and Jeannie Yee.

*Linda S. Fazio*

# *Introduction*

This workbook will provide a basic guide to the development of occupation-centered programs in the community. It offers what the novice needs to know to initiate and further develop programs for community populations. Only a few programs and populations are selected as examples to showcase the process as it has provided primarily service learning opportunities for entry-level occupational therapy students at both the occupational therapy and occupational therapy assistant levels of education. The populations selected are available everywhere, to every student; in many ways they reflect needs that are global.

It is intended that you read Part I and complete the exercises in order to frame your thinking about community populations you may choose to serve. It is not enough to "do;" the "doing" is ever so much more effective if one operates from a paradigm of knowing "why." Knowing why, or establishing the theory to support the actual doing, comes from the best work and ideas of many researchers and disciplines. In addition, Part I will help to stimulate your personal assessment of what you, the programmer, can and do bring to the process—how you can bring a personal perspective that will make your program unique.

Parts II, III, and IV explain the process of community program development step-by-step and intend that you use your own programming example in the exercises. Just as one learns to cook by following a recipe, so does one learn to efficiently and effectively design community programs. To continue the metaphor . . . few experienced cooks continue to rely on a written recipe but go on to creatively enhance the basic instructions with new ingredients and variations in the mix. So will you.

Part V provides brief snapshots of programming for children through older adulthood. The programs have been selected to best illustrate the processes outlined in earlier sections, as well as highlight important elements that are central to all community programming. Of course there are many ways to program for the needs of children and adults; they are infinite, but the process of program development remains the same.

The workbook format may be used in two or perhaps more teaching approaches. One approach occurs in the classroom, with a lecture/participation format, aided by the accompanying instructional materials. With this approach, students may work on the development of one program or several, perhaps where service learning or Level I fieldwork already exists. The workbook also provides an effective self-teaching guide for the student or practitioner who is engaged in independent community program development.

It is important to remember that this workbook is for those who are learning the process of occupation-centered community programming. For those who wish to extend their learning, there are multiple references and Web sites provided within the content and following the description of each process, and within each program scenario in Part V.

# Reviewers

## Second Edition Reviewers

**Deborah Amini,** MEd., OTR/L, CHT
Director, Occupational Therapy
  Assistant Program
Cape Fear Community College
Wilmington, North Carolina

**Rebecca A. Barton,** OTR, DHS
Assistant Professor and Director of
  Fieldwork
School of Occupational Therapy
University of Indianapolis
Indianapolis, Indiana

**Ron Beebe,** MS., OT, LMFT., Psy.D
Assistant Professor
University of Indianapolis
Indianapolis, Indiana

**Kathy B. Bruner,** MEd., OTR/L
Program Director
Salt Lake Community College
Salt Lake City, Utah

**Sherrilene Classen,** Ph.D., MPH, OTR/L
Assistant Professor
College of Public Health
Gainesville, Florida

**Tina Gelpi,** OTD., OTR/L
Assistant Professor/Chair
Florida Gulf Coast University
Fort Myers, Florida

**Susan Gregitis,** Ed.D., OTR/L
Assistant Professor
Florida Gulf Coast University
Fort Myers, Florida

**Sherrill Harnish,** MA., OTR
Coordinator, Clinical Education
COTA-to-MOT Bridge Program
  Coordinator
Interim Associate Coordinator,
  Houston Center
Texas Woman's University
Denton, Texas

**Angela Hissong,** DEd, OTR/L, CAPS
Occupational Therapy Program Director
Penn State University-Mont Alto Campus
Mont Alto, Pennsylvania

**Steve Hoppes,** Ph.D., OTR/L
Associate Professor
University of Oklahoma
Tulsa, Oklahoma

**Jennifer Johnson,** Ph.D., OTR/L
Assistant Professor
University of Central Arkansas
Conway, Arkansas

**Kathleen Matuska,** MPH., OTR
Associate Professor/Program Director
College of St. Catherine
St. Paul, Minnesota

**Irene Phillips,** Ed.D., MA., OTR/L, MPA
Associate Professor
Winston-Salem State University
Winston-Salem, North Carolina

**Leslie Roundtree,** MBA., OTR/L
Acting Program Director
Chicago State University
Chicago, Illinois

**Jennifer J. Saylor,** MEd., OT/L
OTA Program Director/Fieldwork
    Coordinator
New Hampshire Community Technical
    College-Claremont
Claremont, New Hampshire

**Anne Shordike,** Ph.D., OTR/L
Associate Professor
Eastern Kentucky University
Richmond, Kentucky

**Vicki Smith,** Ed.D., MBA., OTR/L
Professor and Chair of
    Occupational Therapy
Keuka College
Keuka Park, New York

## First Edition Reviewers

**S. Kay Ashworth,** MAT., OTR/L
Chair, Occupational Therapy Assistant
Sinclair Community College
Dayton, Ohio

**Shirley Jackson,** MS., OTR/L, FAOTA
Associate Professor/Chair
Howard University
Washington, District of Columbia

**Deane B. McCraith,** MS., OTR/L, LMFT
Associate Professor
Boston University
Boston, Massachusetts

**Judith Melvin,** Ph.D., OTR/L
Chair, Occupational Therapy
Arizona School of Health Sciences
Phoenix, Arizona

CHAPTER 1

# Community: What Do We Mean?

## Learning Objectives

1. To appreciate the many definitions and meanings associated with *community*
2. To understand the distinction between *community* and *the community*
3. To understand *community* as an organizing theme in our development of occupation-centered programs
4. To appreciate the potential role of occupation-centered practitioners as community change agents

## Key Terms

1. Community
2. Locale
3. Social Capital
4. Reciprocity
5. Cultural Shifting
6. Change Agent
7. Gatekeepers
8. Key Informants
9. Chaos Theory
10. Change Curve

# How Do We Define Community?

## Early Foundational Work: Sociologists and Anthropologists

**Community**, with its accompanying definitions and scope of investigation, has long been a central theme in the study of sociology. In fact, most of the earlier, foundational work was done by sociologists. When we review the sociological literature, we find that this discipline has established a number of definitions for the term. Lyon (1987) noted some ninety-four in the sociological literature of 1955 (p. 5). Although there were many definitions noted in his review of the literature at the time, he was able to establish three common characteristics: **locale**, common ties, and social interactions. Other sociological researchers, including Park (1936) and Bernard (1973), concurred with these common characteristics. In general, though, the use of locale or reference to place as a central definition and descriptor for community has been widely accepted across disciplines.

Anthropologists have also long shared an interest in community, particularly as defined by locale. Although Hillery (1955) supported the view that locale is a central characteristic of community, he proposed that groups of people differing in place and time may also differ in their interpretations of meaning surrounding locale. He distinguished between community and *the* community. His distinction separated the idea of common ties and social interactions from locale. In his view, community is the most powerful of the two concepts, emphasizing moral commitment, social cohesion, and continuity in time, or what might be described by the German term *Gemeinschaft*. In his examples, which are based on modes of subsistence, agricultural peoples attach a fixed settlement to their meaning of locale, while hunters/gatherers who subsist by traveling over large geographic areas define locale as a less identifiable place. It is likely that even hunters and gatherers, along with nomadic groups who also travel over wide areas, designate locales and attach significance to them (that is, sources of water, ceremonial/burial sites, and so on). These locales may be designated sites where nomadic bands or groups join together to form communities, albeit a looser definition of community than that of an agricultural group. Those who have studied the transitions from hunter/gatherer to agriculturist have noted that when groups first begin to tend plants and then to grow them, they become locked to a site, or locale (Childe, 1953; Heiser, 1973). Perhaps these groups then become locked to a broader concept of community as well.

Also discussing community from an anthropological perspective, Moore (1996) reminds us that in biology, community refers to a breeding population. His discussions center around bands as the elemental human communities of hunters and gatherers (Moore, 1996; p. 105). As biological creatures, humans also have breeding-population communities. But community means a good deal more to humans than a group with which one may breed. According to Moore, community is "the unit that orchestrates individual movements in space over time," and in our cultural world, "community is the setting in which, from one generation to the next, human beings learn how to be fully human" (Moore, 1996; p. 96). In fact, this community unit is also where cultural creativity and innovation take place.

McKnight (1988) emphasized a common goal as the motivating reason people come together. For him, community was a collective association driven toward a common theme or goal. Green and Kreuter (1991) focus on common values and mutual concern for "their" group (pp. 504–505). And Nisbet (1972) emphasized that community thrives on self-help and equal consent. He suggested that people come together to do something that cannot be done in isolation. These are all important points for those of us who wish to encourage change in the individual, the group, and the larger community as well.

## Exercise 1

We have introduced several foundational terms to assist in our understanding of how and why people come together to form communities. Locale, common ties, and social interaction are three. Make some notes and discuss with others how these terms may be translated into your own motivation for joining a particular community. Maintaining contact with your family, organizations you joined as a child or adolescent, and your college "community" may be starting points.

_____

_____

_____

_____

_____

# What Does Community Mean Today?

The previous, more historical discussions may shed light on our understanding of the present-day metropolitan and urban communities in which we want to establish programs. Many people today relocate frequently during their lives; most reside far from their communities (locales) of origin. It is likely that more transient attachments may be formed for those who move from one locale to another in pursuit of career and economic opportunity, and a sense of community, with accompanying commitments and responsibilities, may be more tenuous. Of course, any privileges or rights attached to community might also be forfeited—at least those that are offered following a period of investment, or tenure. This view of community would appear to place more responsibility for the attributes and privileges of community as described by Moore (1996) on the family and/or the individual.

## Exercise 2

We might ask ourselves, do these individuals and families have the information and skills to establish communities for themselves? Is this an area we might wish to consider as we develop programming? Consider some of the earlier discussion highlighting historical elements associated with community. Can you think of individuals or groups that appear to be without connection to a community? Note and discuss what information and skills you might offer those who appear to be isolated from your understanding of community:

_____

_____

_____

_____

Metropolitan communities where many cultures come together may also redefine our interpretation of community. Consider these questions in your discussion with others: Will these communities provide stress and disengagement, or will they offer us new definitions of cultural creativity and innovation?

_____

_____

_____

_____

Will we evolve new ways of learning to be "human"? If so, will occupation-centered practitioners have a role in facilitating this new learning? What might be some examples?

_____

_____

_____

_____

How will we identify what kinds of services a community might need, want, and value? It is likely that desired services may vary considerably from one locale to another and from one constituency to another. Cognizant of this potential dilemma, Warren (1987) has proposed that we must understand and appreciate that community, particularly the urban community, represents a "local web of relationships around the locality-relevant functions" (p. ii). In his interpretation, various formal and informal networks within a community are connected to others outside the locality. When one seeks to establish a program in and/or for a community, it will be necessary to appreciate and understand what likely will be an intricate and complex series of relationships "between" communities. Even if we may be planning a program that appears fairly isolated in locale or in conceptualization, we must consider extended and overlapping communities and systems, particularly in the present era of heightened communication and access to information.

Most members of established and formative communities in the United States have at least one or more computers in their households. Individuals and families who may once have been isolated now have access to the virtual community, its' resources, and its' potential liabilities. Parsons (1951) reminded us that even within a community there may be substantial complexity displayed by the interplay between cultures and the varied levels of society. In fact, by establishing a program within a community, we are introducing yet another layer of complexity that may cause temporary shifts in balance. However, these potential shifts can be tempered by establishing the program in developmental increments, as we will describe in this text.

The foregoing is important information as we are designing relevant and meaningful programs for our service populations. As you develop your community profile in Chapter 7, you will consider the following questions:

1. What can we learn about the community itself?
2. Is the community one that appears well established or is it one that is in process?
3. What is the nature of common ties, and what are the patterns of social interaction?
4. Are children part of the community of families?

In fact, do we know how the presence of children impacts on our understanding of community? Are the interactions, communications, and expectations influenced by the presence of children? By the presence of elders? These are provocative questions to be investigated, and they may influence and impact our understanding of so-called specialized communities: older adults; young, childless adults; and institutions serving specific populations.

## Locale, Unity, Technology, and the Future

We know that a community may be represented by no fixed locale at all, and yet Nisbet (1967) suggests that such communities may provide the presence of a strong sense of unity. This may be a significant point of understanding in what we have described as the transient world of today. Nisbet's interpretation of community may help us understand such questions as how and why retirees who move from their long-established homes to high-rise senior residences can either feel that they are part of a community, or feel that they are not. And his interpretation can further help us, as care providers, encourage the building of community for those who feel excluded.

Shifting paradigms responsive to the fluidity of attachment to locale by present-day populations heavily invested in technology may, in fact, define a new, more global sense of community. There are very few people in the world today who are not aware of the virtual community created by the Internet; and many avail themselves of the information and connections it provides as a component of their daily round of occupational engagement. For those who wish to know more, Rheingold (1993) provides an extensive account of living in a virtual community in *Virtual community: Homesteading on the electronic frontier*.

Present and future community practices will certainly correspond with and within virtual worlds. However, we might question this reliance on technology; is it one that encourages a perceived and real sense of community, or does it contribute to isolation and despair? Does the *information highway* take us *home*? Does it establish the boundaries of community in a way that we find comforting and satisfying? Or does this global thinking and loss of attachment to locale prompt individuals today, more than ever before, to lust more for the real and assumed benefits of community? Nisbet (1953, 1967) suggested that this was the case decades ago. Perhaps we are simply redefining and reframing locale to be without boundaries (and restraints), and perhaps we are placing our emphasis on other aspects of community that we deem to be more significant.

## Exercise 3

Consider the above questions. Note your thoughts and discuss the potential impact on community (both positive and negative) resulting from reliance on technology and expansion of virtual worlds; begin by considering how technology and virtual communities have impacted you and your network of social connections:

_____

_____

_____

_____

Community may also be conceptualized in a way that negates both locale and emotional investment; this refers to those communities defined by common interests, intellectual bonds, and/or professional bonds (Goode, 1957; Nisbet, 1953). The community of occupational therapy practitioners, the medical community, and the community of women/men are all examples. We may now also include the evolving "community" of community-practitioners representing many disciplines, interests, and areas of expertise.

Etzioni (1995) describes strengthening connections within and between communities with attention to "communitarian design, architecture, and planning"? (p. 113). In a very practical sense, we can make our physical environments as well as all of the contexts of practice more community friendly; both in private and public spaces. The author goes on to suggest that people be provided with shared space to mingle; and that development be planned in ways that enhance rather than hinder the sociological mix that sustains a community (Etzioni, 1995; p. 314). There are many American and European communities being developed today that offer the opportunity of community-building through meticulous design, as Etzioni (1995) has suggested. It remains to be seen whether these communities sustain older adults as they now sustain young families. Occupational therapy practitioners have long been interested in ensuring access and space for everyone; we can now incorporate the interests of encouraging and sustaining community in our plans as well.

Campbell (1995) offers us one of the most engaging discussions of contemporary community. She describes attributes that, to her, demonstrate a "sense of the whole" (or) community. Most notably: a sense of community ownership, engagement in meaningful work, ecological sustainability, and respect for differences (Campbell, 1995; p. 189). In her observations, these principles or attributes promoted a shared experience of belonging and contributing to something larger than oneself. This is the essence of community and we can find evidence in our programming examples. We may need the author's definition of "ecological sustainability" to see just how this concept may fit what we do. For Campbell (1995), the tenets of ecological sustainability suggest that a "sustainable way of life recognizes that the Earth's resources (food, water, air, etc.) are finite and the growth of all living systems is limited" (Campbell, 1995; pp. 193–194). Campbell (1995) suggests that when our lifestyles are aligned with principles of sustainability, we feel more secure and self-respecting. When they are not, we often feel vaguely uneasy. I commend students who design programs with an interest in ecological sustainability . . . and I'm seeing more of these, many providing service learning opportunities to high school and college students. Roots and Shoots Clubs environmental preservation programs are the most notable examples described in this text, but there are others designed to sustain the human system through meaningful engagement in occupation and activity. It is, perhaps, the health and well-being of the human occupants of this planet that may be the most vulnerable to extinction; and it has always been a core value of occupational therapy to preserve and protect the individual person and his or her engagement in a life of choice.

## Community Centered Practitioners: Who Are They?

As we make our way into the present century, it appears that the pendulum of patient/client care is again swinging away from the institution toward the community. This is true not only for occupational therapy, but also for many health care providers. Just as mental health and illness and the concerns of humane care established our origins as occupational therapists, these same concerns have ushered our return to the community as a favored site for practice—and we are not alone.

## Nurses

Arguably the first practitioner to consider community as a point of service as well as investigation has been the nurse. Early on, home and community-based practices of conventional nursing were recognized as some of the most efficient and effective ways to deliver service to individuals and to families (Clark, 2003). Initially, as was the case with occupational therapists, the community was recognized as a place where a nurse might live, work, and play and it was within this natural environment that services were delivered. But beyond individual care, the concerns of nursing have always actively included public health issues. From the late 1800s, the nursing profession has concerned itself with altering unsafe physical environments, addressing health threatening hygienic conditions of individuals and populations, and with the immunization of children (Stevens and Hall, 1992). These authors also note that, more recently, nursing is devising theoretical structures to address additional community-centered issues such as oppressive social arrangements, economic impoverishment, and political disenfranchisement—all recognized as threats to the safety and well-being of aggregate communities. These practices are referred to as emancipatory, freeing individuals and groups from oppressive situations through education, practice, and action. Clark (2003) discusses the concern of community-centered nursing with the recognition and prevention of societal violence. Her discussions include not only physical and sexual abuse of children and adults, but also concerns of critical incident stress, elder abuse, intimate partner violence, and neglect (Clark, 2003; pp. 757–771). Nursing care today is addressing the multiple needs of whole communities as well as target groups within communities. Occupational therapists and occupational therapy assistants are entering this broader perspective of community practice a bit later than nurses but are quickly adapting to the extension of services and concerns to address the health care, prevention, and wellness needs of complex communities as well as general societal concerns.

## Psychologists and Social Workers

Psychologists also include community in their practice perspectives. Orford (1993) refers to theories of person-in-context, social support, and power and control as concerns of community psychology. Recognizing that communities must be empowered to understand and change organizations and conventional ways to access self-help and non-professional help, psychologists in the community are seen as change-makers as well as professional care providers. Social workers, of course, have seated the core of their practices in communities through aggregates of individuals, and individuals and families within the larger community. Drawing from sociological theories, these practitioners have developed their own theoretical constructs to address the needs of individuals within communities, and the structures of organizations that, at times, may assist or impede successful individual and family interface with the larger community (Hardcastle, Wenocur, and Powers, 2004).

### Interpretations of Practice in the Community

For many of the traditional disciplines providing psychiatric and social services (psychology, social work, occupational therapy), the need to embrace the community as a desired and necessary context for intervention seems apparent. It is difficult to know whether this initial shift into the community was in response to the sweeping socioeconomic pressures and resulting deinstitutionalization of the past thirty or fourty years or whether it was simply recognized as the best mode of care. Oseroff, Longo, and Joseph (1998) suggest that all of these choices to establish practices in the community were proactive, not reactive, including those of occupational therapy. According to these authors, the system reform that has taken place over the last decade in psychiatric service delivery, specifically, has challenged institutional models to suggest that the natural setting may be the most effective arena for service delivery. They are particularly supportive of natural treatment environments for children and young adults. This view has been echoed most recently by many practitioners working with children, including occupational therapists, who suggest that the community environments of family, the home, and the school are the most conducive environments for affecting change in the child (Agrin, 1987; England, 1992; Hanft, Burke, Cahill, Swenson-Miller, and Humphry, 1992; Henggeler, 1996; Hyde and Woodworth, 1994; Nelson and Landsman, 1992; Noonan and McCormick, 1992; Schaaf and Mulrooney, 1989; Schultz, 1992).

Other natural settings favored by occupational therapists and others include community centers, housing units, shelters, and work sites (Vanier and Hebert, 1995). Certainly in areas of prevention and wellness promotion, we must go to multiple communities. This renewed attention to the community as a desired context for intervention is also emphasized in one of the profession's recent guides to practice: the *Occupational therapy practice framework: Domain and process* (AOTA, 2002). In establishing broad parameters for context to provide the most comprehensive and successful interventions for all ages, the *Framework* helps establish our practices in the holistic context of *community*. If we are to use this context of community within which to place our programs to its broadest potential then, certainly, we must understand its intricacies and variability. Use of the *Framework* to assist in formulating our community-centered programming structures will be discussed further in Chapter 8.

## The Meaning of Community for Occupation-Centered Practitioners

An appreciation of the early discussions of the meaning of community and the various definitions that have evolved over time establishes a foundation for our work as community-based practitioners, particularly as we first learn to develop programming in the community. As practitioners in the community, we will address not only the needs of the person, but also societal and environmental factors that impact the health and well being of individuals and populations. We may say that, in its simplest form, a community refers to a person's natural environment; but we know that community is more than location or locale as described earlier; it also refers to relationships. To fully appreciate the concept of community; however, it is necessary to consider that it is based not only on relationships, but also on partnerships and coalitions. According to Brownson (1998), inclusion of relationships in the definition of community has implications for occupational therapy practice that go beyond *locations* of practice. Consideration of relationships expands our thinking across and beyond boundaries that the term community may initially suggest. Context, or actual space, may be important as it influences these relationships, but as we've learned, being present in a delimited space is not enough to constitute "community." Neither are communities bound by familiar geography; consider the global nature of the programs described by Kronenberg, Algado, and Pollard (2005).

Warren (1987), studied the functions of community and identified several factors, or functions, of particular interest to occupation-centered program designers: (1) as a "sociability arena" where members are able to develop friendships through regular interaction; (2) as an "organizational base" where members of the community feel a kindred notion of commonality leading to an organization or unique banding together; and (3) as a "reference group" suggesting an identification (preface). Condeluci (2002) reminds us that the term "community" is the blending of the prefix "com" which means "with," and the root word, "unity," which means togetherness and connectedness. He goes on to suggest that when people come together, in unity, for the sake of a unified theme, a community is formed. (p. 11) All of these elements: a dimension for social enactment, the creation of organizations to form a point of reference/identification ("I belong to . . .") result in potential unity and are central to much of our occupation-centered programming.

## Exercise 4

Think of the organizations you've been a member of. How did they provide an opportunity for enacting social connections and bonds for establishing identity and for developing unity? Make some notes and discuss your thoughts:

_____

_____

_____

_____

Can you further think of community programs you may have volunteered with, or perhaps one you're thinking of developing, particularly those intended to empower adults, adolescents and/or children? Discuss how you think such programs help to build a sense of community for the particular population you have in mind.

---

---

---

---

Ray (1995) uses "community" as a metaphor for what he describes as a world-wide paradigm shift. In his analysis, the world is in crisis, offering both danger and opportunity. He sees community-building as the only viable way to maintain as the world is transformed. (Ray, 1995; p. 18). Jarman and Land (1995) suggest that the best of all possible worlds would be: "to live among people without fear, where trust is given and received freely, a place of belonging, where a sense of connectedness and unity provides the foundation for life sustaining and enhancing interactions." (Jarman and Land, 1995; p. 22). The underlying ideal is that everyone in the community is accepted and treated as a valuable, integral member. An ideal, yes, but one not likely to be achieved in its entirety. Can we aspire to create such microcosms in our programming? I would suggest that we can. As Margaret Mead said in the quotation in the preface to this text: "Never doubt that a small group of thoughtful committed citizens can change the world. Indeed, it's the only thing that ever has."

## Elements of Community Reflected in Occupation-Centered Programming

Condeluci (2002) describes elements of community that would include: (1) *a common theme:* all communities share a common theme and for many of our community programs this "shared theme" is expressed in our mission, and in our goals. Sometimes shared theme is also the reason for meeting, as in the structure of clubs discussed in a later chapter; and (2) the element of *membership:* gathering around a theme-purpose provides a structure for membership. Sometimes membership is formal, as in the structure of the *Roots and Shoots Club* program described in Part V, Chapter 17. Sometimes it is informal, as in the gathering of mothers in a pediatric clinic waiting area. Whether formal or informal, both examples offer potential for effective community programming (Condeluci, 2002; pp. 15–21).

Elements of (3) *ritual* are also important to community-building (Condeluci, 2002; pp. 20–23). Again, rituals may be formal or informal. Saying a pledge, establishing the "behavioral" rules of the day, putting on your club T-shirt all may be formal indicators that you are meeting for an agreed-upon purpose. Although more of an informal ritual, gathering for a cup of coffee and conversation before initiating work in a community garden is no less meaningful.

Also important as elements of community are *patterns, jargon,* and *memory* (Condeluci, 2002; pp. 23–27). Patterns refer to the movements and territory of the

An excellent example of programming utilizing components of patterns and memory is the Tule Indian Tribal History Project of Dr. Gelya Frank and occupational therapy students at the University of Southern California. This project involves students and faculty, and younger tribal members, as they assist tribal elders to document their heritage. Pictures and stories are recorded and archived to trace lineage and events; and, in the process, all members of the tribe experience a renewed sense of community (Dr. Gelya Frank, Personal Communication, May 2005).

members, jargon refers to the shared language a group may use to discuss the common theme, and memory occurs over time as the group, the community, creates a shared history. Patterns, jargon, and memory are central to the functions and character of many ongoing programs.

## Exercise 5

Frequently, we enter established communities in an effort to bring about elements of change. Sometimes these communities appear closed to us and are largely translated through established patterns, ritual jargon, and shared memory. These characteristics may be utilized to support programming, as the Tule Indian project suggests, but at other times they may appear to be intimidating and inhibiting. Examples of potentially intimidating layers of established patterns, ritual jargon, and shared memory are encountered when working with street gangs in the community or in the prison systems. Can you think of such experiences you may have encountered? Note how your example(s) demonstrate the above characteristics and discuss your answers.

_____

_____

_____

_____

_____

## Social Capital and Reciprocity

Changing social constructions in today's society, particularly around family, have caused many to feel isolated. Putnam (2000) refers to this phenomenon as a decline

It was the reestablishment of social capital that prompted the Lunalilo Home program for institutionalized elders on the island of O'ahu, Hawaii (Fazio and Lum, in press, 2008). This program was constructed on concepts of empowerment, self-determination, engagement, and social connectedness; contributing factors to the building of social capital. Also see Chapter 20 for further discussion of this program.

in **social capital** or the connectedness between people (the relationships) in their communities. Specifically, Putnam defines *social capital* as ". . . connections among individuals, social networks, and the norms of reciprocity and trustworthiness that arise from them" (Putnam, 2000; p. 19). It is in response to this decline in social capital that many of our community programming goals are established.

Another characteristic implicit to social capital and of importance to programming is that of **reciprocity**. In its simplest form, reciprocity is the act of looking out for each other; of giving and taking. Our most effective programs will build social capital not only between those we help, but with the broader community as well. For many who are differently abled, the relationships that constitute their social capital are with other people who are differently abled. Successful programming will encourage reciprocity between and among the many layers of community. Jarman and Land (1995) suggest that "most communities are very good at identifying and welcoming those who are like them, but fall woefully short in embracing diversity" (Jarman and Land, 1995; p. 22). In further discussions of the concept of social capital, Condeluci (2002) would caution us to carefully consider our programming for individuals with disabilities. By separating them from the greater community, as many of our programs do, we may believe we are creating reserves of social capital or connectedness, building reservoirs, as it were. We may be further contributing to their isolation, however, by not offering programming that enables the building of relationships with others who are not disabled.

## Cultural Shifting: Bringing Communities Together

**Cultural shifting** is a phrase Condeluci (2002) uses to describe the bridging of two or more communities to foster the inclusion of people with disabilities in the mainstream. Our task is to find a "fit" for our clients/patients/members in existing communities, not to establish pockets of isolated communities. Bear in mind, though, that not all programs targeting only your population are isolative; many populations must first be empowered, encouraged to advocate for themselves before inclusion can occur. Empowering our clients also means allowing them to choose the community they wish to occupy; inclusion may not be their choice.

Programs that are intended to blend or bridge cultures require careful design, and in many ways may seem more complex because each program goal is bridging two or more existing communities. Take, for example, the *Ice Cream Cart* program described in Chapter 17. Middle school students who were differently abled learned to operate a small business alongside students who were not identified as differently abled. Selling ice cream during lunch was the venture. When this core of students moved to junior high school, they mentored other students to take up their business and they "all" were mentors, not just the able students.

Condeluci (2002) suggests that all of us have moved people into the community, in fact most of our programs are right in the middle of the larger community. But these programs have not led to inclusion for the vast majority. Condeluci (2002) describes the practice of establishing a program to change the person (with the identified "problem"), as "chasing the wrong butterfly" (Condeluci, 2002; p. 36). We need to remedy what may be the larger problem as well—that of the attitudes, knowledge, and behavior of the larger culture/community. Many programs are responding to this charge today, raising awareness and offering solutions to the larger community while meeting the needs of their selected population. The acts of building collaborations and partnerships are examples of reciprocity in process. By extending notions of reciprocity beyond our immediate population of interest, we are ensuring greater individual connectedness and future successes. We might suggest that *true* community establishes bonds based on the reciprocal sharing of differences. Jarman and Land recommend that this can only happen if individuals and ideas are made to connect in new ways (Condeluci, 2002; p. 30). To be most effective, all of our program designs must factor in goals for creating relationships beyond the immediate boundaries of our population-driven objectives to build coalitions and relationships with many disimilar communities.

# Occupational Therapy Practitioners as Agents of Change

Consider yourself, the occupation-centered practitioner, as the **change agent**. In this capacity, you design and plan a community program that will bring about change. If your goal is to bring about change that will blend communities, before you attend to the needs of your population you must first identify the larger community (this is part of your profile but may require a more in-depth observation than first considered). Remember that this group has established patterns, rituals, and jargon as well. The first step is to find the point of connection. This would likely blend our programming steps of needs assessment, goal, and objective setting. The second step is what Condeluci (2002) describes as finding the venue or play point (Condeluci, 2002; p. 37). For us, this is the actual program and the context within which it will take place . . . where the two communities come together. Remember that, for us, as occupational therapy practitioners, context has a wider meaning than physical space. It also encompasses culture, social dimensions, personal, spiritual, and temporal elements (AOTA, 2002; p. 611). The complexity of this analysis permits opportunities to make a "just right fit."

There is one more critical element necessary to the bridging of communities, that of **gatekeeper**. The "gatekeeper" is the person who will introduce and endorse your programming and may be an indigenous member of the community who has either formal or informal influence. Those of you who may have considered programming with a Native American population or a street gang know the importance of a gatekeeper. For the Tule River project, the tribal elders were strongly identified as the gatekeepers who would introduce the team of researchers and practitioners; and also endorse their project. It was also the endorsement of this group, the gatekeepers, which would release the funds to permit this project to happen. Gatekeepers occupy many positions and may not even be physical members of the local community: funders and legislators are examples. Sometimes known by other descriptions, these are the people you must partner with, often to gain access to the community and, more importantly, to ensure the success of your program.

Clark (2003) refers to **key informants** as those who, because of their position in the community, possess information and insights about the community (Clark, 2003; p. 322). Key informants may be both formal and informal community leaders. Examples may be public officials, school and health care personnel, prominent business people, and local clergy. For the *Ice Cream Cart* program, the gatekeepers were simply the members of the Student Council, and members of the athletic teams. Gatekeepers are not always in leadership roles (formal leaders), however, and it may take some investigation to find the right person or persons.

## Impetus for Large-Scale Change That Will Impact Communities

Pascale, Millemann, and Gioja (2000) present us with another perspective as we continue to investigate the nature of change. They suggest that innovations of any nature rarely emerge from systems with high degrees of order and stability. Systems in equilibrium lose diversity. What they describe as the condition of being "on the edge of chaos" is the precondition for transformation to take place (Pascale, Millemann, and Gioja, 2000; p. 66). In this era of real and potential overwhelming societal problems, every change agent is operating in this unstable zone. If we, as occupation-centered practitioners who understand what we do about the nature of occupation as it is embedded in individuals within their complex communities, can manage to stay afloat (on the surfboard, as it were) we stand a good chance of making positive changes—the world is ripe for them—it has seldom been closer to the "edge of chaos."

Briggs and David Peat (1999) remind us that humans have had to deal with change since the beginning, but only recently has science recognized change as a fundamental force in the universe. **Chaos theory** was, early on, developed to understand the movements that caused thunderstorms, hurricanes, and other similar phenomena. In today's language, it is being applied to almost every body of information including the nature of social dynamics, and particularly in the study of how organizations form and change. Leadership Acumen (2003), a publication that focuses on executive leadership and senior management, devoted an issue to "change, chaos, and globalization" and, in their words, "other windmills." The point of reference to Don Quixote's "windmills" is to point out that the belief that business leaders, or anyone, can manage change is a fallacy (Acumen, 2003; p. 2). What we may do, including those of us who wish to engage in developing community programs, is to understand the "**change curve.**" The idea of a change curve was originally identified by Elisabeth Kübler-Ross in her book dealing with death and dying (1975). The change curve process is a recognition that change is not cyclical but rather an ongoing process that never returns to status quo. Our community programs, to grow and fluorish, must have a built-in understanding that adaptation and re-invention in response to inevitable change will be a necessary working mechanism of the program.

Briggs and Peat (1999) suggest that "chaos" is evolving into a cultural metaphor (Briggs and Peat, 1999; p. 32). When we consider chaos as a metaphor, we can query a wide range of questions relevant to our interest in communities—why they change, how to program when change is most likely, and, perhaps, how to predict the consequences of change. Chaos theory suggests that, instead of resisting life's uncertainties, we should embrace the possibilities they offer.

Young (1994) focuses specifically on change in social systems. He refers to chaos theory as an elegant mathematical grounding for a postmodern social science which affirms variety and change as natural attributes or characteristics of social systems. Of particular interest are his explanations of chaos theory, in his words the "new and evolving science of complexity that offers support and direction for postmodern understandings which honor change, variety, and disorder" (Young, 1994; p. 5). His description of attractors as those agents that compel change is complementary to the work of Pascale, Millemann, and Gioja (2000, pp. 69–75). Attractors are of interest to those wishing to understand change. They are defined as analagous to a compass, "orienting a living system in one particular direction" and "they provide organisms with the impetus to migrate out of their comfort zone" (Pascale, Millemann, and Gioja, 2000; p. 69). These authors provide complex and relevant explanations for the ways in which attractors draw a complex system in a particular direction. What they describe as strange attractors are those that lure systems to the very edge of chaos. There is an interplay between the survival instinct and a hostile environment. We might consider occupational therapy and the changes that have occurred in practice respondent to the complex demands of managed health care as an example. Certainly, all of those working in the community to bring about change are in a position to utilize attractors to shake up the comfort zones of our communities and to make change the desirable outcome for all those involved.

# Community and Occupation-Centered Practice: A Summary

With the words "community" and "occupation-centered practice," we bring together the elements of a theme that will organize our return to the community in the new millennium. Certainly, occupational therapy practitioners have been in the community before (perhaps always), but this time occupation will be at the center of our practices. Centering our practice in occupation frees us to utilize our knowledge and skills in many new, creative, and marketable venues. By locating our programs in the community, defined by locale or spirit, we are accepting the challenge of responding to that community's need with what must be new and innovative "ways of being." We have identified some of the strategies to bring about change, and to provide a map for innovation. Yearly, vast populations are excluded from access to health care; therefore, it is imperative that we do more than ever before to help prevent illness and trauma and that we provide information, access, skills, and caring to "even out the odds" and to empower those who are at risk for becoming new members of the disenfranchised.

Spurred by a desire to extend democracy beyond what she described as its political expression and sensitive to a strong need to extend humanitarian values and concerns, Addams (1893–1990) was dedicated to the community represented by the evolving Chicago location of Hull House. Her commitment and resulting work, which was followed by Slagle (1922); Slagle and Robeson (1933), established our legacy by placing occupation strongly at the center of community. Their combined philosophies and commitment to the community they served provide the cognitive and emotional map that will guide us as we reestablish our presence in service to our communities.

## *References*

Addams, J. (1990). The subjective necessity for social settlements. In *Twenty years at hull house*. Urbana: University of Illinois Press. (Original work published 1893)

Agrin, A. (1987). Occupational therapy with emotionally disturbed children in a public elementary school. *Occupational Therapy in Mental Health, 7*, 105–113.

American Occupational Therapy Association. (2002). *The occupational therapy practice framework: Domain and process* (p. 611). Bethesda, MD: AOTA.

Bernard, J. (1973). *The sociology of community*. Glenview, IL: Scott Foresman.

Briggs, J., & Peat, D. (1999). *Seven life lessons of chaos*. New York: Harper and Row.

Brownson, C. (1998). Funding community practice: Stage 1. *American Journal of Occupational Therapy, 52*(1), 60–64.

Campbell, S. (1995). A sense of the whole: The essence of community. In K. Gozdz (Ed.), *Community building* (pp. 189–197). San Franciso, CA: Sterling and Stone Publishers.

Childe, V. G. (1953). *New light on the most ancient East*. New York: W. W. Norton.

Clark, M. J. (2003). *Community health nursing: Caring for populations*. Upper Saddle River, NJ: Prentice Hall.

Condeluci, A. (2002). *Cultural shifting: Community leadership and change*. St. Augustine, FL: Training Resources Network, Inc.

England, M. J. (1992). Building systems of care for youth with mental illness. *Hospital and Community Psychiatry, 43*, 630–633.

Etzioni, A. (1995). Back to we: The communication nexus. In K. Gozdz (Ed.), *Community building* (pp. 305–317). San Francisco, CA: Sterling and Stone Publishers.

Fazio, L., & Lum, K. (2008 in press). Empowering older adults through the intergenerational sharing of native Hawaiian cultural traditions. In: M. Scaffa, M. Reitz, & M. Pizzi, (Eds.), *Occupational therapy in the promotion of health and wellness*. Philadelphia: F. A. Davis Publishers.

Frank, G. (2005, May). *Tule river project: Personal communication*. University of Southern California.

Goode, W. J. (1957, April). Community within a community: The professions. *American Sociological Review, 22*, 194–200.

Green, L. W., & Kreuter, M. W. (1991). *Health promotion planning: An educational and environmental approach* (2nd ed.). Mountainview, CA: Mayfield Press.

Hanft, B., Burke, J. P., Cahill, M., Swenson-Miller, K., & Humphry, R. (1992). *Working with families: A curriculum guide for pediatric occupational therapists*. Chapel Hill, NC: Frank Porter Graham Child Development Center.

Hardcastle, D., Wenocur, S., & Powers, P. (2004). *Community practice: Theories and skills for social workers*. New York: Oxford Press.

Heiser, C. (1973). *Seed to civilization*. San Francisco: W. H. Freeman.

Henggeler, S. W. (1996). Eliminating (almost) treatment dropout of substance abusing or dependent delinquents through home-based multisystemic therapy. *American Journal of Psychiatry, 153*(3), 427–428.

Hillery, G. (1955). Definitions of community: Areas of agreement. *Rural Sociology, 20*, 194–204.

Hyde, K., & Woodworth, K. (1994). Reforming services to children and families. *The Family Preservation Initiative of Baltimore City, Inc., FY 1994 annual report*. Baltimore: Family Preservation Initiative.

Jarman, B., & Land, G. (1995). Beyond breakpoint: Possibilities for new community. In K. Gozdz, (Ed.), *Community building* (pp. 21–33). San Francisco, CA: Sterling and Stone.

Kronenberg, F., Algado, S., & Pollard, N. (Eds.). (2005). *Occupational therapy without borders: Learning from the spirit of survivors.* London: Elsevier.

Kübler-Ross, E. (1975). *Death: The final stage of growth.* Englewood Cliffs, NJ: Prentice Hall.

Lyon, L. (1987). *The community in urban society.* Chicago: The Dorsey Press.

McKnight, J. (1988). *Beyond community services.* Evanston, Il: Center of Urban Affairs and Policy Research.

Moore, A. (1996). The band community: Synchronizing human activity cycles for group cooperation. In R. Zemke, & F. Clark, (Eds.), *Occupational science: The evolving discipline* (pp. 95–106). Philadelphia: F. A. Davis.

Nelson, K. E., & Landsman, M. J. (1992). *Alternative models of family preservation: Family-based services in context.* Springfield, IL: Charles C. Thomas.

Nisbet, R. (1953). *The quest for community.* New York: Oxford University Press.

Nisbet, R. (1967). *The sociological tradition.* New York: Basic Books.

Nisbet, R. (1972). *Quest for community.* New York: Oxford University Press.

Noonan, M. J., & McCormick, L. (1992). *Early intervention in natural environments: Methods and procedures.* Pacific Grove, CA: Brooks/Cole.

Orford, J. (1993). *Community psychology: Theory and practice.* New York: John Wiley and Sons.

Oseroff, C., Longo, M., & Joseph, I. (1998). Finding our way home: Home- and community-based care. In H. Ghuman, & R. Sarles, (Eds.), *Handbook of child and adolescent outpatient, day treatment and community psychiatry* (pp. 359–368). Philadelphia: Brunner/Mazel.

Park, R. (1936). Human ecology. *American Journal of Sociology, 17*(1), 1–15.

Parsons, T. (1951). *The social system.* Glencoe, IL: Free Press.

Pascale, R., Millemann, M., & Gioja, L. (2000). *Surfing the edge of chaos.* New York: Crown.

Putnam, R. (2000). *Bowling alone.* New York,: Simon and Schuster.

Ray, M. (1995). A metaphor for a worldwide paradigm shift. In K. Gozda, (Ed.), *Community building* (pp. 9–19). San Francisco, CA: Sterling and Stone.

Rheingold, H. (1993). *Virtual community: Homesteading on the electronic frontier.* New York: Harper.

Schaaf, R. C., & Mulrooney, L. (1989). Occupational therapy in early intervention: A family-centered approach. *American Journal of Occupational Therapy, 43,* 745–754.

Schultz, S. (1992). School based occupational therapy for students with behavior disorders. *Occupational Therapy in Health Care, 8,* 173–196.

Slagle, E. C. (1922). Training ideas for mental patients. *Papers on Occupational Therapy.* New York: State Hospital Press.

Slagle, E. C., & Robeson, H. A. (1933). *Syllabus for training of nurses in occupational therapy.* New York: State Hospital Press.

Stevens, P., & Hall, J. (1992). Applying critical theories to nursing in communities. *Public Health Nursing 1*, March, 9: 2–9.

Vanier, C., & Hebert, M. (1995). An occupational therapy course on community practice. *Canadian Journal of Occupational Therapy 62*, 76–81.

Warren, R. (1987). Foreword. In L. Lyon, (Ed.), *The community in urban society*. Chicago: The Dorsey Press.

Young, T. R. (1994). Chaos theory and social dynamics: Foundations of postmodern social science [essay]. In A. Robertson, & A. Combs, (Eds.), *Proceedings of the 2nd annual conference on chaos theory*. Philadelphia.

# CHAPTER 2

# Practicing Occupation in the Community

## Learning Objectives

1. To identify elements of occupation appropriate for guiding community practice
2. To understand the complexity of the practice environment of community, as a system
3. To appreciate the diversity of occupation-centered practice available in the context of community
4. To understand the relationship between community health interventions and occupation-centered community practice
5. To identify the history, and future of occupational therapy practice in prevention of illness and injury; and in the maintenance of health and well-being
6. To distinguish between primary, secondary, and tertiary prevention

## Key Terms

1. Occupation
2. Systems Model
3. Community-based and Community-level Interventions
4. Community Health Interventions
5. Client-centered Rehabilitation Model
6. Community-based Rehabilitation Model

 7.  Independent Living Model
 8.  Prevention and Promotion
 9.  Primary, Secondary, or Tertiary (Prevention)
10.  Lifestyle Redesign
11.  Occupational Dysfunction: Occupational Imbalance, Deprivation, and Alienation
12.  Occupational Therapists Without Borders (SOS—OTWB)
13.  Occupational Justice

The second key concept that accompanies *community* in helping us to define the theme for this text is **occupation**. There is no need for an in-depth discussion of occupation since these core ideas, supporting our professional practices, provide the content for several of your occupational therapy courses. Historically, there were many central ideas expressed by the early founders of "occupation" therapy, among them: moral treatment, balance in occupations, and purposeful activity. These central ideas continue to guide the work of practitioners today.

## Exercise 1

Briefly review your knowledge base regarding our early history as a developing profession and your thoughts regarding each of the above basic tenets underlying the development of the profession. Make some notes and discuss with others the origins of these ideas and how you think these ideas influence practices you've observed. How do these ideas influence practices in the community?

_____

_____

_____

_____

Of course, we must remember that no profession exists in a vacuum, either in its establishment, or in its continued existence. Professions are established to meet the needs of society, however those needs may be translated. The need for engagement in meaningful occupation and its connection to well-being was recognized early in the development of our profession as a core theme that would, in fact, remain timeless.

Through the 1900s, occupational therapists continued to define and refine occupation as an organizing concept for the profession. As researchers investigated occupation as a unifying concept for organizing knowledge in occupational therapy and as they published their ideas, all occupational therapists were able to again explore the potential of occupation for providing the most effective change for our patients and for unifying our profession. The beliefs of the founders were not lost; they were only sleeping and waiting for the time when they could be further developed and matched to other areas of expanding knowledge in the disciplines of philosophy, sociology, biology, and anthropology. Reilly (1962) united the past with the present when in her 1961 Eleanor Clarke Slagle lecture, she proposed that the original hypothesis of occupational therapy can be stated "that man through the use of his hands, as they are energized by mind and will, can influence the state of his own health" (Reilly, 1962; pp. 1–9). This lecture and the writings to follow elaborated an occupational behavior paradigm of practice that renewed our beliefs in the philosophical principles established by the founders. Following Reilly, others continued to develop the tenets of occupation. Yerxa began to explore the development of a basic science of occupation. Her work and the work of her colleagues built on the foundations of many disciplines, and through that work she has reminded us that humans attach meaning to their occupations through their cultures (Clark, Wood, and Larson, 1998; Yerxa et al., 1990). Others remind us that humans are resourceful in mobilizing occupation to act on their world and to manipulate and transform their world (Engelhardt, 1977; Reilly, 1962; Rogers, 1983). In our continued investigations of occupation, we have also developed our knowledge of play, daily living tasks, and work (Kielhofner, 1985, 1995; Reilly, 1974; Shannon, 1970). Kielhofner (1995) has brought all of these ideas together in the definition of human occupation as "doing culturally meaningful work, play or daily living tasks in the stream of time and in the contexts of one's physical and social world" (p. 3).

Over time, others have contributed definitions and these are useful in helping us to establish the parameters of this thing that we call occupation. Pierce (1999) reminds us that many definitions are a sign of a healthy discipline. Recent occupational therapy literature provides us with a few from which to select. Nelson (1977, 1988) defines occupation based on occupational form and occupational performance, and Gray (1998) defines occupation in response to occupation as ends and as means. Some of the most recent work in elaborating occupation is that of occupational science. The definition of occupation particular to this science is "the daily activities that can be named in the lexicon of the culture and that fill the stream of time" (Clark, Wood, and Larson, 1998; Yerxa et al., 1990). Undoubtedly, there will be other definitions forthcoming as we continue to explore and elaborate occupation as the central unifying concept around which we will develop present and future practice. Regardless of definition, there seems to be little doubt that the belief in occupation as well as the dedication to meaningful activity remains strong. Occupation-centered intervention unites us as practitioners.

Kielhofner (1992) tells us that occupational therapy first emerged and continues to exist because "it has an implicit social contract to address the problems of those members of society who have limited capacity to perform in their everyday occupations" (p. 3). The years of epidemic illness (tuberculosis and polio) and the injuries resulting from World Wars served to further establish that skillfully orchestrated therapy, through the utilization of occupation could, in fact, influence an individual's ability to again function in and contribute to his or her community. This belief in occupation continues into the present and is being utilized by practitioners not only to help individuals regain and maintain function but also to act on their worlds in ways that they find most meaningful and satisfying. What Kielhofner (1992) refers to as "our implicit social contract" may be what has maintained our active interest in social justice over time (p. 3). We will return to the ideas of social justice as we examine the needs of present day society a bit later in this chapter.

## Exercise 2

We know that there are many societal issues to confront today. Child and adult obesity and resulting illnesses, childhood and adolescent crime, are but a few . . . can you name others?

_____

_____

_____

_____

What does Kielhofner mean by our (occupational therapists/occupational therapy assistants) implicit social contract? Do your ideas for community programming address societal issues/social justice? How, and in what way will you address these concerns?

_____

_____

_____

_____

_____

The previous exercise explored the connection between society and the individual through the identification of issues of concern to all of us. Individuals act in and on the society and community of which they are members . . . none of us are exempt.

# Understanding Systems as a Way of Thinking About Community Practice

Belief in occupation unites us, and concern for community and the society in general motivates us. But how do we act on these beliefs to help individuals make the changes they desire for themselves, for their families, and for their communities? We first need a way to think about the issues at hand; we need a map. Most certainly, in understanding the community as our context for intervention, we will use a **systems model** to initiate our thinking; this is the beginning of our "map." *General systems theory (GST)* is the term used to describe the scientific efforts to identify the structural, behavioral, and developmental features of living organisms and the ways in which they influence each other (Boulding, 1956; von Bertalanffy, 1968). The use of systems thinking is a way to help us understand things that interact. Gray, Kennedy, and Zemke (1997) suggest to us ways that dynamic systems theory may be applied to occupation, thus blending key components of occupation-centered practice—the components of occupation and the multiplicity of systems that make up community. For our usage in community intervention, we are interested in how the human (an open system) receives and is influenced by information (input), the processing of this information, and the behavioral change that occurs as a result (output). Whether our role is prevention, promotion, or remediation, we are interested in the dynamics of this process within the larger system of environment/community.

If we wish to develop a new way to think about the practice of occupation in the community, then it would likely be from this dynamic systems perspective as a foundation of understanding. We might then adopt or perhaps develop a theory, frame of reference, or paradigm from which to view our practice in the community, that is, a way to think about the community and the relationship of individuals to one another and to the many layers that constitute *the community*. We are not suggesting that this is a simple process. The community is a complex open system with many interrelated levels of function. For our purposes, we would believe that these multiple systems must interrelate in such a way as to produce meaningful occupation. As facilitators of this process, we are active participants and add to the complexity of this open system.

Once we have gained an appreciation of the complexity of the system within which we are practicing, we will want to further develop our "map" to best reach our destination. McColl, Gerein, and Valentine (1997) suggest that the occupational therapy practitioner who is able to assess the situation and choose between a number of models is perhaps best able to meet the challenges of practice (p. 526). These authors are speaking from a "response to disability" perspective, and we might assume that it is even more relevant in the complex "open system" presented to us by the community. In the environment of community we must not only respond to the needs of our clients with disability but also to the needs of those who may require prevention or wellness services. To be eclectic in our choices means that we must have a thorough understanding of all those perspectives from which we may choose to ensure the appropriate and effective delivery of programming.

## Community Health Interventions for Occupation-Centered Practice

Scaffa and Brownson (2005) distinguish between **community-based and community-level intervention**. Community-based practices place the practitioner in the community, a

The Rural Community Empowerment Program (2005, July) represents a series of partnerships between the rural communities of the United States and federal and state agencies, local and tribal governments, private businesses, foundations, and non-profits that engage the resources and commitments of these organizations to carry out portions of the community's strategic plan (http://www.ezec.gov/welcome/index.html). Agendas for the various communities that may be of interest to occupational therapy practitioners, particularly those working in rural areas, include: youth health and employment/creating jobs.

practice venue familiar to occupational therapy practitioners and many other professionals. Community-level interventions are those that attempt to modify the sociocultural, political, economic, and environmental context of the community to achieve health goals (Scaffa and Brownson, 2005; p. 485; Clark, 2003; pp. 148–169). Community health may be viewed as a continuum from community-based to community-level to community-centered (Scaffa and Brownson, 2005; p. 485). Community-centered interventions come from the community itself. Clearly, partnerships and coalitions become ever more important as intervention follows this trajectory. Clark (2003) refers to the building of these alliances or coalitions as a responsibility of the health care practitioner; finding those individuals who may unite to address a common interest and helping them to mobilize their interests (p. 72).

A community-centered intervention occurs when community members come together through partnerships and coalitions to identify common concerns and solve community problems.

According to Scaffa and Brownson (2005), **community health interventions** are "intended to address the physical, mental, social and spiritual health of communities" (Scaffa and Brownson, 2005; p. 477). Perhaps the distinction in emphasis between our understandings of individual clinical practices and those of community health agendas is that community health targets whole populations, or communities within the larger populations, and they do so through emphasis on the role of social and environmental determinants of health (Scaffa and Brownson, 2005; p. 478).

Such ongoing community programs in the Los Angeles, CA area that target childhood obesity, breathing disorders, and delinquency are greatly influenced in assessment of need by social and environmental determinants of health. In these examples, health and well-being are advanced or prevented by complex interactions between the total environment (physical, social, and economic) and the resultant individual and community response. Researchers at the University of Southern California have identified a link between childhood asthma and living within the boundaries of a major freeway or street. Clearly a program targeting only the child with asthma would not alter the significance of the problem. This provides a good example of communities as complex systems. In a community health approach, all concerns must be addressed and included in the intervention. Socio-economic concerns establishing neighborhoods, air quality, and perhaps agendas for safe distance from heavily trafficked roadways; or those for more public transportation or cleaner fuel are all of interest and concern to the coalitions and partnering of community practitioners in this example (USC, 2005).

In identifying a socioecological approach to improving health, Brownson (2001) recognizes the multiple facets impacting health demonstrated by the above example. She recognizes a further layer of complexity demonstrated by the influence of the political environment that may include regulation, legislation, and policy. Of course, interventions within the realm of community health are intended to decrease the incidence rates of disease, disability, and death through prevention activities and to reduce the impact of the disease through early detection and treatment. Such community health initiatives may include both public and private efforts to promote, protect, and preserve the physical, mental, social, and spiritual health of those in a community (McKenzie and Smeltzer, 1997).

## Comprehensive Models for Community-Based Intervention

McColl, Gerein, and Valentine (1997) discuss several models of practice from a disability perspective that we can expand for community use to include multiple roles of

A web-site was designed for an urban Korean community to help explain the symptoms of mental illness, and to offer community access sites for treatment by Korean speaking professionals. The occupational therapist responsible for this Web site was motivated to provide health promotion, health protection, and health services access for an underserved population. Without an understanding of the culture, and of the community, this Web site could not have been successful (Kang, 2000).

prevention, restoration, maintenance of function, and remediation (McColl, 1998). The first model, the **client-centered rehabilitation model**, is one in which clients engage therapists to help them solve the problems they encounter as they seek to achieve their goals (McColl, Gerein, and Valentine, 1997; pp. 511–513). The client is in charge of his or her life and only seeks the therapist's expertise in providing information and guidance. Of course, this is an oversimplification of the process, but it serves to emphasize the importance of a client-driven goal structure. This model recognizes and encourages autonomy and places the therapist in the critical role of facilitator, instructor, advocate, and guide. In the context of community, the therapist will provide the map that will assist the client in traversing his or her way to a meaningful, self-selected place in the community. The therapist helps "clear the way" and also provides direction and instruction when it is needed. The therapist does not do the work of the client but guides and facilitates the work the client chooses to do. Lifestyle redesign programs and life coaching models may be considered in this way.

The second model discussed by McColl, Gerein, and Valentine (1997) emphasizes the social origins of issues relating to disability (McColl, Gerein, and Valentine, 1997; pp. 513–515). As we have learned through earlier discussion in Chapter 1, this particular model defines community as geographical, referring to a particular area or locality, but it also recognizes community as relational, referring to a group with shared interests and values, mutual obligations, a common history, or some other affinity. We are reminded by Kniepmann (1997) that community is always more than a geographic location for our practices, it also includes an "orientation to collective health, social priorities, and different modes for service provision" (McColl, Gerein, and Valentine, 1997; p. 540). For the **community-based rehabilitation model**, the community is first that of persons who are disabled but secondly, persons who are disabled within the context of the larger community.

There are three assumptions associated with the community-based rehabilitation model that are important to our multiple community roles. These include, but extend beyond, the community of the disabled. The first assumption recognizes that people with disabilities do not exist in isolation; rather, they are an integral part of the larger community that also includes their families, friends, and neighbors. There is an assumed relationship, a "system is in place" that supports clients in the community who are disabled and may also benefit from their contributions to the larger economic and social environment. We know from our earlier reading that, although this "system" may appear to be open, in many regards it may also be closed to our clients. The second important assumption is that individuals and communities have available to them the resources needed to influence and enhance their own health, and it may be the practitioners' role to assist these individuals and communities in first identifying and then accessing these resources. The last assumption is that it is not only more possible but also perhaps more important to make small inroads of improvement to the quality of life for all people with disabilities in a community than to select a few for the highest standard of care (McColl, Gerein and Valentine, 1997; pp. 513–514). Together, these assumptions provide us with an orientation for work in the community with all people, whether or not they are disabled or at risk for the onset of disabling conditions.

Another model of interest to occupation-centered community-based practice is that of **independent living**. Independent living is defined by Frieden and Cole (1985) in this way: "control over one's life based on the choice of acceptable options that minimize reliance on others in making decisions and performing every day activities" (Frieden and Cole, 1985; p. 735). They go on to include "participation in day-to-day life in the community, and the opportunity to engage in a range of social roles" (Frieden and Cole, 1985; p. 735). The origins of the independent-living model developed out of a collective political movement of persons with disabilities (Cole, 1979; DeJong, 1979, 1993; Lysack and Kaufert, 1994; McColl, Gerein, and Valentine, 1997). The independent living model is an excellent example of the mobilization of politics and advocacy necessary to prevail and to achieve one's goals, central concepts to occupation-centered practice in the community. Regardless of our client population or our clients' goals, we must be cognizant of the politics that influence the dissemination of resources and we, along with our clients, must assume the role and responsibility of advocacy.

## Exercise 3

Do your programming ideas fit one or more of these community models? If yes, in what way(s)?

_____

_____

_____

_____

_____

# The Community Practitioner in the Roles of Prevention and Health Promotion

We have talked about **prevention** as one of the significant roles of community practice, and this is accurate for both the occupational therapist and the occupational therapy assistant. Kniepmann (1997) discusses the prevention of disability and the maintenance of health from a number of perspectives. It is her contention that as a profession, we must use the knowledge we have to help maintain health—whether it is prevention, health promotion, or building those characteristics we associate with the condition of wellness. Green and Kreuter (1991) emphasize that health **promotion** includes any planned combination of educational, political, regulatory, environmental, and organizational supports of actions and conditions of living conducive to the health of individuals, groups, or communities. In community health today, there are several ways one might work toward prevention as described by these authors. These routes toward prevention may be defined as **primary, secondary, or tertiary** (2000 Joint Committee on Health Education and Promotion Terminology, 2001, p. 101; Kniepmann, 1997, pp. 532–534; Pickett and Hanlon, 1990, p. 81). A brief review of these potential options will be useful to expand our knowledge of practice in the community.

Primary prevention is directed toward the greater society. Efforts to avoid the onset of pathologies might be accomplished by reducing susceptibility in a number of ways, including minimizing environmental factors that increase risk of disease or injury (Tarlov and Pope, 1991). Spraying wetlands for mosquitoes is one common example of primary prevention. The actions of the 2006 Representative Assembly of AOTA to mobilize occupational therapists to address the societal issues of obesity, stress and violence, among others also qualify as primary prevention measures. Occupational therapy practitioners in the community are often instigators and promoters of efforts toward primary prevention. For example, they might consult to town planning boards about architectural barriers or work to get reduced speed limits in recreation areas where children play or support restrictions on unsafe toys, skates, and scooters. There are many varied ways we can engage in primary prevention.

Tarlov and Pope (1991) describe secondary prevention as efforts to target groups in the community who are thought to be "at risk." This can involve early detection of a potential health problem, followed by appropriate interventions to halt, reverse, or slow down progression. Occupational therapy practitioners are certainly involved in secondary prevention, which can run the gamut from parenting classes for teens to the encouragement of condom use for those at risk for sexually transmitted diseases (STDs). Teaching the well elderly how to access public transportation in an effort to widen their options for accessing meaningful occupation and thus maintaining health would also be considered secondary prevention.

The focus of tertiary prevention is to maximize function and to minimize the detrimental effects of illness or injury (Kniepmann, 1997; pp. 532–533). Although this is an area already very familiar to occupational therapy practitioners, we also want to emphasize efforts toward a focus on function, advocacy for social policy as it can influence one's health and ability to be independent, and the direct intervention concerns of the individual.

Most of the programs we discuss in this text that deal with prevention fall under the category of secondary prevention. Some of our programming, however, assumes elements of primary and tertiary prevention as well. Oftentimes it may be difficult to separate one from the other. Associated with prevention but with a different directive, health promotion has been the favored topic of many occupational therapists, including Madill, Townsend, and Schultz (1989) and McComas and Carswell (1994). For occupational therapy practitioners, health promotion or optimization is based in part on our basic belief that a balance of work, rest, self-care, and leisure/play is necessary for optimal health and well-being. Prompted by this belief, occupation is utilized to organize our daily rounds of activity that include this recommended balance. For many of our clients, guidance is first needed in recognizing deficits of balance. This is followed by the offer of assistance in developing the skills, knowledge, and behaviors needed to engage in those self-selected activities that provide "meaningful" balance.

It is not realistic to think that we can separate prevention of illness or trauma and the promotion of health and wellness; one is implied within the other. By providing those aspects of promotion that include information and resources geared to individual needs and wants and through orchestrated changes in behavior and motivation, we will reduce risk and thus help to prevent illness and accidents. Fuhrer (1994) talks of the feelings of elevated health and subjective well-being experienced by people who are engaged in activities they feel are health promoting (Fuhrer, 1994; p. 359). First, we must enlarge our own awareness of community resources, as well as our own programs that promote health, whether these be options for education, medical care, or perhaps exercise/wellness classes. Our awareness of programs is then followed by the sharing of these resources with the client through well-articulated programming that is intended to bring about the desired directive of either prevention or promotion (Dyck, 1993; Finlayson and Edwards, 1995; Jaffe, 1986; Kniepmann, 1997).

Life change as a foundation for occupational therapy practice is realized through what Mandel, Jackson, Zemke, Nelson, and Clark (1999, pp. 12–13) describe as *Lifestyle Redesign*. According to these authors, there are four core ideas of the occupational therapy profession that inform the **lifestyle redesign** programs: "Occupation is life itself; occupation can create new visions of possible selves, occupation has a curative effect on physical and mental health and on a sense of life order and routine, and occupation has a place in preventive care" (Mandel, Jackson, Zemke, Nelson, and Clark, 1999; p. 13). The USC Well Elderly Study is a prime example of the impact of the use of *occupational lifestyle redesign* to offer well-elderly a "customized routine of health promoting and meaningful daily activities" (Mandel, Jackson, Zemke, Nelson, and Clark, 1999, introduction).

Much of our work in the community is directed toward the promotion of health and well-being; however, we cannot assume that all of our clients will be equally engaged in the process, nor will all agree on the parameters of "health." Even though most people would support the idea of seeking better health, oftentimes working toward the goal is received less enthusiastically. A review of those characteristics that influence learning and resulting behavior change will be helpful as you prepare to work in prevention and promotion. If you have previous clinical experience, this kind of practice may not be unlike intervention work that you have already accomplished in the institutional environments of mental and physical rehabilitation. The teaching and acquisition of health-promoting behaviors is not simple, as anyone who has ever failed to maintain an exercise program can attest to. Understanding something of the building of self-efficacy and empowerment is critical to the success of this kind of programming. Kniepmann (1997) provides a useful summary of those constructs for behavioral change that will help in developing successful community programs to include the characteristics of social learning theory, self-efficacy, and perceptions of control as described in the research of Bandura (1977, 1982), Bandura and Walters (1963), and Rotter (1966).

| Exercise 4 |
| --- |

Is your proposed programming directed toward the prevention of disability, or disease? Is it primary, secondary, tertiary, or a combination?

_____

_____

_____

_____

# The Future of Occupation-Centered Practice in the Community: 2000 and Beyond

## Trends in Health Care and in the Practices of Healthy Living

There is little doubt that health care is changing and that, in response, occupational therapy is changing as well. In 1995 the American Occupational Therapy Association commissioned Health Policy Alternatives, Inc. to examine the future of health care and particularly occupational therapy's future within health care. This organization reported numerous markers of the rapid changes in America's health care system, most of them carrying negative implications, and they attributed these changes primarily to escalating costs and the lack of accompanying growth in the population or the underlying economy in order to maintain a balance (AOTA, 1996; p. 1).

It has now been more than ten years since this report was published, and we have witnessed many of the implications in our workplaces. First, there were reductions in institutional administrative structures, particularly in middle management. These were followed by reductions in treatment staff with resulting pressures in maintaining caseloads. The social, economic, and political worlds in which we live and practice have always encouraged, discouraged, or sometimes prevented how and where we choose to practice. Historically, there appears to be cyclical and necessary reversals in exchange systems—fat years and lean years. Restraint is the counterbalance of excess.

Also, in 1996 the Pew Health Professions Commission predicted the pressures on physicians and nurses and also indicated that there would be pressures to consolidate the "allied" health professions. In its 1998 report, the commission asked that health professionals "continue to consider, in fundamental ways, how they best add value to the delivery of health services" (p. i). The Commission suggested that practitioners must contribute to the system in meaningful ways (that is, measure outcomes) or they would risk losing their autonomy. There were messages to educators of future health care professionals as well, which included recommendations to stop preparing students for "yesterday's health care system" and to start preparing students for "emerging systems" (1998, p. iii). It was further suggested that this preparation include broader education with regard to systems, organizational skills, and population skills. Occupational therapists have been articulating these same messages. Baum and Law (1997, p. 280) described a changing health system paradigm that focused on (a) health rather than illness; (b) community approaches rather than medical interventions; (c) abilities and quality of life rather than deficits and survival; (d) personal versus professional control and responsibility; and (e) prevention rather than treatment. Lifestyle redesign is just such an approach focusing on life quality and the belief than an individual may change the way he or she reacts to and interacts with the larger community. The coach/mentor/therapist provides the necessary information for the client to make informed choices in the redesign of his or her life to more effectively function in the world.

In a special issue of the *American Journal of Occupational Therapy*, Baum and Law (1998, p. 7) called on the profession to be "responsive to the needs of our times". There is little doubt that "the needs of our times" include all of society's ills: abuse, violence, joblessness, futility, and ignorance. In addition, there are new ills that result in increased stress, including competition for limited resources, pressure on family and other systems, and the loneliness and isolation that technology can produce. Baum and Law (1998, p. 7) also remind us that in these troubled times, it is through engagement in occupation that people develop and maintain health. We might add that it is also through membership in a shared, supportive community. In her presidential address to the American Occupational Therapy Association Annual Meeting, 2005, President Baum asked the profession what we must do now to position ourselves as the profession that works in both traditional and community health settings to enable occupations and remove barriers that limit participation. In her words, "society is counting on our contribution" (Presidential Address, AOTA, Long Beach, CA, 2005).

Practice in the community that includes intervention, maintenance, and prevention is new for many health care providers, but for occupational therapy it is a reemerging practice arena. Appropriate to occupational therapy practitioners' renewed interests in community-based practice were other recommendations of the Pew Health Professions Commission to include: (1) the encouragement of diversity to reflect the nation's population (that is, our outreach programs to inner-city and ethnic urban population "pockets"); (2) the inclusion of interdisciplinary team competence (that is, our expansion of "teams" to include both professional and layperson community members such as friends and neighbors); (3) efforts to continue to move toward ambulatory practice (our extensions of ambulatory practice to include not only intervention but also maintenance of health and wellness and prevention of injury and illness); and (4) the encouragement of public service for all health professional students and graduates (that is, our service learning opportunities in the community).

The Pew Health Professions Commission's fifth recommendation is particularly significant to this text, and pertinent quotes from it follow:

... Health professional programs should require a significant amount of work in community settings as a requirement for graduation. This work should be integrated into the curriculum.

... Students should assist in the design and development of such programs.

... Communities and the health agencies that serve them should actively participate in the partnerships through which these service programs can be built.

... Existing programs of national service tied to debt forgiveness should be expanded and enlarged in order to incorporate more health professional graduates.

... Professional associations should actively incorporate the idea of public service into regulation and professional development activity (1998, pp. iii–vi).

The Pew summary report *Healthy America: Practitioners for 2005* extends the above directives to include prevention in its set of recommendations to educators. The report notes that the "largest share of our graduates will spend their careers in home- and community-based settings . . ." (Pew Commission, 1992, p. 5; Shugar, O'Neill, and Bader, 1991). The recent national report, *Healthy People 2010* echoes many of these ideas with its prevailing message of responsibility for health becoming the task of the individual. (http://www.healthypeople.gov/default.htm), however, we must ask the question: how will individuals gain the necessary knowledge and skills to maintain and protect their own health? In part, it is the responsibility of our profession, as well as others in health care, to close this potential gap.

One of our emerging roles in today's society will be to build healthy communities. Baum and Law (1997, 1998) suggest that occupational therapists must understand how people interpret and practice occupation, how they apply structure to their daily lives, and how they assign meaning. This can best be done in their natural, self-selected environments—in other words, in their community. Community therapists, according to these authors, must not only be attuned to the intervention needs of their client, but they also must be equally attentive to the ecological, physical, social, cultural, and health environments of the community in order to improve the client's options for healthy living (Baum and Law, 1998; p. 8). Many of the program examples described in this text do just that; they are very responsive to environment. Some of them, such as the program embedded in the philosophies of the Jane Goodall "Roots and Shoots" Club, have preservation and protection of the environment as a central theme (See Chapter 17 for more information on "Roots and Shoots" Clubs). Baum and Christiansen (1997) refer to a changing paradigm in medicine and health care from a biomedical, acute-centered, and provider-driven approach to one that places more responsibility on the consumer (Baum and Christiansen, 1997; p. 31). We might conclude that this places more responsibility on us as occupational therapy practitioners to guide the consumer in how to facilitate healthy habits and behaviors and in how to navigate the community systems to obtain the information and services that they require.

## Globalization of Occupation

Wilcock (1998) broadens our perspective of community to include global concerns in her call for occupational therapists to be responsive to the objectives of the World Health Organization and potential roles in what she describes as the "new public health" (Wilcock, 1998; p. 221). She advocates for a strong foundation in occupation that would prepare the therapist for practices in wellness, preventive medicine, social equity, community development, and ecological sustainability. Her discussion includes risk factors for **occupational dysfunction** that include occupational imbalance, deprivation, and alienation. According to Wilcock (1998), **occupational imbalance** is a lack of balance among work, rest, self-care, and play/leisure that fails to meet an individual's unique physical, social, or mental health needs, thereby resulting in decreased health and well-being. **Occupational deprivation** may include circumstances or limitations that prevent a person from acquiring, engaging in, or enjoying occupations. Such things as less-than-optimal health, isolation, poverty, and homelessness are examples. **Occupational alienation** represents a lack of satisfaction in one's occupations and a general sense of estrangement. Engagement in such tasks that the individual perceives as stressful or meaningless may result in occupational alienation.

The works of Kronenberg, Algado, and Pollard (2005) are perhaps most representative of the directions that occupational therapy can go in a humanistic mission to support social justice for all people. In 1997 Salvador Simo' Algado launched the work of the Dolphin Association to help people who appeared to be neglected or underserved by occupational therapy practitioners. Survivors of war, prisoners, immigrants, prostitutes, and people living with HIV/AIDS were all seen as part of this group (Kronenberg, Algado, and Pollard, 2005; preface). The Dolphin Association was renamed 'Spirit of Survivors' in 2002; **Occupational Therapists Without Borders (SOS—OTWB).** Dialogues and collaborations between occupational therapists and other professionals are encouraged in global communities representing both developed countries and developing countries. The authors view the SOS—OTWB as a catalyst for movement within the international community of occupational therapists. The goal is to "develop, implement and promote occupational therapy practice, education, and research initiatives with marginalized people, inspired and guided by a vision of overcoming occupational apartheid and working toward **occupational justice**, while raising critical awareness about and facing up to the political nature of occupational therapy" (Kronenberg, Algado, and Pollard, 2005; preface). Many of the programs described in this text speak to occupational justice. In all of our communities we have people in need for whom we can advocate. Our urban and rural communities in the US are home to children and adults who are disenfranchised or at great risk for becoming so. Global concerns are often first addressed in our own communities with the same energy and caring we would extend to others around the world.

## Exercise 5

Occupational therapy students around the world have been instrumental in designing and, along with academic faculty and clinicians, implementing outreach programs and Level 1 and 2 fieldwork experiences for underserved populations in many third world countries. Examples include the development of community playgrounds in Haiti and sensory stimulation and play programs for orphans in Ghana.

Note ideas you may have for such programs, and discuss with classmates and your instructors. Programs of this nature provide excellent opportunities for occupational therapy and occupational therapy assistant academic programs to work together on community program development. You may wish to further investigate some of the references mentioned in this section to expand your thinking regarding the globalization of occupation-centered practices.

_____

_____

_____

_____

_____

Since the above recommendations and directives target all health care practitioners, we are not alone in considering ways to practice in the community setting. Occupational therapists, however, have an ongoing history of practice in the community, with a body of published information to help those who may be new to explore their options. You should review the extensive list of publications at the close of this chapter and examine those that interest you. Many occupational therapists have always practiced with an awareness of the community or directly in it. Those who have know that it can be a significantly rewarding practice. It is virtually impossible to practice in the direct environment of the client—in the community system—without being aware of the need for maintenance of health, wellness, and prevention. The community system invites, and likely demands, a comprehensive array of services that includes all that we know and more. We must be practitioners, educators, skill-builders, politicians, health promoters, and advocates.

Not only is our community practice history an advantage as we prepare for return to the community, but our unifying belief and dedication to occupation as a way to orchestrate our practices is also a substantial strength. Few professions have an agreed-upon belief system strong enough to organize their interventions without losing their sense of purpose in what can be a complex and demanding care environment—that of *the community*. It is time for us to embrace the values and ideals of our founders and to meet the challenges of community head-on through our belief in the power of *occupation*.

# *References*

American Occupational Therapy Association. (2002). *Occupational therapy practice framework: Domain and process*. Bethesda, MD. American Occupational Therapy Association.

Bandura, A. (1977). Self-efficacy: Toward a unifying theory of behavioral change. *Psychological Review, 84*, 191–215.

Bandura, A. (1982). Self-efficacy mechanism in human agency. *American Psychologist, 37*, 122–147.

Bandura, A., & Walters, R. H. (1963). *Social learning and personality development*. New York: Holt, Rinehart, and Winston.

Baum, C., & Christiansen, C. (1997). The occupational therapy context: Philosophy, principles, practice. In C. Christiansen, & C. Baum, (Eds.), *Occupational therapy enabling function and well-being* (pp. 28–43). Thorofare, NJ: Slack.

Baum, C., & Law, M. (1997). Occupational therapy practice: Focusing on occupational performance. *American Journal of Occupational Therapy, 51*, 277–288.

Baum, C., & Law, M. (1998, January). Nationally speaking: Community health: A responsibility, an opportunity, and a fit for occupational therapy. *American Journal of Occupational Therapy, 52*(1), 7–10.

Baum, C. (2005, May). Harnessing Opportunities and Taking Responsibility for Our Future. Presidential Address, American Occupational Therapy Association, 85th Annual Conference, Long Beach, CA.

Boulding, K. E. (1956). General systems theory: The skeleton of science. *Management Science, 2*(3), 197–208.

Brownson, C. (2001). Program development for community health: Planning, implementation, and evaluation strategies. In M. Scaffa, (Ed.), *Occupational therapy in community-based practice settings* (pp. 95–134). Philadelphia: Davis.

Clark, M. J. (2003). *Community health nursing: Caring for populations*. Upper Saddle River, NJ: Prentice Hall.

Clark, F., Wood, W., & Larson, E. (1998). Occupational science: Occupational therapy's legacy for the 21st century. In M. Neistadt, & E. Crepeau, (Eds.), *Willard and Spackman's occupational therapy* (9th ed., pp. 13–21). Philadelphia: Lippincott.

Cole, J. A. (1979). What's new about independent living. *Archives of Physical Medicine and Rehabilitation, 60*, 458–461.

DeJong, G. (1979). Independent living: From social movement to analytic paradigm. *Archives of Physical Medicine and Rehabilitation, 60*, 435–446.

DeJong, G. (1993). Health care reform and disability: Affirming our commitment to the community. *Archives of Physical Medicine and Rehabilitation, 74*, 1,017–1,024.

Dyck, I. (1993). Health promotion, occupational therapy and multiculturalism: Lessons from research. *Canadian Journal of Occupational Therapy, 60,* 120–129.

Engelhardt, H. T. (1977). Defining occupational therapy: The meaning of therapy and the virtues of occupation. *American Journal of Occupational Therapy, 31*(10), 666–672.

Finlayson, M., & Edwards, J. (1995). Integrating the concepts of health promotion and community into occupational therapy practice. *Canadian Journal of Occupational Therapy, 62,* 70–75.

Frieden, L., & Cole, J. A. (1985). Independence: The ultimate goal of rehabilitation of spinal cord injured persons. *The American Journal of Occupational Therapy, 39,* 734–739.

Fuhrer, M. J. (1994). Subjective well-being: Implications for medical rehabilitation outcomes and models of disablement. *American Journal of Physical Medicine and Rehabilitation, 73,* 358–364.

Gray, J. M. (1998). Putting occupation into practice: Occupation as ends, occupation as means. *American Journal of Occupational Therapy, 52,* 354–364.

Gray, J. M., Kennedy, B. L., & Zemke, R. (1997). Application of dynamic systems theory to occupation. In R. Zemke, & F. Clark, (Eds.), *Occupational science, the evolving discipline* (pp. 309–324). Philadelphia: F. A. Davis.

Green, L. W., & Kreuter, M. W. (1991). *Health promotion planning: An educational and environmental approach,* (2nd ed.) Mountainview, CA: Mayfield Press.

Health Policy Alternatives, Inc. (1996, November). *Health care and market reform: Workforce implications for occupational therapy.* Limited Publication: No. 444 Capitol St., N.W., Suite 821, Washington, DC. *Healthy People 2010:* http://www.healthypeople.gov/default.htm.

Jaffe, E. G. (1986). Nationally Speaking: The role of occupational therapy in disease prevention and health promotion. *American Journal of Occupational Therapy, 40,* 749–752.

2000 Joint Committee on Health Education and Promotion Terminology. (2001). Report of the 2000 Joint committee on health education and promotion terminology. *American Journal of Health Education, 32*(2), 90–103.

Kang, D. (2000). Web Site for Korean Speaking Persons Seeking Mental Illness Information. Personal Communication. Los Angeles: CA.

Kielhofner, G. (1985). *A model of human occupation: Theory and application.* Baltimore: Williams and Wilkins.

Kielhofner, G. (1992). *Conceptual foundations of occupational therapy.* Philadelphia: F. A. Davis.

Kielhofner, G. (1995). *A model of human occupation: Theory and application* (2nd ed.). Baltimore: Williams and Wilkins.

Kniepmann, K. (1997). Prevention of disability and maintenance of health. In C. Christiansen, & C. Baum, (Eds.), *Occupational therapy enabling function and well-being* (pp. 531–553). Thorofare, NJ: Slack.

Kronenberg, F., Algado, S., & Pollard, N. (Eds.). (2005). *Occupational therapy without borders: Learning from the spirit of survivors.* London: Elsevier.

Lysack, C., & Kaufert, J. (1994). Comparing the origins and ideologies of the independent living movement and community based rehabilitation. *International Journal of Rehabilitation Research, 17*, 231–240.

Madill, H., Townsend, E., & Schultz, P. (1989). Implementing a health promotion strategy in occupational therapy education and practice. *Canadian Journal of Occupational Therapy, 56*, 67–72.

Mandel, D., Jackson, J., Zemke, R., Nelson, L., & Clark, F. (1999). *Lifestyle redesign: Implementing the well-elderly program*. Bethesda, MD: American Occupational Therapy Association.

McColl, M. A. (1998). What do we need to know to practice occupational therapy in the community. *American Journal of Occupational Therapy, 52*(1), 11–18.

McColl, M. A., Gerein, N., & Valentine, F. (1997). Meeting the challenges of disability: Models for enabling function and well-being. In C. Christiansen, & C. Baum (Eds.), *Occupational therapy enabling function and well-being* (pp. 509–527). Thorofare, NJ: Slack.

McComas, J., & Carswell, A. (1994). A model for action in health promotion: A community experience. *Canadian Journal of Rehabilitation, 7*, 257–265.

McKenzie, J., & Smeltzer, J. (1997). *Planning, implementation, and evaluating health promotion programs: A primer* (2nd ed.). Boston, MA: Allyn and Bacon.

Nelson, D. (1977). Why the profession of occupational therapy will flourish in the 21st century, 1996 Eleanor Clarke Slagle lecture. *American Journal of Occupational Therapy, 51*, 11–24.

Nelson, D. (1988). Occupation: Form and performance. *American Journal of Occupational Therapy, 42*, 633–641.

Pew Health Professions Commission. (1992). *Summary: Healthy America: Practitioners for 2005. A Beginning Dialogue for U.S. Schools of Allied Health*. San Francisco: The Center for the Health Professions, University of California.

Pew Health Professions Commission. (1996, November). *Critical Challenges: Revitalizing the Health Professions for the Twenty-First Century. Third Report, First Release*. San Francisco: The Center for the Health Professions, University of California.

Pew Health Professions Commission. (1998, December). *Recreating Health Professional Practice for a New Century. Fourth Report*. San Francisco: The Center for the Health Professions, University of California.

Pickett, G., & Hanlon, J. J. (1990). *Public health: Administration and practice*. St. Louis, MO: Times Mirror/Mosby.

Pierce, D. (1999). Putting occupation to work in occupational therapy curricula. *Education special interest section quarterly, 9*(3). Bethesda, MD: American Occupational Therapy Association.

Reilly, M. (1962). Occupational therapy can be one of the great ideas of 20th century medicine. *American Journal of Occupational Therapy, 16*, 1–9.

Reilly, M. (1974). *Play as exploratory learning*. Beverly Hills, CA: Sage.

Rogers, J. (1983). The study of human occupation. In G. Kielhofner (Ed.), *Health through occupation: Theory and practice in occupational therapy*. Philadelphia: F. A. Davis.

Rotter, J. B. (1966). Generalized expectancies for internal versus external control of reinforcement. *Psychological Monographs: General and Applied, 80,* 1–28.

Rural Community Empowerment Program (07/22/2005). http://www.ezec.gov/welcome/index/html.

Scaffa, M., & Brownson, C. (2005). Occupational therapy intervention: Community health approaches. In C. Christiansen, C. Baum, & J. Bass-Haugen, (Eds.), *Occupational therapy: Performance, participation, and well-being* (3rd ed., pp. 478–492), Thorofare, NJ: Slack.

Shannon, P. (1970). The work-play model: A basis for occupational therapy programming. *American Journal of Occupational Therapy, 24,* 215–218.

Shugar, D. A., O'Neill, E. H., & Bader, J. D. (Eds.). (1991). *Healthy America: Practitioners for 2005. An agenda for action for U.S. health professional schools.* Durham, NC: Pew Health Professions Commission.

Tarlov, A., & Pope, A. (1991). *Disability in America: Toward a national agenda for prevention.* Washington, DC: Institute of Medicine, National Academy Press.

USC. (2005). *Research agendas for the community.* Los Angeles: University of Southern California.

von Bertalanffy, L. (1968). *General systems theory.* New York: Braziller.

Wilcock, A. (1998). *An occupational perspective of health.* Thorofare, NJ: Slack.

Yerxa, E. J., Clark, F., Frank, G., Jackson, J., Parham, D., Pierce, D., et al. (1990). An introduction to occupational science: A foundation for occupational therapy in the 21st century. *Occupational Therapy in Health Care, 6*(4), 1–17.

You may wish to review the following recommended occupational therapy literature describing earlier community-based programming of the 1960s, 1970s, and 1980s; the "needs" for many of the programs described here are still with us today:

Auerbach, E. (1974, May–June). Community involvement: The Bernal. *The American Journal of Occupational Therapy, 28*(5), 272–273.

Bartlett, M. (1977, September). A community therapist in Alaska. *The American Journal of Occupational Therapy, 31*(8), 485–487.

Braun, K. L., & Wake, W. (1988). Community long term care: PT/OT involvement in patient rehabilitation and maintenance. In E. Taira, (Ed.), *Community programs for the health impaired elderly* (pp. 5–19). New York: The Haworth Press.

Broekema, M. C., Danz, K. H., & Schloemer, C. U. (1975, January). Occupational therapy in a community aftercare program. *The American Journal of Occupational Therapy, 29*(1), 22–27.

Burnett, S., & Yerxa, E. (1980, March). Community-based and college-based needs assessment of physically disabled persons. *The American Journal of Occupational Therapy, 34*(3), 201–207.

Cantwell, J. L. (1970, November–December). The community-junior college: Challenges to occupational therapy education. *The American Journal of Occupational Therapy, XXIV*(8), 576–578.

Cermak, S. (1976, March). Community-based learning in occupational therapy, *The American Journal of Occupational Therapy, 30*(3), 157–161.

Christiansen, C. H., & Davidson, D. A. (1974, July). A community health program with low achieving adolescents. *The American Journal of Occupational Therapy, 28*(6), 346–350.

Coleman, W. (1975, August). Occupational therapy and child abuse. *The American Journal of Occupational Therapy, 29*(7), 412–417.

Covey, S. (1970, October). Occupational therapy in the community. *The American Journal of Occupational Therapy, XXIV*(7), 508–509.

Cromwell, F. S., & Kielhofner, G. (1976, November–December). An educational strategy for occupational therapy community service at the University of Southern California. *The American Journal of Occupational Therapy, 30*(10), 629–633.

DeMars, P. K. (1975, January). Training adult retardates for private enterprise. *The American Journal of Occupational Therapy, 29*(1), 39–42.

DePoy, E. (1987, July). Community-based occupational therapy with a head-injured adult. *The American Journal of Occupational Therapy, 41*(7), 461–464.

Fazio, L. S. (1988). Sexuality and aging: A community wellness program. In E. Taira, (Ed.), *Community programs for the health impaired elderly* (pp. 59–70). New York: The Haworth Press.

Finn, G. L. (1972). The occupational therapist in prevention programs. *The American Journal of Occupational Therapy, 26*, 59–66.

Grossman, J. (1971, November–December). Community experience for students. *The American Journal of Occupational Therapy, 28*(1), 589–591.

Grossman, J. (1977, July). Preventive health care and community programming. *The American Journal of Occupational Therapy, 31*(6), 351–354.

Hasselkus, B. R., & Brown, M. (1983, February). Respite care for community elderly. *The American Journal of Occupational Therapy, 37*(2), 83–88.

Hightower, M. (1974, May–June). A part of the community—rehabilitation—or apart from the community. *The American Journal of Occupational Therapy, 28*(5), 296–298.

Hoff, S. (1988). The occupational therapist as case manager in an adult day healthcare setting. In E. Taira, (Ed.), *Community programs for the health impaired elderly* (pp. 21–31). New York: The Haworth Press.

Holmes, C., & Bauer, W. (1970, April). Establishing an occupational therapy department in a community hospital. *The American Journal of Occupational Therapy, XXIV*(3), 219–221.

Howe, M., & Dippy, K. (1968). The role of occupational therapy in community mental health. *The American Journal of Occupational Therapy, XXII*(6), 521–524.

Howe, M., Weaver, C., & Dulay, J. (1981, November). The development of a work-oriented day center program. *The American Journal of Occupational Therapy, 35*(11), 711–718.

Hurff, J. M., Poulsen, M. K., Van Hoven, J., & Olson, S. (1985, April). A library skills program serving adults with mental retardation: An interdisciplinary approach. *The American Journal of Occupational Therapy, 39*(4), 233–239.

Johnson, J., & Smith, M. (1966). Changing concepts of occupational therapy in a community rehabilitation center. *The American Journal of Occupational Therapy, XX*(6), 267–273.

Laukaran, V. H. (1977, February). Toward a model of occupational therapy for community health. *The American Journal of Occupational Therapy, 31*(2), 71–74.

Llorens, L. (1971, October). Occupational therapy in community child health. *The American Journal of Occupational Therapy, XXV*(7), 335–339.

Magrun, W. M., & Tigges, K. N. (1982, February). A transdisciplinary mobile intervention program for rural areas. *The American Journal of Occupational Therapy, 36*(2), 90–94.

Maguire, G. A. (1979, February). Volunteer program to assist the elderly to remain in home settings. *The American Journal of Occupational Therapy, 33*(2), 98–101.

Maynard, M. (1986, November). Health promotion through employee assistance programs: A role for occupational therapists. *The American Journal of Occupational Therapy, 40*(11), 771–776.

McColl, M., & Quinn, B. (1985, September). A quality assurance method for community occupational therapy. *The American Journal of Occupational Therapy, 39*(9), 570–577.

Neistadt, M., & Marques, K. (1984, October). An independent living skills training program. *The American Journal of Occupational Therapy, 38*(10), 671–676.

Neistadt, M., & O'Reilly, M. (1988). Independent living skills groups in a level 1 fieldwork experience. *The American Journal of Occupational Therapy, 42*(12), 782–786.

Nochajski, S. B., & Gordon, C. Y. (1987, January). The use of Trivial Pursuit in teaching community living skills to adults with developmental disabilities. *The American Journal of Occupational Therapy, 41*(1), 10–15.

Shalik, L. D., & Shalik, H. (1987, April). Cluster homes: A community for profoundly and severely retarded persons. *The American Journal of Occupational Therapy, 41*(4), 222–226.

Stein, F. (1972, September). Community rehabilitation of disadvantaged youth. *The American Journal of Occupational Therapy, 26*(6), 277–283.

Tickle, L. S., & Yerxa, E. (1981, October). Need satisfaction of older persons living in the community and in institutions, Part 1: The environment. *The American Journal of Occupational Therapy, 35*(10), 644–649.

Tickle, L. S., & Yerxa, E. (1981, October). Need satisfaction of older persons living in the community and in institutions, Part 2: Role of activity. *The American Journal of Occupational Therapy, 35*(10), 650–655.

Walker, L. (1971, October). Occupational therapy in the well community. *The American Journal of Occupational Therapy, XXV*(7), 345–347.

West, W. A. (1967). The occupational therapist's changing responsibility to the community. *The American Journal of Occupational Therapy, XXI*(5), 312–316.

West, W. A. (1969). The growing importance of prevention. *The American Journal of Occupational Therapy, 23*, 226–231.

Wiemer, R. B. (1972, January–February). Some concepts of prevention as an aspect of community health. *The American Journal of Occupational Therapy, 26*(1), 1–9.

Wiemer, R. B., & West, W. A. (1970, July–August). Occupational therapy in community health care. *The American Journal of Occupational Therapy, 24*(5), 323–328.

You may wish to review the following recommended readings relative to community-centered occupational therapy practice published in the 1990s.

Brownson, C. A. (1998). Funding community practice: Stage 1. *American Journal of Occupational Therapy, 52*(1), 60–64.

Bumphrey, E. E. (1995). The role of occupational therapy in health promotion. In E. E. Bumphrey, (Ed.), *Community practice: A text for occupational therapists and others involved in community care* (pp. 68–78). London: Prentice Hall.

Burkhardt, A. (1997, June). Occupational therapy and wellness. *O.T. Practice*, 28–35.

Camardese, M. B., & Youngman, D. (1996). H.O.P.E.: Education, employment, and people who are homeless and mentally ill. *Psychiatric Rehabilitation Journal, 19*(4), 45–56.

Collins, L. F. (1996, October). Perspectives on your private practice: Starting an individualized practice. *O.T. Practice*, 26–27.

Collins, L. F. (1996, October). Moving on when private practice no longer works for you. *O.T. Practice*, 28–29.

Collins, L. F. (1996, February). Thriving in a rural setting. *O.T. Practice*, 40–44.

Collins, L. F. (1997, April). Connecting the community: Shared housing of New Orleans, Inc. *O.T. Practice*, 40–47.

Crist, P., & Stoffel, V. (1992). The Americans with disabilities act of 1990 and employees with mental impairments: Personal efficacy and the environment. *American Journal of Occupational Therapy, 46*(5), 434–443.

DeMaus, P. (1992). An occupational therapy life skills curriculum model for a Native American tribe: A health promotion program based on ethnographic field research. *American Journal of Occupational Therapy, 46*(8), 727–736.

Devereaux, E. (1991). The issue is: Community-based practice. *American Journal of Occupational Therapy, 45*(10), 944–946.

Dunn, W., Brown, C., & McGuigan, A. (1994). The ecology of human performance: A framework for considering the effect of context. *American Journal of Occupational Therapy, 48*, 595–607.

Gage, M., & Polatajko, H. (1994). Enhancing occupational performance through an understanding of perceived self-efficacy. *American Journal of Occupational Therapy, 48*(5), 452–461.

Giles, G. (1994). Editorial: Why provide community support for persons with brain injury? *American Journal of Occupational Therapy, 48*(4), 255–296.

Grady, A. P. (1995). Building inclusive community: A challenge for occupational therapy: 1994 Eleanor Clarke Slagle Lecture. *American Journal of Occupational Therapy, 49*, 300–310.

Greene, D. (1997). The use of service learning in client environments to enhance ethical reasoning in students. *American Journal of Occupational Therapy, 51*(10), 844–852.

Hurff, J. M., Lowe, H. E., Ho, B. J., & Hoffman, N. M. (1990). Networking: A successful linkage for community occupational therapists. *American Journal of Occupational Therapy, 44*(5), 424–430.

Ingstad, B. (1990). The disabled person in the community: Social and cultural perspectives. *International Journal of Rehabilitation Research, 13*, 187–194.

Kari, N., & Michels, P. (1991). The Lazarus Project: The politics of empowerment. *American Journal of Occupational Therapy, 45*(8), 719–725.

Knis, L. L. (1997, March). O.T. and the community: Helping those with mental illness to transition. *O.T. Practice*, 36–41.

Lysack, C., Stadnyk, R., Paterson, M., McLeod, K., & Krefting, L. (1995). Professional expertise of occupational therapists in community practice: Results of an Ontario survey. *Canadian Journal of Occupational Therapy, 62*, 138–147.

Oliver, M. (1990). *The politics of disablement*. London: MacMillan.

Parker, M. G., & Thorslund, M. (1991). The use of technical aids among community-based elderly. *American Journal of Occupational Therapy, 45*(8), 712–718.

Pizzi, M. (1992). Hospice: The creation of meaning for people with life threatening illness. *O.T. Practice, 4*(1), 1–7.

Reitz, S. M. (1992). A historical review of occupational therapy's role in preventive health and wellness. *American Journal of Occupational Therapy, 46*, 50–55.

Robnett, R. (1997, May). Paradigms of community practice. *O.T. Practice*, 30–35.

Ryan, S. (1993). The role of the COTA as an activities director. In S. Ryan, (Ed.), *Practice issues in occupational therapy education* (pp. 193–204). Thorofare, NJ: Slack.

Schelly, C., Sample, P., & Spencer, K. (1992). The Americans with Disabilities Act of 1990 expands employment opportunities for persons with developmental disabilities. *American Journal of Occupational Therapy, 46*(5), 457–460.

Siebert, C. (1997). A description of fieldwork in the home care setting. *American Journal of Occupational Therapy, 51*(6), 423–429.

Special issue on community health. (1998). *American Journal of Occupational Therapy, 52*(1).

Special issue on occupation, spirituality, and life meaning. (1997). *American Journal of Occupational Therapy, 51*(3).

Special issue on occupation. (1998). *American Journal of Occupational Therapy, 52*(6).

Spencer, J. (1991). An ethnographic study of independent living alternatives. *American Journal of Occupational Therapy, 45*(3), 243–250.

Vanier, C., & Hebert, M. (1995). An occupational therapy course on community practice. *Canadian Journal of Occupational Therapy, 62*, 76–81.

Voas, R. (1997). Drinking and driving prevention in the community: Program planning and implementation. *Addiction, 92*(Supplement 2), S201–S219.

Welberding, D. (1991). The quarterway house: More than an alternative of care. *O.T. in Mental Health, 11*(1), 65–91.

The following may be a useful resource to community practitioners in rural settings: Breaking New Ground Resource Center, Purdue University, 1146 Agricultural Engineering Building, West Lafayette, Indiana, 47907-1146 (assists people with disabilities who are employed in agriculture through written resources and contacts in the community).

# CHAPTER 3

# Identifying Trends and Forecasting Futures

## Learning Objectives

1. To learn how to identify current events reported in the media and in professional literature that may impact you and your potential program
2. To explore how historical events and eras have impacted health care and the occupational therapy profession
3. To analyze trends to make forecasts regarding the potential success of your planned program

## Key Terms

1. Trends
2. Forecasts

What is happening in the community, region, state, country, and world today that will impact us and our ideas and plans for the future? As we venture into the design and development of new programming, it becomes critical that the practice of following trends becomes a part of daily and weekly routines. This is not to suggest that each of us should construct a sophisticated statistical *trends analysis;* rather, we should use the existing information in the literature and the media to chart the direction in which things will likely go (**trends**). According to Celente,

### A Programming Scenario

A community program can be designed to encourage positive parent-child communication through activities and experiences that focus on shared occupations. Such
a program prepares the child for a successful academic future. The planning and
funding of such a program may be greatly influenced by current trends in public
sentiment prompted by recent school bombings and shootings; and a general media
concern for violence. This results in a resurgence of parental concern regarding
children's use of unstructured time and the lack of positive parent-child experiences.

A later example of a parent-child community program will help to demonstrate
how an issue impact tree can be used to forecast possible futures for a potential
program.

a "trend is a definite, predictable direction or sequence of events," and "tracking
trends shows us how we got here, where we are, and where we're going" (1991,
pp. 4–5). We then should use these *trends* to make *forecasts*. These **forecasts**, or scenarios of the probable future, will permit us to make more critical judgments
regarding our own futures relative to practice and, particularly, to new or continued community programming.

Examples of shifting trends may include the change from "national economic
systems (to) an international economy" and the shift from "the management of
illness via the management of medication (to) the genetic treatment of illness"
(Ramsey and Robertson, 1993; p. 28). In addition, computer technology and elec-
tronics, transportation systems, and educational technology have all experienced
shifting trends.

In fact, today we really do not have much choice in the matter of considering
and responding to trends. In the preface to the original edition of *The Temporary
Society*, Bennis and Slater (1968) comment that to engage in the forecasting of social
trends "in a world of unprecedented complexity during changes of unparalleled
rapidity" is probably as absurd as it is necessary.

At least on a weekly basis (and preferably daily), web-based news and/or
major newspapers should be read to ferret out events that may impact us as we
practice "occupation-centered" interventions. For example, what are the current
political events at the international, national, and state levels? By perusing current
events, we can determine where the public sentiments lie and where the state and
federal dollars are going, and we may be able to forecast where these funds are
likely to go in the future. Wars, political intrigues, and adolescent or young adult
fads may appear to be vastly remote from our concerns for therapy, wellness, and
health, but if we remain alert, these things can, and likely will, impact the programming we might propose and the funding available to make it possible.

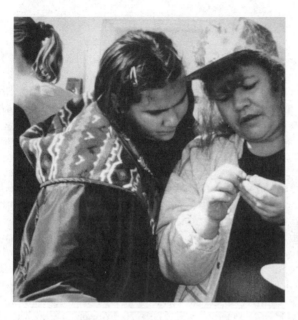

Strengthening the bonds between children and their parents through cooperation in meaningful activities creates partnerships for future change.

## Analyzing Trends by Reviewing History

Our analysis of current and developing trends must also include our awareness of history. We all know of the tremendous impact World War I and World War II had on the history of occupational therapy. The first clinic-community program developed by the author of this text was for veterans of Vietnam. Although this programming was in response to numbers and need, it was initiated with inadequate preparation that an earlier event/trends review might have offered. The programming met the immediate need in something of a crisis mode, but it could have been more proactive had the insights and advanced preparation from (an) analysis of trends been utilized. An analysis or analyses of the social trends and the characteristics of the developing counterculture might have encouraged the design of programming that would have helped Vietnam veterans reenter the community and avoid the emotional trauma that many encountered. This would be true of any programming designed to meet the needs of persons experiencing crisis situations and programming designed to assist in the process of cultural/environmental assimilation (such as for refugees).

Current best-selling books in the popular marketplace give us information regarding the interests, needs, and wants of the public—the public that we, too, are a part of and seek to serve. Often, novelists of both fiction and nonfiction, screenwriters, song writers, and other representatives of popular culture can provide a window to trends or perhaps even set them.

# Finding Trends in Professional Literature

Certainly we must read our own professional literature and that of other health care practitioners, but program descriptions likely will be responding to trends rather than setting them. Those who are setting trends probably will not know it for some time, and even then they may not make a publishable record of such events. We must, however, remain aware of the actions our professional organization is taking at both the state and national levels with regard to the requirements for education and practice. Many of our leaders have been and are courageous trendsetters, but the profession of occupational therapy historically has been conservative; it has moved toward the future tentatively, avoiding uncharted territories. Whatever stance you prefer, our professional affiliations offer us both freedoms and restraints, and neither can be ignored.

Practice in the community does not mean practice outside of our discipline or our profession but in many ways requires an even closer relationship to our values and ethics than in the more institutional-based environments. We may find it difficult at first to open our thinking to entertain innovative arenas from which practice may originate. Certainly legislative decisions, public laws and reforms, and state and local budgeting are factors that may specifically influence our practices, but we most likely learn of these while we are feeling their effects. Often our reactions are prompted either by not being prepared (and "missing the boat" while another, more savvy, provider steps in) or, sadly, by preparing and investing in a rigid service model that is rapidly becoming obsolete.

# Global Trends

There may be circumstances where tracking global trends will strengthen your perception of need, and help establish the parameters of your program. The World Health Organization website (http://www.who.int/en/) can provide statistics and information for countries around the world. WHOLIS is the WHO library database and from this database you can search any country or topic; for example, *Health Topics: Obesity*. You may then access articles of interest free of charge. Accessing the *World Health Report* can provide information such as "life expectancy" which will offer charts for most countries with figures for birth rates, variations in life expectancy for males and females, population figures, etc. Global trends are particularly useful to validate the need for both domestic and international programs in the areas of primary prevention.

# The Impact of Trends—Generating Questions to Consider

Sometimes events, perhaps predictive of trends, appear to have little to do with us and are ignored. Certainly no one can doubt that health care in the United States is rapidly changing. Could these changes have been predicted? An analysis of the large expenditures incurred in the therapy provisions of the 1980s and 1990s likely would have at least partially predicted the inevitable downsizing we are presently experiencing. Even now there are regional changes that are predictive of changes that have occurred or will occur across the country. What are professionals doing to prepare for the changes that may occur? This prompts some interesting questions. Should health care providers seek more or less regulation? With what disciplines should we form alliances? Is it time for new liaisons?

It would appear that people are becoming more responsible for the state of their health. At least we can concur that they are generally more aware and likely worry more about it. Is this a trend? Did the changes in the perceived quality of health care prompted by the corporate entry into an arena thought to be humanistic cause us to become responsive to the need to care for ourselves? Are young adults learning to place their trust exclusively in their own actions? Will the next generation be even more internally controlled than the last one? How will they prepare for shrinking resources and diminished health care and retirement dollars? There is little doubt that they will live longer than their predecessors. Grasping control of your health and life without sacrificing quality and meaning requires skills. Who will provide those skills? Will the trend become a frenzied desire to protect your physical and emotional health and the health of your children in order not to use resources for illness? Or will there be a growing number of drug, alcohol, and accident victims? Will the rich expect to pay for their own services and everyone else be without access to services?

Therapists entering the workforce in the 1950s, 1960s, and 1970s witnessed the ebb-flow cycling of reimbursement and salaries, programming styles, and resources; in response, they have had several turns at the reinvention of the profession. It would appear that the time is right for yet another such reinvention. What about the so-called Generation X, or Y? Apparently these groups are already engaged in the quest for meaning outside the traditional domains of institutional prerogative. What better groups are there to engage in the health care practices of tomorrow, both as givers and receivers? Will these groups require new modes of skill and information provision?

The above discussion is a series of questions prompted by a cursory review of trends—trends that promote forecasts and trends that, assuming we listen, will help us to outline future practices.

The following exercises will help you learn the initial steps to the process of forecasting the direction of future practice.

## Exercise 1

### Identifying Trends by Tracing History

1. To begin this exercise, review your knowledge of history, including occupational therapy history. Under the categories provided, note those things and occurrences that have impacted the nature of our profession today (think broadly, and add

categories if you choose). You may wish to go to the Web to obtain the information or use other references of your choice. You will discover that in some eras you will find more outstanding events of a political nature (i.e., wars, notable presidential elections) and their accompanying philosophies (i.e., optimism/lack of optimism for the economy). Attitudes may, as well, be optimistic, pessimistic, or uncaring (i.e., anti-government/establishment views in the 1960s). Research agendas that have impacted life-threatening diseases through medication, surgeries, and vaccinations are present in some degree in all of these time frames and may be marked by significant events and/or technological advances. Last, technology as a category has evolved from the telegraph and light bulb to the almost daily changes in telecommunications that we live with today.

You may wish to consider the transfer of this grid to a transparency, flip chart, or to the board to facilitate group work.

|  | Events | Philosophies | Attitudes | Technology |
|---|---|---|---|---|
| Pre–1930 | | | | |
| 1930–1950 | | | | |
| 1950–1970 | | | | |
| 1970–1990 | | | | |
| 1990–Present | | | | |

From your position in the present, review the previous exercise, and highlight those things/events that have, in your observation, made a *positive* impact on the profession of occupational therapy and those things/events that may have had a *negative* impact.

Is there anything happening in the profession today that your analyses of events might have predicted with regard to practice, legislation, education, or reimbursement?

If you wish, discuss with your classmates, colleagues, or others, and note your comments below:

_____

_____

_____

_____

_____

## Exercise 2

**Identifying Recent Trends**

1. Since identifying trends may be a new process for you, it may be helpful to do a sorting activity to begin. Either by placing labels on a large table or by writing on a board, note the following categories of events that may be responsive to trends:

1. Events reflective of *public attitudes*
2. Events reflective of *economics*
3. Events (local, regional, national, international) reflective of *politics*
4. Events reflective of *public interests*
5. Events in *education*
6. Events in *medicine*
7. Events in *health*
8. Events in scientific *research*

Can you think of other categories?

Provide yourself with not only your local newspaper but also copies of such newspapers as *The Washington Post*, *The New York Times*, *The Wall Street Journal*, and any others that you believe will help you create a view of the future. What is happening in Europe, for example, may certainly be significant. (Look at the impact the English had on the history of American rock and roll!) However, the above-mentioned newspapers will likely highlight events for you that may be of significance. Watch local and national news programs for at least a week before you begin this exercise. Also use the Internet to determine what people are interested in and what they are chatting about. Remember that not everything you see on the Internet is factual. Although fiction can tell us a lot when we are looking for trends, we must learn early on to separate fact from fiction or conjecture, particularly when doing research (Garretson, 1997). (See the references at the end of this chapter for sources to help you evaluate Internet information.)

2. As you go through your newspapers, news journals, and notes gleaned from newscasts and the Internet, clip those you have selected and place them under the categories noted previously. If this is done as part of a class exercise, do it first without discussion. When everyone is finished, discuss your findings. Is there agreement? Disagreement? While this is an equally valid exercise when done alone, having other opinions and perspectives broadens your observations.

3. As a class or with colleagues, review your selections and separate those you think may represent a trend that could impact occupation-centered intervention, either therapy-based or health-wellness promotion models. Remove all of the news items that you decide are *not* likely to impact occupation-centered programming.

4. Working with those items remaining, separate your selections to make two categories—one category of those trend predictors that may have a *positive* impact

on occupation-centered intervention and another category for those that may have a *negative* impact.

# Steps to Identifying Trends and Forecasting Futures

The following list summarizes the steps to identifying trends and forecasting futures:

1. Find resources such as newspapers, Internet, television, and others.
2. Clip pertinent articles and notes, and place them under one of the identified eight categories.
3. Review your categories and clippings.
4. Remove any news item(s) that you feel *will not* likely impact the practice of occupation-centered interventions.
5. Make two categories of those items remaining—one category of those items that may have a *positive* impact and one category for those items that may have a *negative* impact on occupation-centered programs.
6. Review your categories, and try some forecasting. What is likely to happen next? From the identification of *trends* come *forecasts*. Forecasts are what you might anticipate or predict will come of the reviewed trends. Forecasts can supply answers to questions such as: what impact will these apparent trends have on you professionally and personally?
   From the work you have completed in the previous exercises, can you make forecasts or predictions as to how those things you have identified will likely have an impact on present and/or future occupation-centered interventions, either therapy-based or health maintenance/promotion/wellness practices? How will they impact you personally? How will they impact your professional expectations?
5. Note your forecast(s) or prediction(s) below.

_____

_____

_____

_____

_____

_____

   a. What do you anticipate will be the impact of your forecast(s) or prediction(s) on occupation-centered intervention in general?

_____

_____

_____

_____

_____

    b. What do you anticipate will be the impact on you, personally and professionally?

_____

_____

_____

_____

6. Considering what you have found, note below any identified trends/forecasts that may influence your interests in community programming (either positively or negatively).

    a.  Presently, my community programming interests are:

_____

_____

_____

_____

    b.  Trends that *may* have a positive impact:

_____

_____

_____

_____

    c.  Trends that *may* have a negative impact:

_____

_____

_____

_____

_____

Remember that even if you identify negative trends, this does not necessarily mean that you give up your ideas; rather, it means that you use the present information to make adaptations to your future plans or at least to develop contingency plans.

7. If you have identified negative trends in the previous exercise, how might you wish to adapt your planning, or what contingency plans will you adopt in order to be better prepared for your future?
   Continue to be aware of events and trends, and continue to make forecasts. You may wish to begin charting your forecasts to see how accurate you are. Organize a file that categorizes your interests; when you see something (such as a newspaper article or a news story), clip it and drop it in your file. Review the contents periodically, and examine for developing trends. Always look for social, economic, and political significance. Use a separate category for anything dealing specifically with occupational therapy and with other health professions.
   Ramsey and Robertson (1993) suggest the use of an "Issue Impact Tree" to help in the identification of trends. The following exercise is an adaptation of their work.
8. Select an issue that may be reflective of a trend, such as technology-based distance education, reductions in medical-based health care financing, affordable home-based technology, or another of your choice. Write the issue you've selected in the largest of the circles represented in Figure 3–1. Working alone or with a group, brainstorm on what you think may be major implications of this issue. Write these implications in the next larger circle immediately adjacent to the largest one.

Now think about second-level implications that may grow from the first level. Place these in the next group of circles. Either alone or as a group, come to consensus to determine which of the implications you believe are most likely to occur. Score them as follows:

1. Most likely to occur
2. Might occur
3. Least likely to occur

# Resulting Implications for Future Occupation-Centered Programming

The parent-child community program scenario introduced earlier will help to demonstrate how an issue impact tree can be used to forecast possible futures for a

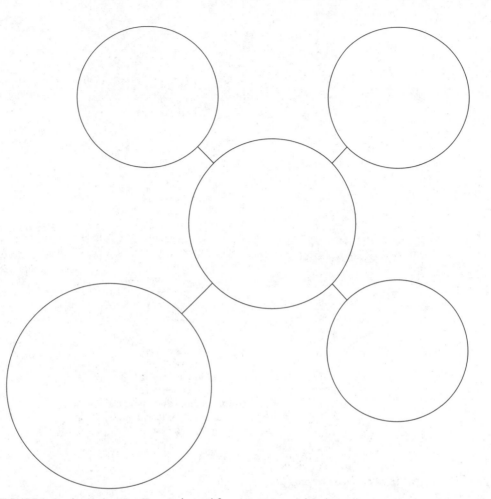

**FIGURE 3–1**  Issue Impact Tree (adapted from Ramsey and Robertson, (1993).

program. As you review Figure 3–2 you will see that the primary issue: violence in schools has a number of primary implications, and several second level implications that may be reflected in the development of future programming.

It is likely that the present and the next few years will welcome community- and school-based prevention programming and research targeting 1) violent behavior exhibited by children and adolescents, 2) the nature of and time spent on computer games by children, and 3) the nature of parent-child communications and time spent in shared activities.

As we develop this scenario and others in future chapters, you will see how we continue to return to the information provided by trends analyses and the resulting futures forecasts.

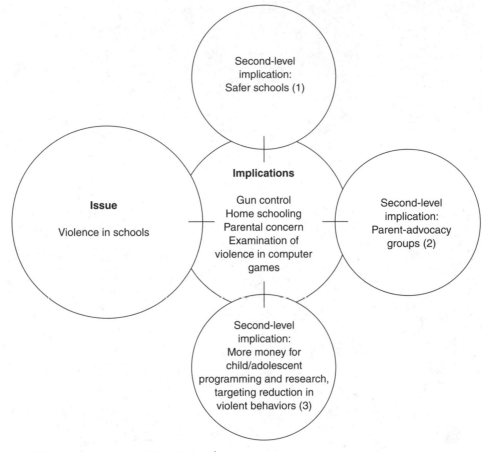

**FIGURE 3–2**    Issue Impact Tree, Example

## Summary

The planning of occupation-centered programs does not occur in a vacuum. An identification of trends based on past and present information will encourage the planner to anticipate the future and make forecasts regarding the potential successes of his or her proposed programming. Envisioning the future will prompt the planner to be prepared for changes in population, funding, and market demands.

The previous exercises are intended to help you plan your future program(s). As a practitioner and program development specialist, it will be critical to your progress that you continue some ongoing analysis of trends. As a leader and as a manager, you may wish to place *futures forecasting* on a yearly retreat agenda; without it an organization cannot successfully complete five-year to ten-year planning. Skillful and sometimes intuitive futures forecasting can place you and your organization in the position of setting trends and designing futures rather than scrambling to keep up with those that are occurring. Begin now to establish habits that will place you in the forefront of futures forecasting.

## *References*

Bennis, W., & Slater, P. (1968). *The temporary society.* San Francisco: Jossey-Bass.

Celente, G. (1991). *Trend tracking.* New York: Warner Books.

Garretson, C. H. (1997). *Factors affecting Webmasters' sense of responsibility for information accuracy.* Unpublished thesis, Georgia Southern University.

Ramsey, D., & Robertson, S. (1993). *Breaking into new markets: Expanding roles in mental health.* Workshop resource book. Bethesda, MD: American Occupational Therapy Association.

### Audio Transcripts

*Evaluating the quality of information on the Internet.* (1997). General Conference Session at the 12th Annual Computers in Libraries Conference, Arlington, Virginia. (Available from Alexandria, Virginia)

Tillman, H. (1996). *Advertising/marketing sources on the Internet.* Denver, CO: National Audio Video.

### Internet Site

WHO (http://www.who.int/en/)

# CHAPTER 4

# Program Development: What Skills Will I Need?

## Learning Objectives

1. To develop a personally meaningful definition of occupational therapy
2. To appreciate the skills of effective/active listening
3. To develop the skills of effective verbal communication
4. To develop the skills of collaboration and negotiation
5. To learn to recognize the distribution of personal time in balancing daily occupations
6. To explore the characteristics of an effective leader and manager
7. To assess personal knowledge and skills relative to community program design, development, and practice
8. To identify personal qualities, attributes, and behaviors in preparation for potential leadership roles in community programming

## Key Terms

1. Program/Programming
2. Communication
3. Effective/Active Listening
4. Negotiation
5. Persuasion
6. Clinical Reasoning

7. Partnering/Collaboration
8. Leader/Leadership
9. Manager/Director

The focus of this chapter is to learn how to identify the skills and information the planner will need to design and develop a *program*. Youngstrom (1999, p. 129) defines **program** as "a specifically designed service that is aimed toward a specific goal and is designed to achieve clearly defined outcomes or results". Specificity is important to this definition, for through specificity we are able to produce program results that are clear and measurable. A program designed by an occupational therapy practitioner may take several directions. For example, it may be therapeutic in its intent; that is, designed to provide therapy for those in need of *therapeutic intervention*. This intervention, the provision of occupational *therapy*, may include identification of specific needs (or screening), assessment, treatment, and evaluation for individuals of any age. Of course, programming of this nature may be developed to provide a new service not offered previously, or it may be developed to extend service in an existing occupational therapy department. Extending new service for an existing program; or, enhancing present programming is often the first venture for programmers.

You will find the term **programming** commonly used in this text to denote the step-by-step orchestrated process of designing and developing a program. Although occupation-centered programs may be intended to solve problems, the order followed in planning programs for *people* is not always linear and, at times, may seem less than logical.

Occupation-centered programs may also be developed for individuals who are not candidates for *therapy* as defined by the need for treatment of disability or disease. Rather, because of life circumstances largely beyond their control, they are considered to be at risk for developing destructive life patterns that may diminish their opportunities for quality experiences. While programs for these populations may also involve screening and assessment, the intention is not to offer therapy. Screening and assessments are conducted to determine where the development of skills and the acquisition of knowledge and information will be required in order to reduce or diminish the potential for problems. Programs targeting the acquisition of skills, knowledge, and information neutralize risk. Whether our intentions are to provide therapy, to prevent problems by reducing risk, or to maintain health and wellness, the belief in *occupation* connects us.

Programs may also be designed to enhance and reinforce already present positive development. Because of occupational therapy practitioners' educational foundation and experience, programs can be carefully tailored to the specific needs of the individual. The understanding of occupation as an outcome of an intricate system comprised of the individual's values, interests, needs, and wants offers a unique perspective to programming not found in other professions. The appreciation of the intricacies of *occupation* coupled with a practical foundation in the analysis of tasks permits the occupational therapy practitioner to match the teaching of skills with the acquisition of abilities for positive occupation-centered outcomes. An occupation-centered perspective offers a particularly unique contribution to the development of programming for "at-risk" populations as well as programs targeting the maintenance of health. Programs designed by those with education and experience in occupation-centered perspectives, then, can be successfully adapted to any population in need of services.

The actual process of program development is a bit like solving a puzzle—one piece placed at a time, and the placement of each piece demanding our knowledge, skill, and expertise. To help select the first piece of the puzzle, we might ask, "just what do I need to know to begin the process of designing and developing a community program?" The answers are fairly simple. To begin, we need to know

- How to communicate clearly and effectively
- How to listen
- How to collaborate and negotiate
- How to serve as a role model of occupational balance
- How to provide occupation-centered services
- How to provide leadership
- How to manage systems

And to complete the package, we need

- A solid occupational therapy professional education
- Strong professional and personal ethics
- Good common sense
- Energy and motivation to try something new

# The Skill of Becoming an Effective Communicator

The first skill—or perhaps we should say the prerequisite skill—is to be an effective communicator. Most of us can communicate well enough to get the things we need and sometimes the things we want, but all of us can use some help in communicating effectively in many and varied situations. Effective **communication** is a skill to be learned, and we need to identify and practice the skills of finding and utilizing efficient and sufficient language to communicate ideas to anyone with optimal results. This is the key to marketing our program first to the agency or facility we may wish to have sponsor our program and then, ultimately, to the consumer.

## Exercise 1

### Communicating to the Listener: Your Definition of Occupational Therapy

It is likely that on many occasions you will have to explain who you are and what you do as an occupational therapy practitioner. Perhaps you will first explain this

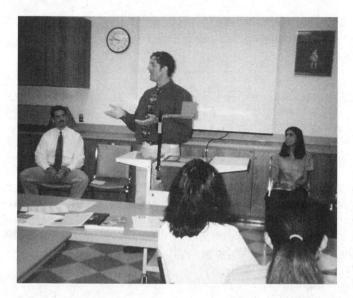

Developing confidence through presentations of proposals helps students first discover and then build skills for effective marketing of occupation-centered community programs.

to those whom you hope will welcome your program in their facility, second to other professionals, and third to consumers. Although many of the people with whom you come in contact or wish to collaborate with will have an idea of what occupational therapy is (perhaps from the roots of the words themselves or from personal experience), it is unlikely that many will appreciate the diversity in practice exhibited by the profession. This may particularly be the case if you choose to develop community-based programming targeting prevention or maintenance.

If one of your student assignments provided the opportunity to explain occupational therapy to a group outside of the profession, you have a head start on this exercise. Experienced practitioners have likely developed their own definitions of occupational therapy; however, these definitions are usually tailored to a particular practice niche. If you, as the practitioner, are entertaining thoughts of designing and developing a program for a new niche, you may want to expand or change your definitions.

1. In your textbooks or the professional literature, find a definition or definitions of occupational therapy. Write the definition(s) below (use additional paper if you need more space):

_____

_____

_____

_____

_____

2. Using a highlighter, note *key words* that you find *meaningful* in the definitions of occupational therapy. Write those words below:

_____

_____

_____

_____

3. Review the *key words* you selected. Use these words to write your own definition of occupational therapy—a definition by which *you*, as a practitioner, would like to be identified. Remember to keep your definition broad and not specific to only one kind of practice or to one kind of practitioner (for example, occupational therapist or occupational therapy assistant). Write your definition below.

_____

_____

_____

_____

4. Write your definition of what occupational therapists or occupational therapy assistants *do* (what *you* wish to do). Again, keep your perspective broad, and avoid listing specific skills or roles. Begin to think of yourself as an *occupation-centered practitioner*. Write your definition below.

_____

_____

_____

_____

_____

5. Using the definition you developed, translate it to use in the following scenario:
    You wish to start a summer day camp for children who have been identified by parents and/or educators as emotionally-socially immature. It is not your expectation that any of the children will carry a diagnosis; but all may be seen to be "at risk." You have been asked by a mother who is interested in your program, "What does an occupational therapist do?"

Have a classmate, colleague, or friend role-play the question. Briefly write your response below. (You should also provide a verbal explanation. Remember to use the definition you developed in question 4 to structure your answer.)

_____

_____

_____

_____

6.  Continue the exercise by applying the following scenario:

You have at least partially won the trust of the mother who now invites you to the Parent-Teacher Association (PTA) meeting to talk about occupational therapy. You can assume most of the audience will be interested in what occupational therapy can do for children, so you may wish to focus on this aspect. Consider how and why the above-mentioned children may be "at risk" and what kinds of assistance your camp might offer. This is likely your first opportunity to begin marketing your proposed camp program for "at-risk" children to a large audience, so you might also wish to include how mothers might recognize if their children would be good candidates for your camp.

This one may be a bit challenging, for there are several considerations that may be presently outside your experience. You may wish to first discuss it with classmates. Share your earlier definitions. When you are ready, briefly write below what you might say differently to this group and how your presentation style might be different. When you have written your responses, role-play your brief presentation to the group.

_____

_____

_____

_____

7. Try different groups with different interests, and critique each other in your responses. Maintain the essence of what occupational therapy is and what occupation-centered practitioners do.

You may want to follow your preliminary response with some specific purposes related to the different groups you are targeting, but resist the temptation to drift into splintered definitions appropriate to only very specific populations. Rather, think about your definitions in a broad way: *What does all of occupational therapy have in common? What do all occupational therapy practitioners strive to do regardless of their clientele?*

Certainly you may wish to direct some of your responses to the specific concerns of your audience; however, if you find yourself explaining how to evaluate joint range or reciting the basic tenets of sensory integration, start again! Use the space below to make any notes you may need to structure your brief responses to new scenarios.

_____

_____

_____

_____

_____

Although critical, learning how to express our ideas and thoughts in a clear and succinct manner is only one aspect of communication. Often when we are new to practice, we become so concerned with trying to communicate our ideas (particularly to patients, clients, and caregivers) that we forget to or are unable to listen.

# Learning to Listen

In *Effective Coaching* (1999), Cook tells us that perhaps the best thing we can do for another person is to give that person our full, undivided attention. We all have attempted to talk with someone who was shuffling through papers, talking to someone else, or gazing somewhere over our head. If you are unable to drop everything to listen to someone who needs your attention, then it is best to be honest and ask that person to return when you are able to listen. It is a human tendency to engage in overlapping occupations, but the listening aspect of communication requires and deserves full attention, whether the speaker is a child, adult, client, coworker, or friend.

In his discussion of **effective listening**, Cook (1999, pp. 70–77) goes on to say that we must let the speaker finish before responding. It is easy to interrupt when we *think* we know the intent of the communication. In therapy environments, where we often hear similar questions and concerns from our patients/clients, the tendency to believe we know the outcome of the communication may be particularly troublesome. Often we manipulate speakers when we interrupt or finish their sentences, particularly if they are not assertive enough to stop us. For many cultures, the therapist/professional represents a powerful authority position, and it would not be easy (or, perhaps, possible) for the patient/client to redirect the communication. Of further note, listening to the needs of a "community" or population is critical to an effective assessment of programming needs and successful outcomes. Individuals may reflect this information, but often the listener must be attuned to a larger, collective voice to ensure that all members are equally represented.

Other characteristics of effective listening include hearing, reflecting, and rephrasing. In the counseling professions, the term **active listening**—that is, listening for the emotional-feeling content as well as the information that is being provided by the speaker—might be used to collectively describe these characteristics. Active listening might include

- Hearing the words,
- Reflecting on and rephrasing what was communicated, and
- Hearing the emotional-feeling content as well as the information.

If you would like to practice, there are many exercises to encourage active listening that your instructor may choose to provide; or these may be included in other aspects of your curriculum.

In summary, active listening describes the ability to hear and to *listen with total consciousness* not only to the words that are being spoken but also to the meaning and emotional content our speaker is expressing. Not only does this ability make us good friends and desirable companions, but also it is absolutely critical to our varied roles as therapists and as programmers/planners.

Whether speaking to an employee, a consumer, the owner of a building we would like to lease for our program, or a granting agency board, we must express our ideas clearly, *and* we must listen fully. It is a skill to be learned.

## Using Your Communication Skills to Negotiate

According to *Webster's Dictionary* (1975), to *negotiate* means "to confer or bargain, one with another, in order to reach an agreement." It is unlikely that you will move through your program design and development process without some **negotiation**. Negotiation does not necessarily mean compromise, and it is important to keep this in mind as we develop our goals and objectives for programming. Our identified need for services and our related goals will continue to remind us of our directive to provide quality programming in ethical ways. If some compromise must occur, it will not be within these dimensions. Shapiro and Jankowski (1998; p. 3), authors of *The Power of Nice*, put a bit of a spin on *Webster's* definition of negotiation by stating that "The best way to get what you want is to help the other side get what they want." The multilevels of the needs assessment (to be discussed in Chapter 7) will give us at least the surface characteristics of what is "wanted" for our targeted population by the community, the organization, or facility for whom we may provide services and then for those who will actually receive the services. Our ability to actively and effectively listen will allow us to identify the more subtle wants that may not necessarily be articulated by either group.

Conger (1998, p. 25) adds another characteristic of communication to the negotiation mix—the art of **persuasion**. He states that *effective persuasion* "is the ability to present a message in a way that leads others to support it." In our interests, to persuade someone is to first influence and then to convince them to support our ideas and plans for a community program.

Interestingly enough, as we expand our ideas regarding negotiation in the design and development of community programs, we are also talking about the skills that are relevant, even critical, to our clinical relationships with clients/patients. This refers to a therapist's abilities to negotiate the selection of treatment goals with the client/patient, or what in the past we may have referred to as "motivating" the recipient of services. We probably cannot truly *motivate* patients/clients for they must do that for themselves; rather, we negotiate and persuade.

Mattingly and Fleming (1994) provide another window of understanding for this intricate and delicate client/patient-therapist negotiation in what they describe as interactive reasoning, or collaborating with the person. They provide numerous examples of how therapists demonstrate skill in learning to interact with their clients/patients, that is, how they "collaborate." The therapist's ability to interpret what a person wants from therapy and the meaning that person attaches to the progress he or she wishes to make is perhaps the highest level of communication-based negotiation we could identify in our therapy process, and it is significant in our understanding of what Mattingly and Fleming (1994) describe as **clinical reasoning**. Clinical reasoning is a complex process involving at least three approaches: procedural reasoning, interactive reasoning, and conditional reasoning. Fleming (1994, p. 119) collectively refers to the mobilization of these processes in collaboration and treatment as the "therapist with the three-track mind." As mentioned previously, it is likely interactive reasoning that best engages the therapist and the patient/client in the negotiation process through a true collaboration. Successful collaboration is at the root of effective intervention, whether with one person, or many.

## Partnering: Developing Collaborative Relationships

We know that collaborating with other professionals and community members strengthens our ability to provide programming that is relevant, efficient, and effective; however, in today's climate that may not be enough. The term **partnering** better describes what must occur in order to work effectively, and to obtain funding. Karsh and Fox (2003, p. 150) tell us that to turn a good idea into a winning program (that will be funded), the right partners must be actively involved. **Collaboration** is a term that we're all familiar with, but in reality it's a concept and set of behaviors that most of us find quite difficult. In his book *No More Teams!* Schrage (1989) suggests that most Americans support the idea of being a "team player," but they often prefer to be the "captain!" Rugged individualism begins, for most of us, in kindergarten. Very few people have much experience at true collaboration . . . sitting down with the intent of working with others (individuals, groups, organizations) and making a commitment to finding the best possible solution to the problem. However, the more people with expertise and varying points of view who are sincerely committed to developing a solution to a pressing problem, the more likely it is that the solution (the program) will be developed and developed with quality. In community programming, our *partners* may include other health care practitioners, teachers, school administrators, universities, museums, city parks and recreation, the police department, the fire department, the Chamber of Commerce, parents, and consumers to name but a few. Negotiating collaborations and partnerships will likely challenge our communication styles, our ability to listen, and our knowledge base, but the rewards will be well worth the extra effort.

# Leading and Managing

All of the previously mentioned skills come together in helping us to identify ourselves as **leaders** and **managers**; two qualities significant to the role of community program planner and facilitator. We will first examine your present management skills and your potential to become a manager. The first task of good managers is to manage themselves and their own round of daily occupations.

## Managing "Yourself" First

Do you currently represent yourself as a model for a healthy balance of occupations? Take a moment to reflect on your response and perhaps those of your classmates or colleagues. In particular, students are likely to say that they do not have enough time in the day or week and that they find themselves studying to the exclusion of leisure and self-care. Time, of course, is not infinite. It is likely that we do not manage time; rather, time manages us. But we are not victims. If we begin by making a daily, weekly, or monthly *map* of the way we spend our time, then we can learn to manage ourselves within the time we have available. These skills need to be learned as students. If we do not manage to balance our occupations today, it is not likely that we will later; and our future as managers may be in jeopardy.

### Mapping Time for Engagement in Daily/Weekly Occupations

On a separate piece of paper, using the *pie* in Figure 4–1 to represent the time available to you in a day or a week and using colored markers or pencils to separate work/productive activity, play/leisure, and self-care, draw a slice in the pie to represent the percentage of time you require for each of these categories.

We have not attempted to define meaning in daily occupations, but this is implicit as we move on with this exercise. Which occupations/activities have meaning for you, and which do not? It is likely that we feel more balanced when we have

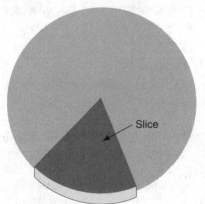

Slice

**FIGURE 4–1**    Pie Graph of Daily Occupations

a distribution of meaningful and meaningless activities in our day. After all, most of us can't attend to a totally meaningful existence. It would be exhausting!

What about play/leisure? Is it important to you to play everyday? Do you need that balance? It does not matter what activity you choose to represent play; that will depend on your values and interests and how you establish meaning in your life. Play may mean tossing a ball against a wall or rolling it to your cat; perhaps play means running three miles, engaging in sex, cooking, or another activity of choice. Although it may commonly be considered self-care, taking an uninterrupted bath or a shower is pure leisure for some, particularly for those with small children. If it is important in order for you to feel balanced, then draw in the time you spend doing it. If it is not important, if it does not hold meaning for you, or if you do not consider it true play/leisure, then leave it out of your map under this category. After all, one person's play may be another person's work. When mapping time for work, again, it is important to recognize how much overlap plays a part in assigning meaning to occupations. For many people, their work is also their play; and even though to others they appear to work to the exclusion of play, in reality they may feel quite balanced.

Review your "pie," and take a careful look at what you have. Is there any activity in which you regularly engage that is missing? Is there anything you deem truly meaningful missing? Evaluate your map critically. You probably look more balanced in your daily/weekly occupations than you might have expected, and you probably have some empty space to use as you choose (play, self-care, and/or work). The human animal is fairly self-protective. We are skilled at balancing our occupations even when, at times, we believe ourselves to be balance-impoverished.

Remember this exercise, and complete it whenever you feel stressed regarding your balance of occupation(s). You may need to reexamine your priorities. Priorities change frequently when we are goal-directed and as we move from one context to another. Are your priorities appropriate to what you wish to achieve? If so, you likely feel balanced, and you can maintain your health and well-being. If not, you may feel stressed, and it is time to make adjustments.

Now that you have completed the previous exercises, you should have a better sense of your *priorities* and how these priorities influence your personal *balance of occupations*. You have identified your *communication* strengths as well as those areas where you may need to do a little work on your communication skills. You now have a much better grasp of what it means to *manage yourself*.

# The Characteristics of a Manager/Director

There are many resources available to you for the fundamentals of management (such as budgets, staffing, billing, and daily operations), and you will find them referenced in several chapters of this text. If you are aspiring to start a community program and to manage/direct operations then you must either be familiar with all of the expected operations of an occupational therapy department, or have access to the services of someone who does. If you are a student, then this book is intended as a supplement to an occupational therapy professional education management and supervision course or courses rather than as a replacement for such courses.

If you are a professional but have not had the opportunity to manage a department or program, then taking the time to closely observe the manager of your place of practice is strongly recommended. Also, if possible, spend time with a mentor who is successfully operating a program such as the one you are contemplating, with the goal of understanding the management of day-to-day operations. Arranging an additional internship or externship in management would be beneficial to students who are seriously considering developing and managing programs. Of course, the intent of a community program is to offer a service or services to a targeted population. The skills involved in delivering an occupation-centered service are implicit in your professional education and any advanced coursework, specialty practice, and/or credentials you may have earned beyond your professional courses and fieldwork.

Management involves managing complex whole *systems* of both things and functions, but often those who are considered to be the best managers are known for their demonstrated abilities in the management of people. In his book *Winning 'Em Over*, Conger (1998) talks about a revolution in management that is occurring in the business world. This revolution is marked by a shift from a management model strongly anchored in the power of authority and hierarchy to one of persuasion and teamwork. Shapiro and Jankowski (1998) echo these thoughts in their book *The Power of Nice*. If such a shift is actually taking place in the world of business, then we might expect similar shifts in the business of health care. It seems likely that the upper tiers of health care management, the tiers that represent the transition to business and corporate influence, may be struggling with the shift from power-dominated authority to a friendlier model as well. Though these shifts are probably not entirely voluntary, Conger and others would suggest that Generation X was a strong part of the mix, forcing a more interactive management style that continues today.

The actual providers of health care—in our discussions, occupational therapy practitioners—have long extended their care-giving styles to blend with their management styles. In recent years, which have been marked by competitive and challenging times in health care, it would seem that many occupational therapy managers/directors have felt apologetic for this more caring, people-centered management style and have aspired to be more authoritative and tougher (what they may have perceived to be more "business" oriented). It is interesting to note, at least according to Conger, that business may now be moving toward a more "people-friendly" model, a management model occupational therapists have long demonstrated and probably have developed from their therapeutic *ways of being*.

As mentioned earlier, in his discussions of the "new management," Conger (1998, pp. 43–46) elaborates on persuasion as a central concept for managers in developing relationships with their personnel/teams. He feels that the components of successful persuasion include "Building your credibility; finding the common ground; developing compelling positions and evidence; and connecting emotionally". We might pose the question, "who knows more about persuasion than the occupational therapy practitioner?" These concepts are also core to successful therapy, and the core skills we use as therapists are central to our abilities as managers, directors, and leaders. The same is true of teamwork and collaboration; occupational therapy practitioners have always seen themselves as participants in teams. For the students, working in groups represents the beginning of the belief in teamwork as the most effective way "to get the job done." Therefore, the profession of occupational therapy has already acknowledged the importance of management by persuasion, teamwork, and collaboration. The goal now must be to solidify and refine these already-acquired professional skills and to avoid the authoritative, more linear model that is generally unresponsive to the needs of today's employee and appears to be rapidly moving toward obsolescence.

# The Characteristics of a Leader

In his discussion of leadership, Townsend tells us that "leadership is unique to each person" and that in his estimation, "leadership is a matter of character" (Bennis and Townsend, 1995; p. 13). Both Townsend and Bennis delineate the qualities of a good leader to include controlled personal ambition, intelligence, and a clear and well-articulated communication style. Many current writers on leadership and management styles agree with these characteristics, particularly those centered around effective communication (Bennis and Goldsmith, 1997; Capodagli and Jackson, 1999; Conger, 1998; Cook, 1999; Shapiro and Jankowski, 1998). Writing about leadership from an occupational therapy perspective, Gilkeson (1997; pp. 3–4) describes the successful leader as someone who is unique. Yet she also notes that common traits that all leaders possess are "values, vision, communication skills, persistence, self-confidence, optimism, empathy, and observation."

Drawing a distinction between leaders and managers, Bennis and Goldsmith (1997, p. 4) note that "managing is about efficiency," and "leadership is about innovating and initiating." In their words, "leaders conquer the context" (p. 4), and the *context* of concern to occupational therapy practitioners—the environment of health care and health maintenance—is most certainly a flying carpet these days; to conquer it, a leader must be agile, visible, and clever.

Can the leader and the manager exist in one person? Perhaps, but it is more likely that the most comprehensive leadership is produced by a team. This team must include a charismatic and visionary leader and managers who are effective and efficient in the understanding and control of multiple systems. The team members must be ethical, loyal to their cause, skilled, and above reproach. Bennis and Goldsmith (1997, p. 4) note that the profound difference between a manager and a leader is that a "good manager does things right and a leader does the right things."

In some circumstances, the development of a community program may pose a risk for the developer. The luxury of taking such a risk alongside a good manager may not be financially realistic. Therefore, the programmer often must acquire the skill sets of both a leader and a manager, at least in the beginning. Certainly the programmer is a leader; starting a new programming venture in the community, whether for-profit or not-for-profit, would not likely occur to anyone else.

But often the skills needed to manage the developing program have to be learned. Perhaps the true leader and the true manager cannot ever really exist in one person; the personalities, the *ways of being*, and the *ways of thinking*, are likely different. The wise leader, though, will certainly appreciate the intricacies of management. If not able to employ a management team early on, he or she will at least consult with one as development occurs.

Early in this chapter, we discussed the importance of clear and efficient communication. The first task of the leader is to sell himself or herself and the proposed program, which requires the ability to engage others in the venture. Most likely the planner/leader first will need to obtain support for his or her potential program from those outside of occupational therapy; beginning the processes of collaboration and partnering. The nature of these early communications may be different from those that will follow. Soon after, though, the planner must engage the support of the team that will be carrying out the programming; the planner must gain the team members' trust and must encourage them to share in the excitement that comes with such an undertaking. The task of the leader/manager is first to recognize and then to supervise and manage the knowledge and skills of others in such a way as to form a successful and productive goal-directed team. Whether program personnel are aides, occupational therapy assistants, occupational therapists, other professionals, students, or volunteers, the planner's skills as a leader/manager will make the difference in the success of the program. A leader must clearly communicate his or her goals for a program and accompanying expectations for the performance of employees and others. It is also critical that a leader provide honest, direct, and open feedback regarding performance while not losing sight of the larger goals. A successful communicator will be able to provide honest and supportive feedback that will strengthen and empower the employee and the program.

## Exercise 2

### Reinventing Yourself as a Leader

Now that you are on your way to becoming a more effective communicator and you are developing an awareness of what skills are necessary to be an effective manager/director, you must begin the process of reinventing yourself as a leader. If you consider yourself to be a leader now, look at strengthening your capacities. Young, less experienced leaders are likely to have difficulty in delegating responsibility to a team. Not trusting anyone but yourself to do a job will lead to rapid burnout and, eventually, failure. Learning to delegate wisely is a skill that is initiated when the leader/manager first establishes a goal or goals for the program; from these foundational goals, he or she can then build a multiskilled team. The trust that is established around this team makes the process of delegating responsibilities much less hazardous. Comfort with the process comes with each successful experience. The following exercise is adapted from Bennis and Goldsmith (1997):

1. What do you personally consider to be the qualities, attitudes, and behaviors of a leader? You may wish to think of those people who are considered leaders. List the

characteristics below, and beside each one, note your skills and/or attributes in that particular area:

Qualities
(for example, personal honesty)                Your Qualities

_____                    _____

_____                    _____

_____                    _____

Attitudes
(for example, open/friendly)                   Your Attitudes

_____                    _____

_____                    _____

_____                    _____

Behaviors
(for example, working hard)                    Your Behaviors

_____                    _____

_____                    _____

_____                    _____

   Carefully assess your strengths with regard to the above. Do you have leadership qualities that will assist you in the development of new occupation-centered programs? You may wish to discuss the results of your personal assessment with others. Most people have trouble identifying their own leadership qualities and tend to minimize their strengths in this area. Your friends, colleagues, and perhaps family may be able to help.

# What Knowledge and Skills Will I Need?

We have discussed ways to develop our abilities to communicate clearly and effectively, how to identify daily and weekly time use in prioritizing for occupational balance, and how to recognize and develop the characteristics that make a good leader and manager, but there is one more thing we must do. We must recognize that what we must know (knowledge) and what we must do (skills) are the foundation upon which leadership and management develop; without them we have little about which to communicate. Although we have briefly touched on the importance of meeting the needs of our targeted community population, it is imperative that we avoid soliciting needs and wants that we cannot realistically hope to satisfy. Not only would this be unethical, it would also be enormously stressful and foolish. Experienced professionals have a good idea of their knowledge base and their skills, but often still need to do some self-assessment homework with regard to the information and skills necessary to successfully design and develop a community program. This certainly does not mean that if you identify a need in your target population but find yourself lacking in knowledge or skills, you must give up the idea for the program. What it does mean is that you must acquire the knowledge and the skills yourself (mentorships/continuing self-instruction/education) or that you must engage the services of other professionals, paraprofessionals, or volunteers (partnering/collaboration).

Students bring a variety of skills, expertise, and experience to the learning environment, and these skills need to be identified. For students, prior experience and resulting knowledge and skills are the foundations upon which occupational therapy principles, philosophy, and practice will be placed. Unique skills, expertise, and experience oftentimes produce the entrepreneur.

Occupational therapy practitioners as well as students may overestimate or underestimate their expertise and may often fail to anticipate the need for adequate resources. Thus, before you initiate program design and planning, complete the following checklist. This exercise will be helpful in achieving a good sense of what you can offer to any potential program, and as you develop your ideas for specific programming, it will help you to identify areas where you may need some assistance.

## Exercise 3

### Self-Assessment of Knowledge and Skills Relevant to Designing and Developing Community Programs

1. Assessing What You Know: Your Present Knowledge Base

   a. Your *academic* knowledge base. Consider what you have studied, including your professional occupational therapy education and other disciplines you might have studied previous to or following occupational therapy that you think might assist you in designing, developing, and working in occupation-centered community practice. Highlight your academic knowledge base below.

   _____

   _____

   _____

   _____

   b. Your *experiential* knowledge base. Consider any previous or present experience that contributed to your present knowledge base that might assist you in designing, developing, and working in occupation-centered community practice. Such experience might include clinical practice, outcome/evaluation research, sales, managing, marketing, interacting with communities, or other areas. Highlight your knowledge gained through experience below:

_____

_____

_____

_____

2. Assessing Your Skills

Consider what you can do. Do you have expertise with particular modalities, tools, equipment, or assessments used in occupational therapy practice or other clinical practices? Consider any particular credentials you may have earned, certifications, or, for the practicing COTA, service competencies. Do you have particular expertise with arts and crafts? A sport? Perhaps music? Do you have any other skills that may not be directly related to clinical practice but that might be useful when working in the community? Remember that we are also interested in prevention and maintenance of health. (*Note: Of course the above-mentioned skills are interrelated with knowledge; but for the purposes of this exercise, we will separate them.*) Highlight any skills you may have below.

_____

_____

_____

_____

In later chapters, when you have selected your target population and have begun to discuss the service needs they may have and the kinds of programming that will help you meet those needs, you will want to revisit the above lists of knowledge and skills from your new perspective.

In conclusion, when you have selected your target population and know its needs, you will:

- Determine the knowledge and skills required to successfully meet the needs of the target population
- Revisit the knowledge and skills of the planner and others that may be involved in developing the program

The difference between these two items will tell you where you must acquire additional knowledge/skills (if realistic and if time permits) or where you must find others to partner with (professionals, paraprofessionals, volunteers, or others).

# Summary

To return to our original question, we must ask ourselves, "what do I need to know to develop a community program?" Through the course of this chapter, we have identified the following areas of personal responsibility in preparing the foundation for program development:

- The development of clear and effective communication styles
- Knowing how to effectively and actively listen to others
- Developing the skills of collaboration and negotiation
- Recognizing the responsibility to serve as a role model of occupational balance
- Knowing how to provide occupation-centered services for our patients/clients/consumers
- Knowing how to provide leadership
- Knowing how to manage and direct systems

The above characteristics, which are established on a firm base of professional ethics and personal integrity and sound occupation-centered practice knowledge and skills, will provide a foundation for the continued development of any additional expertise that may be needed to become an insightful and effective planner, leader, manager, and director. The resulting "package" will not be difficult to market!

# References

Bennis, W., & Goldsmith, J. (1997). *Learning to lead: A workbook on becoming a leader*. Reading, MA: Addison-Wesley.

Bennis, W., & Townsend, R. (1995). *Reinventing leadership: Strategies to empower the organization*. New York: William Morrow.

Capodagli, B., & Jackson, L. (1999). *The Disney way*. New York: McGraw-Hill.

Conger, J. (1998). *Winning 'em over: A new model for management in the age of persuasion*. New York: Simon and Schuster.

Cook, M. (1999). *Effective coaching*. New York: McGraw-Hill.

Fleming, M. (1994). Therapist with the three-track mind. In C. Mattingly, & M. Fleming, (Eds.), *Clinical Reasoning: Forms of inquiry in a therapeutic practice* (pp. 119–136). Philadelphia: F. A. Davis.

Gilkeson, G. (1997). *Occupational therapy leadership: Marketing yourself, your profession, and your organization*. Philadelphia: F. A. Davis.

*International Webster new encyclopedic dictionary*. (1975). Chicago: The Language Institute of America.

Karsh, E., & Fox, A. (2003). *The only grant-writing book you'll ever need*. New York: Carroll and Graf.

Mattingly, C., & Fleming, M. (1994). *Clinical reasoning: Forms of inquiry in a therapeutic practice*. Philadelphia: F. A. Davis.

Schrage, M. (1989). *No more teams! Mastering the dynamics of creative collaboration*. New York: Doubleday.

Shapiro, R., & Jankowski, M. (1998). *The power of nice: How to negotiate so everyone wins—Especially you*. New York: John Wiley and Sons.

Youngstrom, M. J. (1999). Developing a new occupational therapy program. In K. Jacobs, & M. Logigian, (Eds.), *Functions of a manager in occupational therapy* (3rd ed., pp. 129–142). Thorofare, NJ: Slack.

CHAPTER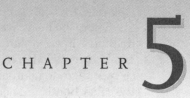

# Developing a Time Line for Program Design, Planning, Preparation, Implementation, and Evaluation

## Learning Objectives

1. To appreciate the importance of a time line in the accomplishment of program design, implementation, and review/evaluation
2. To define the three phases of program development to include: 1) the design and planning phase; 2) the preparation and implementation phase; and 3) the review and evaluation phase
3. To identify tasks associated with each phase of the program-development process and to develop a time line to reflect these tasks

## Key Terms

1. Time Line
2. Design and Planning Phase
3. Preparation and Implementation Phase
4. Review and Evaluation Phase

One of the first critical steps of the program design and development process is to establish a firm calendar of what is to be done in order to accomplish the program and when it must occur in order to initiate the program at the anticipated time. This calendar, or **time line**, ensures that nothing is forgotten and that there are no surprises that cost time and often add expense.

There are many ways to develop a time line, and much of the design and detail depends on the organizational style of the individual. For planners who are sufficiently organized in their work routines, a sketchy time line is generally enough to permit them to maintain a schedule; those individuals who are less organized, on the other hand, will need to include everything.

# Designs for Time Lines

Time lines may be organized according to the full process of designing, developing and evaluating a program. For example, one might prefer to develop the time line according to the three phases of program development

1. Design and planning phase
2. Preparation and implementation phase
3. Program review and evaluation phase

## The Design and Planning Phase

The **design and planning phase** may include the following: 1) identifying trends and needs to develop and support program ideas; 2) research of established and existing programs similar to the one you are designing or expanding; 3) researching and developing the community profile; 4) researching and developing the service population profile; 5) conducting the Phase I and Phase II assessment of need; and 6) consideration of a tentative goal or goals for the program.

This preliminary phase would include the detailed calendar for interviews and on-site visits to collect needed information such as the mission and philosophy of the sponsoring facility, data for the community profile, and the needs assessment. You should also block out time for the research that may be needed to develop the service population profile, to explore other established and existing programs that may be similar to the one you are designing, and to obtain evidence that similar programming is effective. In addition, scheduled time to review and chart trends on a daily or weekly basis would help to ensure that this program will likely be viable now and in the future. If you are a practicing clinician and you find that you will need to obtain new practice skills or knowledge, then you must anticipate this on your time line as well. For those working in a group or as part of a team of collaborators, a coordinated time line/calendar will balance the workload.

## The Preparation and Implementation Phase

The **preparation phase** will include: 1) review of all data collected in the preliminary phase; 2) establishment of a firm goal or goals and accompanying objectives; 3) selection of a theoretical orientation or frame(s) of reference to guide the development of the programming; 4) development of detailed, day-to-day program plans to enable goal achievement; 5) matching of potential staff, furnishings, equipment, supplies, and space to the goal and objectives; 6) specifying a budget of needed funds; 7) identifying potential funding sources, their specific time lines, and securing the funding; and 8) selection of program-evaluation methods.

Although there may be some blurring between the **preparation phase and the implementation phase**, knowing that some of the planning has already occurred, our time line for the implementation phase will include the following: 1) more detailed and specific budgeting related to actual acquisition of funds; 2) hiring of staff; 3) acquisition of all equipment and supplies; and 4) active marketing. The completion of this phase would then signal actual start-up and continuation of the programming.

## The Program Review and Evaluation Phase

The program **review and evaluation phase** would be initiated with the formative evaluation of objectives on a weekly basis, or at the end of a programming cycle. This information will assist us in fine-tuning goals, objectives, programming, and evaluation measures. This first phase of evaluation would establish the foundation for measurement of longer-term outcomes, perhaps measured in six months, a year, or continued for several years. This early phase would include critical review of all data collected, including data provided by any individual assessments that may have been done, as well as formative and summative assessments of the program. As mentioned above, this data would then be evaluated against the program's goal or goals and objectives. The results of these evaluations would prompt the examination of program content and mode of delivery to determine if either or both would require change to better satisfy the goal(s). Finally, resultant changes might be initiated in the actual measurement of the goal or goals and the objectives; objectives might be altered (we would assume goals would not be); and programming content or delivery might be changed.

At the one-year review, it would be appropriate to again review the ongoing collection of trends, to update the community profile, and perhaps to revisit the assessment of need. At earlier intervals—perhaps monthly and certainly at three-month intervals—the budget, staffing, furnishings, equipment, supplies, space, and marketing would require scrutiny.

For the above phase planning, some program planners prefer to keep a large, lined calendar where they record what has to be done each month and each week of the month for the full length of the process. If they were also the recipient of grant or foundation funding, they would include any reporting and resubmission deadlines on this calendar as well as the collection dates for required program data. It should be noted that your funding sources may require program evaluation and review on differing schedules.

Other planners who may not require a detailed calendar might prefer to develop lists of what must occur each month. For example, if a planner wishes to establish a private practice, a monthly list calendar might look something like the following:

Month 1

1. Investigate trends
2. Meet with financial planner and/or small business attorney
3. Conduct market analysis
4. Complete community profile

Month 2

1. Investigate site location
2. Network the professional community; perhaps seek partners and collaborators
3. Initiate Phase I needs assessment with professional community

Although the style you choose to form a time line will depend on personal preference, some form of time mapping must be included to ensure that no detail is forgotten. Some sites, and many insurers, will require inspections by fire and safety personnel or perhaps licensure or credentialing before a program is permitted to open. Both of these requirements could take months, so they must be anticipated. Another consideration is equipment, which could arrive in a matter of days but sometimes can take six months. If it only takes a few days for delivery, then it cannot be ordered until you have a space for it. Finally, ask yourself the following questions as you continue to develop your time line: if you're remodeling space, what is the projected time for completion? If remodeling or building is initiated in the winter or spring, how will weather affect your projected opening? When will you hire staff? How will the staff be paid before you generate revenue or receive funding? In anticipating responses to all of these questions, it is far better to be proactive than reactive; answers to these questions are necessary and must be represented on your time line.

## Exercise 1

### Establishing Your Time Line

As you anticipate your full program plan, group the tasks to be completed according to the three phases included below. As you continue to work on your programming, through the chapters of this text, you will provide more detail for the time line.

1.  Design and Planning Phase

_____

_____

_____

_____

_____

2.  Preparation and Implementation Phase

_____

_____

_____

_____

_____

3.  Program Review and Evaluation Phase

_____

_____

_____

_____

_____

_____

_____

If you are designing and planning a program as a student group, then your calendar will reflect the tasks that must be done to develop your *proposal* over the course of your academic semester, quarter, or year. However, you will still develop the full time line for the remainder of the tasks even though you may not actually be implementing the program as part of your assignment.

4. When you have completed the above exercises and have defined all of the tasks that will be necessary to take your program from initial design through

implementation to review and evaluation, transfer the specific tasks to a calendar of your choice. The time line is a work-in-progress and will need to be revisited frequently as you continue your work.

## Summary

Regardless of the style, developing and following a time line is the key to accomplishing all of the tasks of program development in a timely and efficient manner. Several recommendations have been made for ways to develop your time line calendar. Organizing your time line around the three phases of program development has been identified as a preferred method of organization. These phases include: 1) the design and planning phase; 2) the preparation and implementation phase; and 3) the program review and evaluation phase.

It will be important to make your calendar as functional as you can. If working alone initially you may prefer to keep your calendar on the computer. Devising a method to note when a task has been completed (perhaps using a colored marker on a wall calendar) can be encouraging for a group and will keep you motivated during the months when things may slow down more than you would like. A wipe-off calendar that you can post on the wall is another option since you may have to frequently move things around (for example, acquisition of funding or a loan, staff hiring, arrival of equipment, and progress on developing a space).

CHAPTER **6**

# *Getting Started: Developing the Design*

## Learning Objectives

1. To explore ideas for occupation-centered programs
2. To discover a variety of avenues for developing programs
3. To learn how to locate a site for your program
4. To identify the purpose of your program and to begin to develop goals and outcomes

## Key Terms

1. Community Profile
2. Target Population
3. Member/Client/Consumer
4. Advocacy Groups

The following brief illustrations suggest several avenues for potential programmers that will lead to the design, development, and implementation of a program in the community. The success of all of these will ultimately be based on the match between the needs of a population, the needs of the general community, and the interest and expertise of the programmer in bringing together partnerships, collaborations, resources, and effective programming for the participants. One may begin with personal interest and expertise followed by the search for a population who can

## Scenarios for Potential Program Designs

A successful program utilizing the occupation of "gardening" could begin with any one of the following scenarios:

1. Recent trends in professional and community-oriented literature suggest that there is considerable interest in, and civic and government funding for, programs to assist persons with severe and persistent mental illness to find a productive niche in their local communities. A further review of the pertinent literature finds evidence to support gardening as a suitable pre-vocational venue to establish long-term skills for continued employment in the community. A specific profile and needs assessment of the planner's local community will help determine if local demographics and needs are reflective of the larger trends.

2. "I love to work outdoors, and I think gardening is very therapeutic, so I'd like to start a gardening program for persons with severe and persistent mental illness who reside in the community, or are homeless. . . . I'd like to staff it myself (an occupational therapist or an occupational therapy assistant) but might want to include the assistance of retired volunteer gardeners; as well as collaborate with the local garden club. All would help to raise vegetables, herbs, and flowers for local restaurants, and maybe someday we would have a restaurant attached to the garden."

3. A network of advocates for young adults with developmental disability living in a community group home in a small rural town is seeking someone with knowledge of pre-vocational skill development and vocational services and resources to help these young adults find a productive niche in their community. The tasks involved in maintaining the group home may include carpentry, painting, landscaping, and gardening, as well as the daily and weekly household tasks. A planner who has familiarity with task analysis, developmental disabilities, pre-vocational, and vocational skills is needed.

4. A day treatment facility for older adults with varying stages of dementia wishes to expand programming to include use of adjoining property. Suggestions for additional programming have included: an aviary, care of small animals, a garden, and other similar suggestions for out-of-doors occupations geared to the interests and abilities of the clients. The programmer is a consultant to the facility and will be responsible for the development of the new and expanded programs.

benefit through a comprehensive assessment of need. Or, the programmer may first identify a population with need, and match this need to his or her interest and expertise. The beginnings may differ but the process of development, implementation, and evaluation will remain the same.

# Getting Started

But just how do we begin establishing an occupation-centered program? We might start by asking why programs are needed in the first place. In reply, we would suggest that a program is responsive to need. Programs are designed to focus effort and activity in meeting the needs of an identified group. For us, as occupation-centered practitioners, these needs may be to develop knowledge and to provide information and skills in order to help our clients/patients/members/consumers first identify and then engage in meaningful occupations. These are our areas of expertise.

Ideas for programming are seldom spontaneous. As the aforementioned examples illustrate, impetus for new or expanded programs comes from a number of sources that may include: 1) other occupational therapists such as the manager of your department (for example, when an outpatient clinic for pain management clients is needed, or a camp for children with learning disabilities); 2) patients and their families (for example, Parkinson's patients and spouses requesting an exercise program that they can enjoy together); 3) other health care providers/professionals (for example, dentists/orthodontists who wish to help their patients manage temporal-mandibular-joint, or TMJ, pain); and 4) advocates for populations in need of services (engagement in work or balanced occupations). In addition to the sources listed previously, the changing health care environment itself may be the impetus for ideas (for example, post-surgical hand therapy clinics or cardiac maintenance and wellness programs), as well as changes in funding for health care (managed care directives that have pushed for service continuation in other areas). Finally, the recognized need to bring together services for clients in a new or more efficient way that is more readily understood and accessed by the community may generate ideas for new programs (for example, child day care and therapeutic programming for children with disabilities coordinated with child day care for siblings; or intergenerational programs coupling retirement facilities and schools). New programs may certainly come as the result of a structured marketing plan originated by the insightful leader/planner.

An example of sources for programming ideas can be seen in the parent-child program to be discussed in Chapters 8 and 9. The program came about as a result of networking with other professionals (teachers and education coordinators) who were familiar with other occupation-centered after-school programs originated by occupational therapy students. The expressed need was for some kind of programming that would strengthen parents' involvement in their children's educational pursuits, particularly in science. It was clear that the need was strongly occupation-centered and appropriate to our interests and abilities.

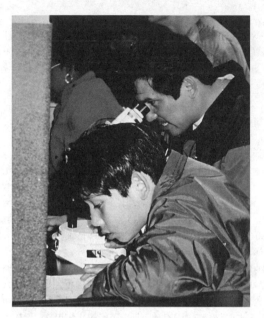

Meeting parent-child partnership goals while learning about marine science is an example of combining occupations in the design of effective programming.

When we come up with ideas ourselves, most often they are based on something that we enjoy or something we think would be fun. The gardening program is a clear example of this kind of motivation. But the interest and accompanying skills motivating the development of a program could just as easily be horseback riding, keeping and caring for pets, arts and crafts, river rafting, surfing, scuba diving, or anything else for which we feel a profound affection. We also must harbor a belief in the activity's potential as therapy or as prevention. Israel "Izzy" Paskowitz's successful surfing program for children with autism was initiated through an intense love of surfing as a sport, a belief in the healing power of the ocean, and love for his own son with autism (www.surfershealing.org).

As a psychologist, Jolkowski (1998) speaks of the power of utilizing our interests in developing and marketing programs. He encourages the exploration of what he describes as niche markets. In his case, he extended his personal interest in music to develop group programming for musicians who were experiencing performance anxiety (Jolkowski, 1998; p. 5). Occupational therapy practitioners interested in music could develop similar programming but perhaps could target musicians with stress-related hand injuries or those musicians who wished to prevent hand injuries. Clearly, an understanding of occupation and the meaning invested in such an occupation as that practiced by the professional musician would place the occupation-centered practitioner firmly in the marketplace. In the same article, R. Phillips (also a psychologist) found his particular niche in the sport of golf, but the programming was similar in that it targeted performance anxiety (Jolkowski, 1998; p. 5). Again, for occupation-centered practitioners, the niche might be expanded to help golfers avoid or treat golf-induced or golf-related injuries. Personal interest and skill in the occupation of golfing will certainly be advantageous in developing such a practice.

As mentioned earlier, a need might be expressed by persons in the community, advocates or advocacy groups, family members, or potential clients or groups of clients. If we think we can fill that need, the beginnings of a new program may emerge. Ideas are also generated when we recognize a potentially lucrative endeavor. Although this may be one of the seminal ideas for a private practice, it, alone, is not enough to design a program that will achieve results. Meticulous research and continued work will be necessary to ensure a successful program in the present, and over time.

In summary, ideas for programs may come from:

- Other occupational therapy practitioners
- Patients/clients and/or their families
- Other health care providers/professionals
- Advocates or advocacy groups
- The changing health care environment
- The program developer's interests and skills coupled with a good marketing plan

# Revisiting Scenario #2: The Community Garden Example

Let's return to the idea of a community garden for homeless persons with severe and persistent mental illness. What happens after we've generated the idea? Even if gardening is not new to our experience, there is still research to be done. Since community gardening is an idea that has come to fruition in many and varied ways, there are resources available to us. The occupational therapy-managed horticulture program at the Veteran's Administration Medical Center in Brentwood, Los Angeles, referred to as the "vet's garden," is one of the longest running and successful ventures of its kind (Strege, Molina, and Jewell, 1991). Gardening as a pre-vocational and vocational skill and knowledge set is utilized in this program. Substantial information describing horticulture therapy and the therapeutic aspects of gardening is available on the Internet. There are also many resources for the occupation of gardening in general. Regardless of your selected modality, you can further your research at the library or on the Internet. The Internet has made the process of program development much more efficient than it was even a few years ago.

It is important to note that, although our second community garden scenario was greatly influenced by personal interest in gardening as therapy, it was also facilitated by the concerns of citizens who felt that persons with severe and persistent mental illness ("idle" and homeless persons with severe and persistent mental illness) present problems for the city. Perhaps this interpretation seems a bit brutal, but there are many and varied motives for the practice of good works, and the astute planner will stay abreast of these motives, mobilizing them toward positive outcomes for the clients.

In Part V we describe some of the characteristics of the urban homeless. We know that persons with severe and persistent mental illness are a large part of this group. The development of programming for this population is challenging, even to the most experienced therapist. Clients are extremely varied in their interests, values, and skills, and it is not easy to find meaningful occupations for them.

The idea of a community garden in our example may be a possible solution. Our task, then, is not only to develop a garden in the community but also to *build a community* around a garden.

# Where Do You Locate a Gardening Program?

To expand on our second scenario, the location of the targeted population was an urban, downtown setting. The planning process was initiated by exploring the ways for people to garden in a large city, assuming that they have no property of their own. This exploration can be facilitated by contacting the botanical gardens, the city's Park and Recreation Department, or local nurseries. In some cities, community gardens are sponsored by a University Cooperative Extension—Division of Agricultural Sciences. All of these resources offer potential for future partnering. To find a site for your program, you can also:

■   Contact city or regional agencies for collaborative ventures
■   Contact the Chamber of Commerce, churches, or local businesses
■   Go to the telephone book, the library, and/or the Internet
■   Check posted notices at the local market; or Town Hall
■   Ask people in the community

Another way to find a site is simply to walk around the neighborhood where you wish to provide your program. This is part of what we describe as developing the **community profile**, or getting to know as much as possible about the community/ neighborhood where your program is expected to take place. The detailed procedure of developing the community profile is provided in Chapter 7.

If most people reside in apartments or public housing, there is likely to be an empty lot set aside for a garden or an empty lot that could be developed in that way. Some of the urban garden sites are quite restrictive and, of course, the garden site in our example needed to be where the population to be served was located. It was not likely that the client/members would board a city bus and travel to the garden daily (although once the garden was established, perhaps they would). This ability to navigate the community, in fact, could have been one of the goals for the programming.

As we think about our program participants in this stage of the planning process, we must clarify the rather liberal use of terms we have employed to describe them. During our planning process, and before they actually become participants, we refer to potential participants as our **target population**, or those we have targeted to receive our services. When the members of our target population become involved in our program, we may refer to them in several ways. In general, those participants who are not paying for services (that is, community gardeners) prefer to be referred to as

**members**, and a club structure designating membership may be useful for many types of community programs. Although the term outpatient may be used in some cases, the more medical term patient is less used in community settings. **Client** or **consumer** are the common terms used to designate the participant of services for prevention, maintenance, and general wellness programs. Third-party payers may have a preferred terminology that you will certainly want to use if you are relying on them for reimbursement. Finally, when in doubt, ask the consumers how they prefer to be known. Often it may just be a term such as camper, gardener, craftsman, etc.

# After Locating the Site, What Comes Next?

## Planning in a Nutshell

If you are planning a gardening program such as the one described, some negotiation will likely occur as you select a site. Of course, early on you will have done your preliminary homework. You will have researched existing programs and found evidence that they are successful. Initial need will have been established by others, but you will have verified that need through your own assessments and you will have drafted a detailed plan for how you will proceed. Although not incorporated into this phase of planning, you may still be entertaining the possibility of a small restaurant or maybe a vegetable/flower stand. If you have not already located it, you have a good idea what kind of site/location you require (for example, slope, sun, shade, water, accessibility, and so on), how large it should be, and zoning requirements. You will have honed your communication/negotiation skills, determined how many client/members you can accommodate, and developed a preliminary list for what equipment/supplies you will need to begin and an estimate of what they will cost. Certainly, your supply and equipment list, staffing, and client/member selection will require additional work, but you will have done enough to have an estimate of costs. Your credibility as a planner likely will be matched to the specificity of these early estimates, so be as accurate as you can be.

You might encounter the scenario, as in our case example, where urban leaders want something done but do not want to spend any money in order to do it. In addition, you might not know how much they will provide until you have presented your proposal. Thus, it is advisable to identify some potential small, private granting organizations (such as garden clubs or family sponsors of local gardens and parks). These private granting organizations can be delegated to a secondary plan to be identified if you are not able to get the monies you need from your first organization.

## Attracting the Volunteers

A significant challenge for a project such as the one we are describing is in attracting the potential clients/members to the site to begin the work of gardening and to get the volunteer help that will be needed to develop the program. You must begin by contacting the local gardening clubs to solicit the assistance of volunteers who have a strong commitment to gardening (this, of course, was included in the draft plan to the city or other decision-making group). Perhaps you will also have access to students. Although they might not be gardeners, enthusiasm is an equally strong attribute. We cannot overlook the fact that the presence of youth and free food have assisted in the marketing of a number of community programs.

While accessing volunteers to supervise the gardening seems simple enough, helping them feel comfortable with your client/member population may not be so easy. You must now market your idea and your targeted population to your volunteers, and you will need to know the needs of both groups. Finding a confidante on the garden club board may help, or perhaps you know someone who has an established relationship with your proposed volunteers. The intention is to utilize any networks you have established in order to help you get started . . . collaborate, collaborate, collaborate!

First, you need to explore any preconceptions your potential volunteers might have regarding persons with severe and persistent mental illness and the homeless. You will need to know how to present factual information so that it will be heard in the most productive way. Although statistics regarding the population of homeless persons with severe and persistent mental illness will be critical in establishing need, they will not necessarily be convincing information for this group. An **advocacy group** can provide a strong incentive to your potential volunteers based on realistic information and an emotional investment. Advocacy groups advocate for particular groups of people—generally people with disabilities and/or those with special needs. Advocates may be persons who are disabled themselves, relatives or friends of these persons, and professionals. You might wish to contact local advocacy organizations such as Parents of Young Adults with Schizophrenia, Persons with Severe and Persistent Mental Illness, or other advocacy groups with similar interests. Utilize community resources such as Directories of Social Services for your city or county to find the groups that might be best able to assist you.

You may have years of experience working with persons who have various forms of psychiatric illness, or you may have little or no experience, but a critical skill in marketing to nonprofessionals is to understand their experience and their views and not to minimize either. The average person knows about psychiatric illness from the media or from brief personal encounters with a delusional and hallucinating person living on the streets. Neither image presents all there is to know, but your marketing task is to skillfully distinguish between the realities and the myths. Further, you must provide an incentive that is meaningful to your volunteers. Assuming you accepted this challenge because it has meaning for you, then sharing your commitment to this venture with your volunteers should not be difficult. If you accepted the challenge with little real interest, then it is doubtful that you will be able to mobilize the help you need.

## Attracting Your Clients/Members

Once you have your cadre of occupational therapy personnel and motivated volunteers, you can begin recruiting clients/members from your targeted population. You may want to arrange for a van or a truck to literally drive around and encourage people to come with you. If you have homeless shelters or missions in the area (and you probably do), solicit their assistance in providing transportation for your clients/members. If homeless persons with severe and persistent mental illness are indeed a problem for the city, then the police or volunteer police organizations might assist in marketing your program and in transporting potential members to your garden. Another option is to solicit the assistance of churches or other volunteer groups working in the area.

Once your clients/members have arrived, it will be the enthusiasm and caring of your volunteers and the skills of your occupational therapy personnel that will keep them there. It is important that your first group of participants be involved in the actual building of the garden plots and in the initial development of the gardens, for this group will become your future supervisors, perhaps your board members, and your strongest advocates.

Although our case example was designed for an urban area, you can do the same thing in a suburban or rural area. In these locales you might not find a large population of homeless persons with severe and persistent mental illness or adolescents who are delinquent youth offenders, but you can apply a similar concept with other groups who are in need of your services. Gardening on a smaller scale—even in pots—has been very successful in nursing-rehabilitation facilities, in residential facilities for persons who are developmentally delayed, and in numerous school-based facilities.

If we expand our ideas to residential housing for the well-elderly or adults who are developmentally disabled and living in the community, then a shared community garden is an excellent way to keep these populations connected to their neighborhoods and to meaningful activity. In addition, grouping clients/members of different ages and abilities together with volunteers of different ages

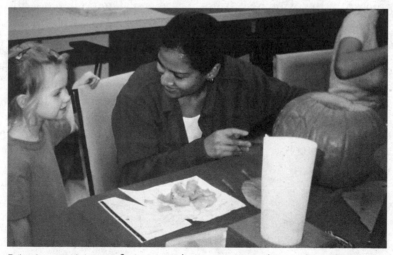

Bringing participants from several programs together to share the carving of the garden "harvest" can meet program goals in fun and creative ways.

and abilities is recommended in an effort to *create community*—something we should facilitate at every opportunity.

Whereas suburban and rural areas often have fewer restrictions on establishing gardens and on selling the produce than urban areas do, finding small granting agencies or donations in these areas may be more difficult than in the city. These are reasonable tradeoffs in many ways, and the opportunities to make the garden a "paying proposition" with the therapeutic rewards of sharing dividends may outweigh the opportunity for donations. However, do not automatically assume that grants and donations are not available in rural areas; start-up monies, in fact, are likely to be there as well.

# Beginning to Think About Tentative Goals for Your Program

Through our garden example, you see how an idea takes shape and grows into a program step by step. Throughout the course of this evolution, it is wise to continue to return to our purpose—the need for our program—and to ask the following questions:

Why is a program needed?
Why this program?
How is it occupation-centered?
How will it have meaning for the client/member?
What do we expect will be the outcomes of the program?

When we begin to define our purpose and think about outcomes (or what we expect will happen), we are beginning to develop the goal or goals that we will use to guide programming. These are early, tentative goals to provide direction as we proceed in the planning process. These goals are not intended to be fully developed, and they are not yet accompanied by measurable objectives—that will come later. For now, they serve to define and structure our purpose.

In our community garden case example, the central idea or tentative goal based on what was perceived to be the need was to establish a *community* for homeless persons and others with severe and persistent mental illness living in the city. Secondly, another tentative goal was to provide a variety of meaningful choices of occupation for those involved in the program. At this point in the process, these goals are very vague statements, and it might be difficult to write objectives that would be measurable or outcome based. They do, however, define our *purpose*, and they provide a good foundation for the more formal goals and objectives that will follow.

## Exercise 1

### Trying Out Your Ideas

Now that you have an understanding of what is involved, try brainstorming some programming ideas of your own. At this point, the ideas do not necessarily need to be practical, and you do not need to know exactly how you will carry them out. You may have a potential need in mind already; and, as in some of our early scenarios, that need may be specific. If so, tailor your ideas to those needs.

1.  Write your ideas below:

_____

_____

_____

_____

_____

2.  Who is your target population? What special needs does this population have that must be considered in your planning?

_____

_____

_____

_____

_____

In our community garden example, the population consists of homeless men and women with severe and persistent mental illness, and there is the possibility of children accompanying their parents. In our parent-child example (to be discussed in Chapters 8 and 9), the population is comprised of inner-city fourth-grade and fifth-grade boys and girls and their parent (mother, father, or other home-care provider). When we think of "special needs" as occupational therapy students and practitioners, we often think of physically, emotionally, or cognitively disabling conditions. Certainly, these things must be considered in our work in the community; however, we must also consider the "special needs" prompted by socioeconomic circumstances. The clues to these considerations in our present example are *homelessness* and *inner-city*. Both of these considerations will require our attention as we address the needs of our case example populations and as we develop their service profiles.

Describe your targeted population and its special needs below:

_____

_____

_____

_____

_____

Will the special needs of this population require specific programming? Adaptations? Other considerations?

_____

_____

_____

_____

_____

Persons who are homeless with severe and persistent mental illness not only must deal with the repercussions of their particular illness, but they also must develop their own adaptive survival measures to remain safe and nourished. The adaptive strategies that permit survival on the street must be understood and appreciated by planners in order for community programs to be successful.

The first "special need" noted by the parent-child program planners was, in fact, their own. To be responsive to several of the participants, it was necessary for some of the planners to speak both Spanish and English. The need to translate the written materials into Spanish was also quickly apparent. There were also other concerns prompted by the inner-city public school environment and the multicultural considerations of the children and parents.

3. Have the earlier scenarios and the gardening example prompted your consideration of any other needs your targeted population may have that will influence your program planning? If so, note those needs below:

_____

_____

_____

_____

_____

4. If you have identified additional needs, what will they require of you and of your program?

_____

_____

_____

_____

5. Stop and ask yourself the following questions, and note your responses in the space provided.

Why this program?

_____

_____

_____

How is it occupation-centered?

_____

_____

_____

How will it have meaning for the client/member/participant?

_____

_____

_____

What will be the purpose? What do we want the outcomes to be? Remember these are outcomes for the *program*—the collective outcome for all of the participants.

_____

_____

_____

_____

_____

What might be a tentative goal or goals relative to the purpose for all participants in your program? What do you want to accomplish for all participants? Note that with the community garden example we stated that the primary purpose, or tentative goal, was to establish *community* for all of the participants. Later you will find that for the parent-child program, the purpose, or tentative goal, is to build parent-child *teams*.

_____

_____

_____

_____

_____

6. What are your ideas for where the programming that you are proposing might be accomplished? Do you have a community site in mind?

_____

_____

_____

_____

_____

The process of locating a site may be very different from one program to the next. In our gardening example, the idea was developed before actually locating the specific population or the site. The program held certain advantages for the city and, in fact, when the plan was proposed, assistance was offered in finding a suitable garden site, without cost, adjacent to an established community garden.

The location of a site for the parent-child program took several turns before resolution. In the early planning stages, where you are now, it seemed obvious that the program should be held at the school. Previous to actually doing the needs assessment, it was believed that the program would be conducted immediately after school and that the children would be joined in one of the classrooms by their parents. This also seemed to be a convenient place and time for the occupational therapy coordinator and students who would be conducting the program. Most of the activities were appropriate to the tables, chairs, and desks of the classroom, so it seemed the perfect place. In fact, much of this early brainstorming was on-target; however, a detailed assessment of need helped the planners to design a program much more appropriate to the concerns of the participants and, therefore, much more successful.

7. Continue your brainstorming by noting some ideas for the following considerations. Remember that these are very early, tentative ideas, however, they will help structure the remainder of the process.

Who might carry out the day-to-day operations?

_____

_____

_____

_____

What equipment/supplies would you need to support the programming you are considering?

_____

_____

_____

_____

8. Have you discovered areas where you will need to conduct more inquiries, do more research, or review previous learning in order to prepare a proposal? If so, what areas are they? List them below, and note where you might go for more information.

Unanswered Questions                    Possible Resources

_____            _____

_____            _____

_____            _____

_____            _____

9.  Have these cursory exercises caused you to alter your initial idea or plan? If so, in what way? Note your response below:

_____

_____

_____

_____

_____

Present your idea or the idea of your working group in a brief proposal to classmates. If you are a professional, or working independently, present your idea to colleagues or others who could provide constructive feedback. Have their suggestions caused you to alter your initial plan? If so, in what way? (Note: making alterations in your initial plan during the development process is almost always necessary, but it should not mean that you compromise your initial idea.) Note your response below:

_____

_____

_____

If classmates or others found your idea amusing, remember that all great leaders and planners were probably ridiculed at least once! Observers of a young midwestern artist in 1923 struggling to start a film-making business based on a "mouse" must have laughed long and hard; but undoubtedly their grandchildren visited Disneyland and certainly recognized Mickey Mouse (Capodagli and Jackson, 1999). And most told Debbi (Mrs.) Fields that she could never survive "just selling cookies." She now not only survives but also has over 650 domestic locations and 65 international locations in eleven countries (http://www.mrsfields.com/the_story/story-bottom.html).

If your idea is larger than your present abilities, save it for the future. This reveals an important point. Begin now to keep a journal or file of ideas for programs. Many great ideas were probably first recorded on cocktail napkins; the same can hold true for great ideas in occupation-centered programming! Your occupational therapy professors and instructors and your colleagues drop interesting ideas for practice and program development all of the time. Occupational therapy journals and publications frequently highlight entrepreneurial practices, as do the journals and newsletters of other helping professions. An idea does not have to be yours alone to be successful. Consider all of these ideas to be "pearls of programming wisdom," and write them down to stimulate your future program-planning ventures.

In a few years, when your practical wisdom and experience match your present creativity, intellect, and enthusiasm, pull out the journal or file and see what interests you. If you are already a practitioner, you probably have lots of ideas; still, take the time to organize them in a file, and when you feel the need for a change, page through the file and take a good look around you. You will most likely find opportunities just waiting to be discovered.

## Summary

Generating your ideas for programs either in expectation of establishing need or in response to apparent need is the first step. This is followed by careful and detailed planning that might include asking lots of questions and pursuing the answers in the community, in the library, and on the Internet. Learning as much as you can about the needs of your proposed population and brainstorming ideas for why, where, and how the program may be conducted will prepare the way for the detailed work that is to follow.

## *References*

Capodagli, B., & Jackson, L. (1999). *The Disney Way.* New York: McGraw-Hill.

Jolkowski, M. (1998, October). *Practice Strategies: A Business Guide for Behavioral Healthcare Providers.* Washington, DC: American Association for Marriage and Family Therapy.

Strege, M., Molina, M., & Jewell, J. (1991, August). Vets' gardeners reap a full harvest. *Advance for Occupational Therapists, 5*(31).

### Internet Resources

Israel "Izzy" Paskowitz: www.surfershealing.org

Mrs. Fields Cookie Company:
  http://www.mrsfields.com/the_story/story-bottom.html
  email: marcelenew@mrsfields.com

Community Gardening:

The American Community Gardening Association provides links to university and college horticultural extension programs; community gardening specific to states and locales; and general community gardening information, including getting started, organizations to assist, and funding. You can contact this association at:
  http://www.communitygarden.org/links/index.html

Children's gardening and community gardening grants (including opportunities for free seed, tools, plants, garden products, and assistance), ideas, projects, products, books, and manuals:
  http://www.hort.vt.edu/human/CGgrants.html
  http://www.hort.vt.edu/human/commgrants.html
  http://www.hort.vt.edu/human/CGmoreres.html
  http://www.hort.vt.edu/human/CGbooks.html

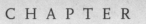

CHAPTER 7

# Profiling the Community, Targeting the Population, and Assessing the Need for Services

### Learning Objectives

1. To recognize the layers of inquiry necessary to determine what services are needed by a population
2. To learn how to profile a community for information to support the need for services
3. To develop a profile of your selected community
4. To identify potential collaborations
5. To understand the characteristics of the service profile as it is used to support the need for specific targeted population services
6. To develop a service profile for your selected population
7. To explore the options for the needs assessment
8. To conduct a needs assessment for your selected population
9. To thoroughly investigate relevant research literature to support program development

## Key Terms

1. Layers of Inquiry
2. Population
3. Condition
4. Context
5. Service Profile
6. Assessment of Need/Needs Assessment
7. Interview/Interview Questionnaire
8. Focus Group
9. Survey
10. Occupation/Occupational Science

At this early stage of the planning process, we are asking a set of fairly straightforward questions. These questions were first entertained by the potential planner during the "idea" stage: are services needed? What kind of services are needed? Are *my* services needed? Walt Disney once said, "You don't build the product for yourself. You need to know what the people want and build it for them" (Capodagli and Jackson, 1999; p. 59). Although he was talking about the design and planning of the first *Disneyland* theme park, this statement by Walt Disney is appropriate to our discussions of need. His statement prompts us, as community program planners, to remember that if we are more responsive to our own personal needs than to the needs of our targeted population, we may have a hard lesson to learn. Sometimes we are so impressed with our idea and so committed to it that it causes us to ignore the results of the assessment of need. Sadly, the resulting program will do little to serve the population.

There are several **layers of inquiry** necessary to determine what programming services are needed by a population. These layers include knowing the community where you will provide services; knowing the targeted population that will receive services; knowing your own potential for providing services; and, if you anticipate working with an agency/facility, knowing what that administration wants for its clients/patients and knowing what the clients/patients want for themselves. If any of these areas are neglected in the early stages of planning, it is likely that you will not be as successful as you could be.

In summary, layers of inquiry to determine what programming services you will provide are as follows:

- Know the community where you will provide services.
- Know the targeted population who will receive services.
- Know your potential for providing services.
- Know what services the agency/facility administration wants for the clients/patients.
- Know what the clients/patients want for themselves.

# Knowing Your Personal Potential for Providing Services

In Chapter 4 we discussed ways to ascertain your present foundation of personal and professional knowledge and skills. If you participated in the exercises provided, you have a good sense of what you can offer a potential program. It is important to remember, regardless of where you are in your occupational therapy program of study or in your career, that you do possess a considerable amount of both knowledge and skills. Many, if not all, students today have had previous work, family/home, and academic experience. Often, these are the experiences that bring a unique perspective to your practice, particularly in the less proscriptive environment of the community. In the context of community, we are truly defining and creating a new practice—not only for the community and the population that resides within it or is transitioning through it, but also for ourselves as practitioners. Whether or not the particular practice has occurred previously, *this community*, coupled with the uniqueness of the programmer, sculpts a totally new practice that cannot be duplicated in other settings.

# Profiling the Community

As discussed earlier in this text, community is a complex concept and one that the potential programmer must explore at many levels. By examining one level at a time, we will investigate the community broadly to create a description of what factors exist that may impact our developing plans. We are referring to this description or brief picture as the community profile. In creating this profile, the Aspen Reference Group suggests that the planner contribute equal attention to both the community demographics (that is, age, sex, ethnicity, education, and so on) and to the social demographics, or those community social and medical services that presently exist as well as those that are lacking (DiLima and Schust, 1997; pp. 73–74). The addition of social demographics will not only help the planner know if his or her services are needed, but it will also help the planner know what services are needed to complement those that may already exist. Forming complementary services to those that are presently being provided is often the most successful way to enter a community.

Youngstrom (1999) offers suggestions for identifying service needs that are appropriate for the experienced professional who may have expertise to offer and who is looking for a community where this expertise will be most needed (that is, establishing a private practice). Youngstrom recommends that the following questions be used to structure the early planning process, or what we are describing as the community and service profiles (Youngstrom, 1999; pp. 197–198):

1. What is the event of the given problem? How often does it occur?
2. How many individuals does it affect?

3. How frequently does it occur?
4. Is it expected to increase? (identification of trends)
5. How and to what degree is the problem currently being addressed within the community? Who is addressing it?
6. What are the factors that contribute to or sustain the problem?
7. Will your proposed program address one or more of the contributing factors?

Collecting demographics that include service dimensions for the community will help us to determine if our proposed programming is presently being offered. With further investigation, we could know if additional services are warranted, perhaps with alternative methods of delivery. The sum of all of the observations and research we conduct will result in a description, or profile, of the community or communities where our targeted population resides and engages in occupation (and the community, if different, where we will provide services).

In many instances the programmer may feel some familiarity with the larger community. Perhaps, for example, he or she has lived in a community such as suburban Denver, Colorado, for some time. If programming is being considered in a downtown Denver sanctuary for runaway teenagers that may be frequenting Laramer Square, then the programmer must explore and understand the specific community—in our example, downtown urban Denver. The next level to be considered is the community of the homeless in urban Denver and the community of runaway homeless teens which is perhaps similar in some ways but likely very different in other ways. Of course, communities are made up of individuals. Each homeless teen in our example brings with him or her the remnants of the cultures and communities from which the teen may have recently sought an exit. These multilayers of community always exist and must be explored and understood in order to define and develop the most effective programming possible .

# Developing the Profile of Your Selected Community

For most of our program designs and plans, we will seek the support of an agency/facility in order to assist us with our work. This does not preclude the possibility that programs can develop without such agency/facility support or sanction (e.g., private practices). However, it is strongly recommended that initial student learning experiences be structured to include work with an agency/facility. First, identify the location of your agency and the neighborhood/community where your targeted population resides. This may be the same community where the agency is located or it may be different. (e.g., a detention center population may come from many communities within an urban city or from the state). At this point, collect as much demographical information as you can. Census data is often the place to begin to establish a foundation for understanding the community or communities. You can obtain such data from the U.S. Census Bureau's internet site: http://www/census.gov. It will lead you to various resources for demographics to assist in understanding your population. Once you have demographics and background, locate the community where your agency is located and the community where your targeted population resides, if different. Mapping will provide you with a sense of where your selected community is located with respect to adjacent communities. The location of landmarks, public buildings, and public services will be useful information as you begin to develop specific objectives for the program and as you identify partners and collaborators. As you develop your program, you may find that you will rely heavily on public services; if this is the case, you will want to obtain more specific and detailed maps such as those of transportation networks and public services. It may be useful to determine the boundaries of ethnic neighborhoods and accompanying services adjacent to your selected community. While these boundaries are sometimes fluid, permitting easy passage of persons and things from one neighborhood or community to another, they also can be fixed by language, social custom, and culture. Either circumstance may affect your targeted population and the range of services your program will provide.

When you have enough information to develop a brief profile of your identified community, it is time for a visit in order to match what you have learned with what you can observe. This is sometimes done enroute to your first on-site appointment, but you can also explore the area before you schedule the appointment to begin the process of determining the programming needs. Either way, this first visit will permit you to make useful observations and to ask yourself questions pertinent to your program design and development. As you begin to explore the community, you might ask yourself the following questions:

What is the standard mode of housing?
Are there playgrounds, parks, and recreation facilities?
Are there adults and children on the streets? If so, what are they doing?
Are police visible?
Are there as many churches and schools as there are liquor stores and convenience stores?
Is there graffiti, including gang signs?
Do these observations match the statistical/demographic information I have gathered?

When you arrive at the site for your first appointment with the administrator or another professional, you have already gleaned substantial information from your demographical research and these early observations. You will have established the foundation for any questions you will wish to ask in order to center your targeted population in the community. Again, it is important to remember that sometimes the population to be served by a program may live in a completely different community or many different communities. This is an important question to ask, and the answer might prompt you to extend your community profile to other communities in addition to the one where services will be located.

Your observations might also prompt the need for community information beyond what you have collected previously. In addition to census bureau data, you might wish to examine national and local marketing and survey data; government documents, reports, and statistics; or data from other agencies. Your collected information may include ranges of income, the incidence of single-parent families, employment, education, religion, ethnicity, crime and police statistics, and other information of specific interest to you as you develop your ideas for programming. Many times the facility/agency can provide you with some of this information since it is often used to justify funding for programs and, in fact, might justify the funding for the one you are proposing. You might also want to consider community newspapers, newsletters, or posted materials describing local interests and events. Items posted on a town hall or grocery store bulletin board can tell you a great deal about the community.

Considering the information provided to structure the dimensions of a community profile; think about how you will develop the profile of the community or communities where your anticipated population resides as well as where the agency/facility is located. As suggested earlier, begin by locating the agency/facility on a map (paper or computer version). In the following exercise, note any generic information the map might provide, such as landmarks, public facilities, and so on. Also determine what route you might wish to take when you make your first visit to the site. Locate a route that will provide you with optimal observational information to assist you as you develop your profile. Even if you are already familiar with the location, locate it on a map to visually center it with regard to surrounding communities. This careful and detailed mapping of communities is likely of greater importance to those who establish programs in large urban areas; however, smaller communities may hold isolated cultures or socioeconomic groupings with which the programmer is equally unfamiliar.

## Exercise 1

**Initiating the Profile of Your Selected Community**

1. Using a highlighter, draw what you presently perceive to be the boundaries of your selected community on a map. Note surrounding communities, locations of freeways, and other points of interest.

2. Record below any information you are able to glean from your map review, including landmarks and public facilities (libraries, parks, and so on). If you are already familiar with the location, use what you know to supplement the map review.

_____

_____

_____

3. Develop a brief profile of the community you have selected using demographic information from the census bureau or other resources of your choice (see web addresses at the close of this chapter). This profile should provide you with a foundation from which you can extend your research as you continue to investigate the community. Record your responses in the space provided.

  a. Socioeconomic data:

_____

_____

_____

  b. Level of education:

_____

_____

_____

  c. Nature of family households (that is, single-parent, extended, and so on):

_____

_____

_____

  d. Ethnicity and religion:

_____

_____

_____

  e. Other data you may wish to collect:

_____

_____

_____

4.  List potential partners in the community who may be able to collaborate in your programming efforts; consider clergy, law enforcement personnel, shop owners, schools, service organizations, and others:

_____

_____

_____

_____

# Profiling Our Anticipated Services

As students, when you are preparing to select an agency/facility for which you wish to design and plan a community program, you are informed of the population that agency serves. Experienced therapists most often wish to expand or extend programming within their area of experience and expertise (that is, public school therapists may wish to extend programming to after-school clubs or day camps; acute care therapists may wish to develop outpatient services). In these examples, the therapist may wish to solicit the assistance of an agency/facility with which he or she is already affiliated. In many instances, the therapist may seek referrals from other agencies as well. In expanding or extending services, conducting an investigation of the services already available, as mentioned earlier, would be important.

It is also important to remember that a relationship in which you are seeking support from an agency/facility is different from one in which a program is developed for an agency/facility. The latter circumstance is suggested as a good first student experience. Of course, students may not have had sufficient experience to develop expertise with a particular population, as we might expect from a practicing therapist. However, selecting a population on the basis of interest and sometimes previous experience in a different context is an equally valid way to begin programming.

Although the potential population cannot be fully explored and understood outside the context of the specific community, we can and should carefully research both before developing an interview format and instrument to facilitate the specific assessment of needs. As we have suggested with the early development of the community profile, it is best to begin with a map or maps. By gathering necessary demographic data, we can also "map" our expected population by finding out all we can before going on site. With some preliminary information about the community and the expected population, we will be prepared to ask the most useful and focused questions when we first meet the administrator or professional who will contribute to the needs assessment.

To return to our earlier Denver example, at the core of the potential program in downtown Denver and composing one level of community, is the adolescent. Our first challenge will be to understand the developmental characteristics of adolescence. Only later, after reviewing what we know of adolescents, do we consider the needs imposed by the complex layers of community. In our example, homelessness may be the next characteristic to investigate. Homeless runaway teens may or may not have the same characteristics in New York City, Denver, Las Vegas, or Los Angeles. While knowing something about one community will likely tell us something about the others, it will not tell us everything. We may know statistically that, nationwide, runaway teens are likely to have attempted suicide, have been abused, and be addicted to drugs and/or alcohol (see Chapter 19). Those characteristics, however, may or may not be present to the same degree in every community of runaway teens. To continue our understanding, we must learn something about shelters, sanctuaries, and transitional centers. These settings may provide the context for programming and are, in themselves, yet another layer of community. This community is sometimes self-selected by the homeless teen, but often it is imposed by social services or the police. Therefore, the population of one shelter-community may represent programming needs differing from another based on whether it was chosen by the teen or ascribed by authorities.

As you can see from the previous example, before even going to a specific site, we have at least three or more areas to research if we anticipate program development to meet the needs of homeless teens. We must develop a profile of the **population**—in our example, adolescents.

We must learn all we can about the **condition** of homelessness and particularly about homelessness during adolescence. We have also mentioned the conditions of substance abuse and abuse by others. Learning what we can about these conditions will further strengthen our profile. We must also investigate the **context** for services: shelters, sanctuaries, and transitional centers. The sum of this information will provide us with the profile of anticipated community-based services for this population, our **service profile** (see Figure 7–1).

Population, condition, and context = service profile.

We know that the population cannot be fully explored and understood outside the context of the specific community. But we also know that the above information will be adequate to assist us as we prepare more targeted questions to ask

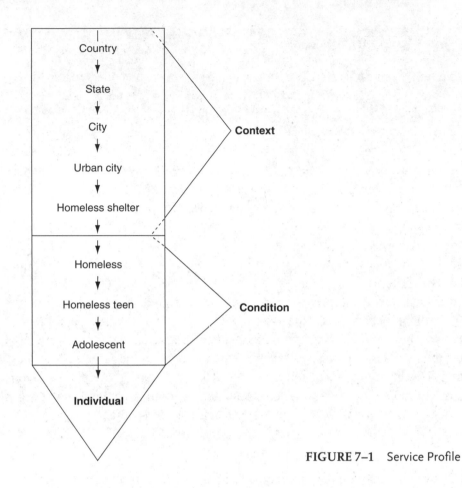

**FIGURE 7–1**   Service Profile

when we go on-site to first visit with those persons (administrators or other professionals and service providers) who will assist us as we continue to develop our program design. We have mentioned credibility as one of the prerequisites for developing a successful working relationship with the agency, with others who may assist us, or with future collaborators. A carefully researched and insightfully written community profile and anticipated service profile will go a long way to establish your credibility. If your anticipated population is one with disability then you must include the disability in your research of conditions. Remember that the service profile we are developing for the population is simply a place to begin. Certainly not all adolescents, or all adolescents who are homeless, or all adolescents who are substance abusers exhibit the same individual profiles, nor do they have the same needs. However, they have many characteristics in common, and those are what we hope to identify with this early research. Later, we will determine where the needs of our specific population may differ from the general population.

It may be useful to mention that the experienced therapist who is considering developing a new program but is not yet ready to target a specific site may wish to postpone the community profile, first observing and researching service populations similar to the one anticipated. The community selected for observation of the population may be different from the one where programming will eventually be developed, but there is still useful information to be gained. By understanding the general needs of the population—developmentally, clinically, and socially—you can develop the community profile when the site has been selected. You will know the parameters of your profiles, and you will know how your knowledge base and skills are matched to what the anticipated need will be. You will also have a much more realistic idea of the resources that will be needed whether you gain the expertise to supply these or you glean them from partners and collaborators in the community.

## Exercise 2

### Developing the Service Profile

The following are examples of populations for whom occupation-centered community-based programs have been designed; use them to practice identifying the population, the condition(s), and the context to develop a service profile. You will likely discover overlap when examining population and condition:

a. Junior high school adolescent girls between the ages of twelve and fifteen who are pregnant or raising an infant while attending school
b. Well-elderly men and women between the ages of 65 and 94 who are living in a low- to moderate-income inner-city transitional apartment complex
c. Young adults with low vision who are living at home and working in the community

1. Discuss the above examples with your instructor, other students, or colleagues. Organize the information provided for each of the above examples into the following categories:

*The population:*

a. _____

_____

b. _____

_____

c. _____

_____

*The condition(s):*

a. _____

_____

b. _____

_____

c. _____

_____

*The context:*

a. _____

_____

b. _____

_____

c. _____

_____

### Developing the Service Profile for the Population *You* Have Selected

2. Review all of the information you have for the agency/facility you have selected and the population it serves. Provide a brief but comprehensive description below (as was done in the previous example):

_____

_____

_____

_____

Discuss your description, and with the help of your student group or colleagues, separate and delineate the following categories as you did in the previous examples:

*Population:*

_____

_____

_____

*Condition(s):*

_____

_____

_____

*Context:*

_____

_____

_____

When you have completed the above exercise, you have the anticipated service profile for the population you have selected. With this profile, you are now ready to research your textbooks, library, and Internet resources to learn as much as you can about 1) the population; 2) the conditions expressed and experienced by this population; and 3) the context in which services will likely be conducted. You will have generated enough information with this recent research and the preliminary community profile to begin a program-development file for this specific program. You can index the file in the same way the chapters of this text are organized, or you can develop your own system. By the end of the process, you will have collected a substantial amount of information and resources from which you will develop your formal program proposal.

When you have completed the research to further develop the anticipated service profile, you are ready to develop the formal needs assessment. The results of the needs assessment will help us identify areas where we may wish to do further research to enhance the accuracy of what will become our specific service profile and to complete the data collection for the community profile.

# The Needs Assessment: Phase I

The preliminary work we have accomplished to develop our community profile and the profile of our anticipated services sets the foundation for what we are beginning to define as the needs of this particular population in this particular community. Until now, however, we have been working with primarily demographic quantitative data collected by others and with qualitative generalizations formed through our observations. Perhaps we also have had brief conversations during an early, informal community visit. For example, from our preliminary research into the demographics of the community we might know that there are a certain number of adolescent girls with infants living in their single mother's households, and we might know that these girls did not finish high school. We might also know that pregnancy prevention, parenting classes, or other such services for these girls are nonexistent (or exist but appear to be ineffective). Perhaps we also have talked informally with a school counselor, a minister, or a teacher who confirms some of this data. In our preliminary research efforts to develop the profiles, we may have identified existing programs for similar populations. These programs may have evidence to support their effectiveness; we will return to them when we develop specific programming.

At this point in our inquiries, we have not formally asked other professionals in the community what kinds of services are needed for these girls and their families, and we have not asked the girls or their families what kinds of services they need (such as for education, skill building, prevention, remediation, and so on). In short, we still must formally or specifically assess or define the needs of our community population. In other words, we now must conduct the formal **needs assessment**.

The formal process of assessing the need for services is generally done in two phases. Phase I determines the needs of the targeted population from those who may be involved with them at some level. Phase II assesses the perceived needs from the target population themselves. Those assessed in Phase I might include other health care professionals, teachers, counselors, police, parents, spouses, and caregivers. It may be that the proposed population is already being seen by an occupational therapist, perhaps in the school system, and you want to extend services to a camp program or after-school enrichment program. If you are working with an agency, the first phase of the needs assessment is initiated with the professional(s) at the site (the facility, institution, or agency). For the above example, this may be the principal or the counselor at the school. If we know that there is a community agency already providing services to meet the needs of this population, we may go directly to the agency. We have indicated that it is advisable to be as familiar as possible with the demographics of the community and with the proposed population before going on-site. From this information, you will develop the structure of this first interview visit with the agency representative(s).

This visit begins with your self-introduction (or the introduction of your group). This interview also includes the purpose of your visit and sometimes includes an explanation of the parameters of your assignment (if a student) and explanations of occupation-centered practice. Much of this will depend on how your instructor elects to structure the experience. Although this chapter focuses on *need* as the starting place for program development, it is worth mention that our assessment of need often becomes complicated by *want*. It is important to distinguish clearly between the two. We certainly do wish to help the agency/facility achieve its needs; however, at the level of the clients/patients, we wish to address not only their needs, but their wants as well. It is through our ability to meet needs and wants that we are able to offer programs that our target population finds meaningful. If programming is not meaningful to our client/patient, there cannot be successful goal development or positive outcomes.

Our first **interview** is semi-structured; it often begins appropriately conversational and consists of a discussion centered around the following core set of questions (the **interview questionnaire**):

1. What is the purpose (that is, the mission and philosophy) of your organization?
2. What group of individuals (that is, your targeted population and others served by this organization) do you serve?
3. What are some of the characteristics (that is, their ages, abilities, and so on) of this population?
4. What kinds of programming (that is, treatment, prevention, group, individuals, and so on) do you offer?
5. What are your funding sources? Are you a for-profit organization, or is your organization not-for-profit?
6. Are there unmet programming needs (from the perspective of the interviewee) that you, as an occupation-centered practitioner, might be able to consider?

We describe this interview format as conversational because the interviewee's responses to our core questions will often prompt other questions. This is also your opportunity to introduce information you have collected from your earlier work developing the foundational community and service profiles. The interviewee can validate and perhaps dispute your information and may direct you elsewhere for more research. It is appropriate to note the responses under each question. In these interviews, you are expected to take notes so you do not miss important information.

When you have completed this interview, you can use the answers to your interview questionnaire to check the accuracy and scope of your preliminary community and service profiles. Based on the information you have received, you might find that you do not need all of the information you have collected to form a comprehensive picture of the population identified by the agency. To this end, you might want to synthesize, from the earlier work, information specific to the group in which needs have been identified by the representatives of the agency/facility. Even if you don't presently need it, retain all the demographic and observational information you have collected for future options, such as the extension of services or alterations in the way services are provided.

# The Needs Assessment: Phase II

There are several methods used to assess the need for services; we already mentioned one of these—the *interview*—in our discussion of Phase I. When this method is used in conducting formal research to obtain quantitative data, the interview instrument (the interview questionnaire) establishes a prescribed, structured set of questions that is given to each participant. There are no open-ended questions.

The interview format we have described for use with the agency/facility or other community service providers is not entirely true to the above definition. We are using a structured set of questions we want interviewees to answer, but we are also hoping to generate more questions. We can appropriately call this approach a semi-structured interview, which is more characteristic of qualitative research methods where in-depth interviews are conducted via probing and open-ended questions. This would seem to fit our more conversational open-ended exchange. Our interest in having a core set of questions answered, and perhaps generating more questions, makes this method very appropriate for Phase I of our needs assessment.

If we decide to again use an interview questionnaire when we prepare our second set of questions targeting the specific needs of the population for whom we wish to develop programming, it is likely that it will not be as open-ended as the first one prepared for the agency or other care providers. We use the results of the first interview to prepare the second interview questionnaire, which is more focused and contains fewer, if any, open-ended questions.

Also very appropriate to assessing the need for community-based programs is a **focus group**. A focus group may be used in Phase I, Phase II, or both. Although a focus group typically is a fairly small group (usually six to ten members), the group can consist of up to approximately thirty members when there are several planners conducting the group. With several planners, one or more may take notes, or one of the group members might be asked to record on a flip chart. If the group agrees, audiotaping is a good way to capture all of the discussion. Members do not usually know each other but probably share some common characteristics that relate to the focus of the group. For successful outcomes, Dumka and Michaels (1998) recommend careful consideration to seemingly simple things such as a convenient and comfortable location and a convenient time. The group *focuses* on a set of questions provided by the facilitator (planner). Like an open-ended interview, the intent is not only to get questions answered but also to generate questions. When used as a Phase I assessment, the planner guides a group of interested community members (such as professionals, service providers, and potential collaborators) through increasingly focused issues related to the core set of questions or concerns and utilizes the same process for a Phase II assessment with potential clients/patients/members. When used as a Phase II assessment, the questions prepared for the focus group will likely have been generated from previous Phase I interviews. In some cases, the process of formalized needs assessment may begin with this group. Generally, the focus group generates diverse ideas and allows members to influence each other by listening and responding to the ideas presented in the discussion. A successful focus group experience can result in a developing network of support for the program.

DiLima and Schust (1997) recommend the use of a focus group when we wish to find answers to the complicated issues of health beliefs and behaviors, barriers to health care, and cultural influences on care. These issues often make the difference in the success or failure of a community program. Using members of such a focus group for a continuing Advisory Council or developing new focus groups during programming can assist in finding answers to programming questions in an efficient and effective manner.

In some cases, when the use of interviews or focus groups is not practical (for example, the population may be quite large or is not readily accessible, or respondent anonymity is desired), a **survey** may be the preferred instrument. A survey is most often conducted via a questionnaire that is distributed on-site, via email, or by surface mail. Its intent, of course, is to collect information from a sample of the population.

In our case, we wish to collect information with regard to the community programming services people may need and want. As in the other methods described, our sample, or those we wish to survey, will be selected from our initial target population.

Our survey questions are developed around the initial identification of need provided by the facility, but they are now developed toward the specific sampling of our proposed population. For those wishing to know more about the sampling method, Fink and Kosecoff (1985) and Fowler (1993) offer in-depth explorations of survey design and development.

Thus, methods that can be utilized in assessing the need for community-centered services include:

1. Structured or semi-structured interviews
2. Focus groups
3. Surveys

All of the aforementioned methods are appropriate for the student programmer as well as the experienced therapist. Depending on the characteristics of the population and the nature of service provision, there are additional mechanisms for obtaining data related to needs. For example, never neglect information that has already been collected, *assuming permission to review can be obtained.* We have already discussed ways to access demographic data but there are other existing data banks that may provide programmers with useful information. Medical charts, institutional survey results, quality-assurance studies, end-of-year reports, and other such institutional information are all examples of existing data banks that may be useful to support the need for occupation-centered services. Local and regional regulatory agencies collect and maintain information on items such as indicators of health status, which may also be useful to preliminary programming work. Collection of data may vary from one region to another, but reviewing what is available in your area is well worth the time.

Remember that the questions designed to structure the needs assessment are prepared within the parameters of the therapist's expertise or that of previously considered resources (that is, other persons, instructional aids, or further training within a realistic time frame). In many cases, one round of Phase II assessment following the first interview with the agency/facility or others may be all that is necessary. Phase II, however, is most often a process involving several formats, each one more specific and more targeted. For example, following the review of survey results, the planner may wish to conduct focus groups or interviews. It is not uncommon to continue to assess need while the programming is being conducted. For example, ongoing information regarding needs and wants may be gleaned from the care provider, patient, parent, child, social service worker, house manager, vocational counselor, and, perhaps others who are in contact with the population for whom you are providing services. This continuing assessment of need may be included in program evaluation if the programmer asks the clients/patients/members and perhaps others questions regarding satisfaction with services and what additional services they might need.

You will use the results of the needs assessment to guide the establishment of goals and objectives for programming. It is important to remember that the needs assessment guides the services that will be provided, but does not establish them. The establishment of programming will require substantial negotiation among everyone involved in the process. For example, the needs identified in Phase I and those identified in Phase II may be in disagreement, or the needs as they are identified may be outside the purview of the programmer. It is the task of the programmer to ensure that once negotiations end, he or she has crafted a program that represents the needs of all those concerned.

In summary, the following are steps to identifying the needs of your targeted population:

- Develop the community profile
- Develop the service profile
- Conduct the first phase of the needs assessment (interview the agency/facility director or others involved with the target population)
- Conduct the second phase of the needs assessment (select a methodology and obtain the needs as identified by your target population)

## Exercise 3

### Developing the Needs Assessment
#### Phase I of the Needs Assessment

Develop the specific questions you will ask in your initial interview according to the parameters recommended earlier: what is the purpose of your organization (mission and philosophy)? Who do you serve? What are the characteristics of your service population? What services do you presently offer? Are there any unmet needs?

1. Based on what you have learned while developing your community and service profiles, write below the questions you will ask when you have your first interview with the representative(s) of the facility/agency where you expect to develop your program. Your questions will provide a structure so that you do not forget anything you wish to know, but they may be altered as you move through the interview.

Drawing from our previous example, the work accomplished in developing the community and service profiles for the homeless adolescents in Denver might prompt the following question to the director of a sanctuary:

I see from your mission statement (hanging on the wall when you entered the building) that you provide free meals, a shower, and a bed in a safe environment for adolescents who are homeless. Are there other services you provide as well?

The answer will satisfy several of your questions and will likely prompt the director to think about other things he or she does or wishes to do at the sanctuary.

Draft the questions you will ask below:

_____

_____

_____

_____

_____

2. Are there others you would like to interview as part of your Phase I assessment? Note below who they might be and what questions you would like to ask them:

_____

_____

_____

_____

_____

3. Following your first interview, are there persons you would like to add to the above list? Are there any you wish to delete? Will you need to alter your questions? If so, note the changes below:

_____

_____

_____

_____

_____

4. Following your first interview, review the answers to the questions you listed previously. Are there any areas you will need to research further before developing your Phase II assessment? If so, note them below:

_____

_____

_____

_____

5. What did the director identify as an unmet need or needs?

The mission of the sanctuary for homeless adolescents identifies the purpose of the sanctuary to be the satisfaction of what Maslow (1970) would describe as basic biological needs—physiological needs and safety. In keeping with this purpose and the characteristics of the population (adolescents), the director might identify an unmet need of programming for "safe sex."

Note below any unmet needs that were identified during your interview:

_____

_____

_____

_____

6. Review all the information you have to date, including the results of any additional research or interviews you may have conducted. Discuss the unmet needs that were identified during your Phase I assessment process. Ask the following questions:

    a. Are the identified unmet need(s) appropriate for occupation-centered programming? Why or why not? If you said no, you might need to return to your definitions of occupation; they may be too limiting. Note your responses below:

_____

_____

_____

_____

"Safe sex" was identified above as an unmet need for our community of adolescents. Is the expression of sexuality **occupation**, and is it, therefore, appropriate to our interests as occupation-centered programmers? To help answer this question, we might turn to occupational science. The activities and behaviors associated with sexual expression lend themselves to the three major research orientations of **occupational science** as described by Larson, Wood, and Clark (2003) and Clark, Wood, and Larson (1998). These activities and behaviors exhibit directly observable aspects of occupation (form); collectively they serve adaptation (function), and they provide significance within the context of the adolescent's life and in the culture (meaning).

If we use the parameters established by occupational science of form, function, and meaning to understand the occupational patterns of developing sexuality in our population, and if we further use them to consider the multiple expressions of sexuality as adaptive responses to the potentially dangerous context of homelessness, we have the scaffold on which to build a significantly meaningful program. If we add to this developing theoretical construct what we know of the adolescent's developmental "window" for cognition, emotion, and morality, we further strengthen the potential for a successful program (Austin, 1995; Cronk, 1992; Garsee and Schuster, 1992; Schuster, Cronk, and Reno, 1992). For the creative occupation-centered programmer, meeting the need for "safe sex" is more than displaying a basket of condoms and a few pamphlets. This seemingly simple need might open a door to multiple programming objectives. It is not likely we could have arrived at the above conclusions without substantial investigation of the relevant research literature. A good programmer is an avid consumer of research.

## Exercise 4

### Phase II of the Needs Assessment

1. Review the recommended methods for assessing the needs expressed by your targeted population. Match these methods to what you know about the population. Discuss the pros and cons of structured or semi-structured interviews, focus groups, or surveys. You might wish to review the references at the end of this chapter or other sources for additional information.

Select the method you wish to use, and begin to develop the instrument. Remember that you begin with the needs that were identified in Phase I (assuming that these were acceptable to you and that you have the knowledge and skills to provide programming to meet them). Also remember that during all phases of assessment, you can negotiate.

In our "safe sex" example, a focus group might be successful with our population of adolescents, particularly if it could be organized at the time of a meal served by the sanctuary. Group process might diffuse some of the suspiciousness that individual interviews would likely prompt. A survey could be tried to supplement the focus group, but it is not likely that this population would fill out even a brief survey unless a substantial reward were offered for doing so. Occasionally rewards (such as food, movie tickets, or concert tickets) are given to solicit cooperation in the types of programs we are suggesting, but if true need is defined, then this should not be necessary. In general, homeless adolescents are not anxious to be identified. Most are running away from a life circumstance they found to be compromising and/or dangerous. They don't wish to be found by a parent, step-parent, foster parent, or care provider. They are more likely to cooperate with programming if their anonymity can be protected.

The first question or questions for our focus group would be designed to determine if the group supported the Phase I identified need for "safe sex." As the answers to this question or questions emerged, we would then develop further questions to identify what sexual behaviors are being practiced and what this population means by "safe sex." If new needs are introduced in the discussion and we feel we could design programming to meet those needs as well, we would take note of them and bring them back to those first interviewed in Phase I to see if there is consensus. This process is what we described as *negotiation*. In many ways we are the arbitrator/negotiator between the agency and our targeted population. We must meet the needs of both in order to receive the cooperation and support that we will need to offer the program.

a. Note below the method you will use to conduct your phase II needs assessment:

_____

_____

_____

b. Draft the questions you would like answered to support the identified Phase I needs. The nature of your questions will likely be different depending on whether you wish to use an interview questionnaire, a focus group, or a survey. You might also wish to offer some programming options based on Phase I needs, particularly if you use a survey instrument. Chapter 15 offers an example of a Phase II survey that defines what kinds of programming the respondent can expect.

_____

_____

_____

_____

_____

When you have your draft of questions, develop your final instrument.

c. When you have field tested your instrument, discuss the responses with your instructor, your group, or your colleagues. Do you have the answers you need to develop one or two goals for your program and related objectives? Do you need to draft another instrument or try a different methodology? It is often the case that you will need to assess your population again for more focused questions. If you have what you need to begin the design of the program, you can always return later with more rounds of focused questions (such as where and when would you like the programming to be conducted).

## Summary

In this chapter, we discussed the multiple layers of inquiry that must be conducted in order to design and develop a community-based, occupation-centered program that meets the needs of our targeted population. Our first layer of inquiry resulted in the development of a community profile. We explored the demographics of our community and, later, matched this information to our on-site observations. To our community profile, we added the profile of our targeted service population. This service profile represented the characteristics of our targeted population through our understanding of conditions and context.

The next layer of inquiry was represented by the Phase I assessment of need. This needs assessment was conducted through a semi-structured interview with a representative of the agency/facility where we would access our targeted population. Through this interview and perhaps others, we determine what services the agency/facility already provides and what needs the agency/facility considers unmet for our targeted population. We then would evaluate the expressed need for appropriateness with occupation-centered programming, and we would evaluate our skills and expertise to determine if we could realistically meet the need as expressed. We would also determine the accuracy of our earlier work and what areas we might need to further research.

Using the Phase I results, we then determine the methodology we wish to use to assess the needs as expressed by the targeted population (Phase II). An instrument format appropriate to the methodology is selected, and questions are developed to determine if the targeted population supports the needs expressed by the Phase I respondents. Depending on the responses of the targeted population, we may then return to those we questioned in Phase I and begin the process of negotiation between the two groups. We may find it necessary to return to the targeted population with more specific questions with regard to how the program will be implemented, and we likely will continue our process of assessing unmet needs throughout the program via our program-evaluation procedures. When we are comfortable that we have identified the needs for which we will develop programming, we are ready to draft our goals and objectives.

## References

Austin, E. W. (1995). Reaching young audiences: Developmental considerations in designing health messages. In R. Parrott, & E. Maibach, (Eds.), *Designing health messages: Approaches from communication theory and public health practice* (pp. 114–143). Thousand Oaks, CA: Sage.

Capodagli, B., & Jackson, L. (1999). *The Disney way*. New York: McGraw-Hill.

Clark, F., Wood, W., & Larson, E. (1998). Occupational science: Occupational therapy's legacy for the 21st century. In M. Neistadt, & E. Crepeau, (Eds.), *Willard and Spackman's occupational therapy* (pp. 13–21). Philadelphia: Lippincott-Raven.

Cronk, R. (1992). Cognitive development during adolescence. In C. Schuster, & S. Ashburn, (Eds.), *The process of human development: A holistic life-span approach* (pp. 513–531). Philadelphia: Lippincott.

DiLima, S., & Schust, C. (Eds.). (1997). *Community health education and promotion: A guide to program design and evaluation.* Gaithersburg, MD: The Aspen Reference Group.

Dumka, L., & Michaels, M. (1998). Marketing prevention services in a community context. Workshop conducted at the American Association for Marriage and Family Therapy, Annual Conference. Dallas, TX.

Fink, A., & Kosecoff, J. (1985). *How to conduct surveys: A step-by-step guide.* Newbury Park, CA: Sage.

Fowler, F. (1993). *Survey research methods.* Newbury Park, CA: Sage.

Garsee, J., & Schuster, C. (1992). Moral development. In C. Schuster, & S. Ashburn, (Eds.), *The process of human development: A holistic life-span approach* (pp. 330–350). Philadelphia: Lippincott.

Larson, E., Wood, W., & Clark, F. (2003). Occupational Science: Building the science and practice of occupation through an academic discipline. In E. Crepeau, E. Cohn, & B. Schell, (Eds.), *Willard and Spackman's occupational therapy* (pp. 15–26). Philadelphia: Lippincott-Raven.

Maslow, A. (1970). *Motivation and personality* (2nd ed.). New York: Harper and Row.

Schuster, C., Cronk, R., & Reno, W. (1992). Psychosocial development during adolescence. In C. Schuster, & S. Ashburn, (Eds.), *The process of human development: A holistic life-span approach* (pp. 532–543). Philadelphia: Lippincott.

Youngstrom, M. J. (1999). Developing a new occupational therapy program. In K. Jacobs, & M. Logigian, (Eds.), *Functions of a manager in occupational therapy* (3rd ed., pp. 129–142). Thorofare, NJ: Slack.

## Related Internet Sites

Center for Disease Control (CDC) (information for incidences of disease, and conditions related to disease processes; eg. obesity). http://www.cdc.gov

Developmental Research and Programs, Inc. (will send free copy of their *Communities That Care Youth Survey* instrument): www.drp.org

KIDS COUNT Data Online (summaries of state and national data regarding educational, social, economic, and physical well-being of children): http://www. aecf.org/

U.S. Census Bureau: http://www.census.gov

CHAPTER 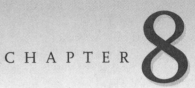8

# Researching the "Evidence," Finding Experts, and Developing Program Goals

## Learning Objectives

1. To review steps to accomplish in preparation for writing goals and objectives for programming
2. To appreciate the process of clinical reasoning as it may be used to describe the complex course of first establishing programming goals, and then helping patients/clients/members reach those goals
3. To identify those individuals who may be able to validate our early goals, objectives, and programming (expert opinion)
4. To identify and locate evidence that supports the effectiveness of programs such as the one we're proposing (evidence-based practice)
5. To appreciate the art of practice and the value of a judgment-based practice
6. To learn to recognize and develop empowering goals for occupation-centered community-based programs
7. To learn to develop measurable objectives to support a program goal
8. To appreciate the complexity in developing a program goal and accompanying objectives to meet multilevel missions and Phase I and Phase II needs
9. To understand the relationship between the program goal, related objectives, and the design of programming

10. To understand the relationship between theories, theoretical frames used to guide practice and intervention strategies, and the program goal and accompanying objectives
11. To explore the relationships between *your* program goal, the accompanying objectives, and your selected theory, theoretical frame of reference, and/or intervention strategies for practice

## Key Terms

1. Expert Opinion
2. Clinical Decision Making
3. Evidence-Based Practice
4. Judgment-Based Practices of Care
5. Goals
6. Objectives
7. Measurable Outcome(s)
8. Mission
9. Theory/Theoretical Frames of Reference
10. Intervention Strategies
11. Occupational Therapy Practice Framework: Domain and Process
12. International Classification of Functioning, Disability and Health (2nd Edition) (ICF)

Using imagination and creativity, occupational therapy practitioners and occupational therapy students develop inventive and creative ways to engage their patients/clients in meaningful occupation. Because they have many ideas and know how to access resources, the development of programs is seldom a problem. It is, however, challenging at times to develop realistic, needs-based, measurable goals and objectives for community-based programming.

Let's consider what we have accomplished. First we explored our knowledge, skills, and experience in preparation for program development. We then identified the population with whom we would work and, in some cases, the agency/facility or site where we would develop programming. Next we developed some ideas for occupation-centered programs that might be appropriate for this population. This was followed by practice in matching these ideas to tentative goals and program outcomes. Next we selected our facility/site and specific population, and we developed our community profile and our service profile. A visit to our facility (or programming site) helped us to obtain the facility's mission and goals, to learn something more about the population, and to gain some sense of the unmet need for services. Through these efforts, we accomplished Phase I of the needs assessment. We then went to the targeted population and conducted Phase II of the needs assessment. Throughout this process, we identified potential collaborators and partners and we explored the research and practice literature to help us learn more about our population and our programming context. Based on the results of these processes, we can now initiate a firm plan for developing an occupation-centered community program. The next step is to write a goal or goals and objectives for the specific community program we are developing, but before this is accomplished we will examine the available "evidence" to support our earlier, more tentative goals, and identify any "experts" who know our population and our anticipated programming better than we do.

To summarize, the steps to accomplish in preparation for writing goals and objectives for programming are as follows:

- Investigate what you can bring to programming—your knowledge, skills, and experience.
- Investigate trends and explore ideas for occupation-centered programs.
- Select your population and identify what you believe will be the purpose of the program (considering tentative goals and outcomes).
- Develop the profiles of the community and the service population where you wish to conduct your program.
- Conduct Phase I and Phase II of the needs assessment.
- Compare the results of your needs assessment and your literature reviews with what you have accomplished thus far:

    Do you need more information? For the community? For the service population?
    Will your skills and knowledge base permit you to meet the expressed need?
    Do your earlier ideas regarding the tentative purpose and outcomes of the program still fit?
    Where will you find published support for your purpose and outcomes? Evidence? Expert opinion?

# Expert Opinion and "Evidence" to Support Programming

We've mentioned several times that you will need to thoroughly examine the available research and practice literature to fully understand your population: condition and context. As you entertain program goals, objectives, and potential programming, there are two other resources to explore. Finding an **expert** who knows your population, or has done similar programming to what you're considering is a beneficial supplement to what you've already accomplished. This may be one of your instructors, or perhaps an occupational therapy practitioner who has published his or her work in *O.T. Practice, Advance*; the *American Journal of Occupational Therapy* or other relevant publications. You may wish to speak with other practitioners who aren't occupational therapists. Although not likely working from a perspective of "occupation," they may provide sound information to validate your present and projected work, or to offer suggestions. Visiting programs similar to the one you're proposing will help you see first hand what works well and what may not. You can match your proposed population and context to the ones observed and discuss the differences with the programmer and personnel.

You will also want to seek any available evidence that your programming goals, objectives and actual program will achieve the results you wish. Searching for accounts of practices that mirror, or strongly reflect the work you wish to do, and that demonstrate its' effectiveness is a necessity in todays practice environment.

What did we rely on before the push for practices supported by evidence of effectiveness? Likely theory, opinion, our experiences, and intuition. In adding evidence-based practice to the mix, these elements of clinical reasoning are not lost, they are simply expanded to include everything available to us that will provide evidence that we're on the right track. Kellegrew (2005) describes an evidence-based approach as a "style of thinking that incorporates research findings as one part of the **clinical decision-making** process" (p. 12). Evidence-based practice supports clinical experience, but does not replace it. The effective therapist combines multiple kinds of research, alongside clinical experience in a reasoning process to shape his or her practice. Law (2002, 2005) is a strong proponent for the integration of individual knowledge and expertise with the best available external clinical evidence that can only be obtained from systematic research.

In the mix of factors that influence clinical decision making, the astute therapist knows that the consumer's values, preferences, and choices are of significant importance (Haynes, Devereaux, and Guyatt, 2002). These authors write from a mental health perspective but, as occupational therapy practitioners, we are all very much proponents of client-centered approaches and the assurance of mechanisms for shared decision making between consumer/client, sometimes family and significant others, and therapist.

## What is Evidence-Based Practice?

According to the Institute of Medicine (2001), "effectiveness refers to care that is based on the use of systematically acquired evidence to determine whether an intervention, such as a preventive service, diagnostic test, or therapy, produces better outcomes than alternatives–including the alternative of doing nothing" (Institute of Medicine 2001, p. 46). In community programming development and practice, where we often rely on grant or foundation funding, we are held to the same standards for evidence to support our designs and programs as practitioners in institution based practices. We must always ask ourselves: will this program produce the desired outcomes, and will it do so over other alternatives, including doing nothing? Generally, we would assume that "doing nothing" is not an alternative, but selecting another trajectory for action might be. We must also remember that there are qualitative measures to consider in our clinical reasoning process, and these studies are not as prevalent in the bank of evidence-based data as are quantitative approaches. This also prompts us to consider our role and responsibility, as therapists and programmers, in generating data to construct evidence.

The movement to make medicine more scientific has evolved over many decades. According to Drake (2005) and Guyatt and Rennie (2002), the term evidence-based medicine was introduced first in 1990 to refer to a systematic approach to helping practitioners to apply scientific evidence to decision-making relative to a specific consumer. According to Relman (1988) the concept of "evidence-based" developed when medical practitioners were charged with greater responsibility for monitoring their practice standards, initiating what would be described as the "age of accountability" ( p. 1).

Equally shared by many occupational therapy practitioners in mental health and illness and in many community practices focusing on prevention and wellness is what Drake (2005, p. 45) describes as the "science-to-practice gap." This phrase describes the gap between what we may know works and what we actually offer clients. We all recognize this gap must close and efforts must be made to inform clinicians of the best and most efficient ways to first find evidence, and then utilize it in developing our practices.

Over time, the need for accountability broadened to include other health care practitioners. The term evidence-based medicine evolved into the more inclusive term of evidence-based practice. Occupational therapy practitioners cannot avoid using evidence to support their practices and to produce evidence-based decision making. Insurance companies are using evidence-based practice guidelines to determine standards of care, including the nature of services they will routinely fund. Hospital and rehabilitation facility administrators support evidence-based measures by advocating for data (evidence) to document client/patient outcomes and Kellegrew (2005) notes that the impetus for accountability of educational systems began with the No Child Left Behind Act that called for evidence-based education in classrooms.

It is not uncommon for health care consumers to research their diagnoses and accompanying treatment to advocate for their own effective and efficient services. It is likely that this trend toward self-advocacy in matters of illness, and in health, will grow stronger over time. Sackett (1996, pp. 71–72), a Canadian physician, and his colleagues proposed early on that "evidence is high quality, current research or high quality information that contributes to a decision about the care of a particular patient." The therapist, generally through his educational background, learns to review and critique research studies. There are generally three parts to a thoughtful critique: (1) What are the study findings? (2) Is this study of sufficient rigor and quality? (3) How can the results help me do what is best for my client/patient?

## How Do I Find "Evidence" to Support My Programming Ideas?

Evaluating research for application to practice takes time, as well as expertise. This is time that a therapist, particularly one engaged in program development, may not have. The systematic review is a way for therapists to utilize research findings without doing a full analysis of individual research studies. The systematic review was introduced by the Cochrane Center, which is now referred to as the Cochrane Collaboration (www.cochrane.org). This organization aggregates multiple studies on many topics to determine the effectiveness of an intervention or practice. The studies selected are current and considered of high quality in their method. The Cochrane Collaboration is a clearing house for a wide array of practice specialists, pharmaceutical clinical trial data, and consumer information. The focus on consumer/client opinions, rights, and preferences in the shared decision-making process assumes that the clients have access to accurate and understandable information (Charles, Gafu, and Whelan, 1999).

In support of the growing importance of evidence-based practice to the practitioners in the broad field of psychiatry and mental health, the Journal of the American Psychiatric Association, *Psychiatric Services*, dedicated 2001 to articles dealing with evidence-based practices. Drake and Goldman (2003) offer most of these in their book *Evidence-Based Practices in Mental Health*. The following topics of interest to occupational therapy practitioners and other providers for clients with severe and persistent mental illness are addressed, among others:

- strategies for disseminating evidence-based practice to front-line providers
- ways to integrate evidence-based practice into the recovery model
- evidence-based practice in child and adolescent psychiatry
- evidence-based practice in services for family members of persons with psychiatric disorders.

Other clearing houses and organizations that provide a research synthesis or critiques are: ERIC Digests (www.eric.ed.gov.); the What Works Clearinghouse (www.whatworks.ed.gov); the Orlena Hawks Puckett Institute (www.puckett.org) dealing specifically with early childhood; and, of similar concern with early childhood, the Center on the Social and Emotional Foundations for Early Learning (www.csefel.uiuc.edu). The latter two are representative of a research-to-practice orientation that includes not only a synthesis of relevant research, but also companion research-based consumer handouts.

Kellegrew (2005, p. 15) recognizes that we must find better and more efficient ways to find evidence and utilize it in our work. She notes that the ability to use evidence-based practice requires some specialized skills and resources. She expands on this further with ideas for how to help the clinician to include Journal Clubs, developing a "favorites" list of evidence-based databases; using software such as *EndNote* to develop a customized database of one's most useful resources; updating critical appraisal skills at evidence-based practice workshops or in a college research methods course; and many other useful suggestions for the practitioner.

## Guidelines and Data Bases
## for Practice Supported by Research

Practitioners can now access evidence-based practice guidelines from national and international health care organizations. The National Guidelines Clearinghouse Web Site (www.guideline.gov) documents the ways in which each guideline was developed, including the quality of the research evidence. Although these may be helpful, they are presently somewhat narrowly focused and one does not find standard practice guidelines that are tailored for occupational therapy implementation from any one group. However, the thoughtful practitioner will not select only one method to obtain evidence for effective practice, but many methods to provide the best care.

Also to be considered are data bases. There are many that now support an evidence-based practice approach to include: Medline and PubMed (www.ncbi.nlm.nih.gov/entrez); the National Rehabilitation Information Center (NARIC) (www.naric.com); Agency for Healthcare Research and Quality (www.ahrq.gov); the National Institute of Mental Health (NIMH) (www.nimh.nih.gov); and the Substance Abuse and Mental Health Services Administration (SAMHSA) (www.samhsa.gov). Currently, SAMHSA is funding an evaluation of evidence-based practices through the Implementing Evidence-Based Practices Project. Some topics of interest to occupational therapy practitioners in mental health are:

- Assertive Community Treatment
- Integrated Dual-Disorder Treatment
- Supported Employment
- Illness Management and Recovery
- Family Psychoeducation
- Medication Management.

This work is available on DVD; see reference at the close of this chapter for ordering information. Describing evidence-based practices specific to mental health concerns, Azrin and Goldman (2005, p. 67) refer to employing clinical interventions that research has shown to be effective in "helping consumers recover and achieve their goals."

AOTA members can access evidence-based practice (EBP) through (www.aota.org). The EBP Resource Directory provides links related to evidence-based practices of occupational therapy. Additional data bases of interest to occupational therapy practitioners are CINAHL (www.cinahl.com), specializing in nursing and allied health related information (for purchase). OTSearch is a subscription service operated by the American Occupational Therapy Foundation (AOTF) through the Wilma West Library. OTSeeker (www.otseeker.com) is an occupational therapy data base housed in Australia and is useful for the entire international occupational therapy community. Another subscription data base, OTD-BASE (http://www.otdbase.org), catalogues twenty occupational therapy journals.

See the list of recommended additional books and internet resources at the close of this chapter for many ways to access evidence for effective practices.

# The Case for Trusting the "Art" of Practice: Seeking Synergy Between Judgment, Experience, and Evidence

At this writing, "evidence-based" practice is all the buzz. Granted, accountability is a good thing, but the pendulum of trusting in evidence to support practice exclusively will likely need to swing back a bit. Polkinghorne (2004, p. 1) makes a convincing case for what he describes as a **judgment-based practice of care**. Over recent decades, the practices of care (teaching, nursing, social work, psychotherapy, occupational therapy, and others) have become part of what Polkinghorne describes as a general cultural shift toward a technified worldview. In his observations, practitioners have been challenged to "substitute a technologically guided approach for determining their practice in place of situationally informed judgments."

The human being is unique and is perhaps the singular variable in the larger dynamic of practice that can neither be controlled, or fully understood. When two of these unique individuals come together, the client and the practitioner, face-to-face, in an interaction focused on reduction of injury, stress, illness, and emotional pain, can the outcome be anything less than limited in predictability? A practice model that will best prepare the practitioner will emphasize what Polkinghorne (2004, p. 2) describes as the "situated judgment of practitioners." Certainly, every practitioner can benefit from scientifically validated knowledge (evidence) to support their practices. This knowledge provides the cushion of confidence for the practitioner; not controlling the nature of the interaction with the client, but permitting the practitioner to fully enter the therapeutic relationship with the freedom to explore and trust in his or her experiences, creative nature, empathetic foundation, and knowledge/skill base. In their discussions of clinical reasoning, Fleming (1994, p. 4), suggest that it is this, which may be described as the "underground practice," most therapists employ in their work.

What is the task of the practitioner, the provider of care? Is it not to work with the adult, the child, the family to establish and accomplish goals that are situational and time-oriented? It is the practitioner who is the preliminary change agent, and it is his or her responsibility to rely on every resource available to orchestrate an effective intervention—certainly tools, techniques, and evidence, but most singularly trust in experience, knowledge, and the motivational impetus of "caring."

## Learning to Write Goals for Occupation-Centered Community Programs

Occupational therapy practitioners and students have spent a considerable amount of time drafting goals. Practitioners familiar with Medicare and other insurers have learned that the key to reimbursement for services is a patient goal that is functional, measurable, and objective. In the language of patient care, the term goal is used to describe what happens following evaluation by the therapist. A **goal** is what you aim to have happen, or your target. In general, a treatment plan developed by a practitioner will establish long-term goals (what will be accomplished at the end of the treatment process) and short-term goals (what will happen along the way to the accomplishment of the long-term goal).

For example, a *long-term goal* for a head-injured patient might be:

1. Patient will be able to shop independently for necessary grocery items. The accompanying *short-term goal* would be:

   a. The patient will be able to generate a shopping list with minimal assistance.

You might have considerable experience writing goals using the above structure; even if you do not, you likely have used "goals" to structure your personal growth and progress. Over time, many of us have had the goal to lose or to gain something. For example, we might aspire to lose weight or to gain friends. Goals are what we often vow to do in the passion of some fairly intense emotion. If these are left as general goals, then nothing much happens. But if we attach a short-term goal—an **objective** that we can measure—results are likely to follow.

In developing language to describe the processes of occupation-centered program development for the community, our use of the term goal will be reflective of the needs of the community of clients/patients/members, and the use of the term objective may take into account the profiles of individual participants. When our goals and objectives are tightly connected and our objectives are measurable, we can determine the first measure of program effectiveness. Of course, it is our interest that the goals of the program benefit all of the clients/patients/members; however, unlike individual goal setting, if not all participants meet their personal objectives, this does not mean that the program is a failure. This distinction between goals developed for ourselves or for individual patients and the goals we will develop for occupation-centered community programs and, most particularly, our expectations for outcome will take some practice. This is quite a different orientation from what we may have become accustomed to in more traditional occupational therapy treatment environments. When writing goals for a community as opposed to an individual, we must consider the needs of the community, and we must write goals for the community (of individuals). By assessing the need from both those who are observing what they believe to be the need(s) of the service population and those who are directly receiving services, we have a good idea of goals that will be meaningful for everyone involved.

Our shared knowledge base and our understanding of occupation permit us to translate the expressed "needs" into goals that are meaningful for occupation-centered intervention. In our earlier community gardening example, the city officials who responded to the Phase I needs assessment expressed the need to find a place other than the street and the city parks for the homeless population, including those who were homeless with severe and persistent mental illness. And something was needed to keep them busy. In the parent-child program example (also discussed in Chapter 9), the children's teachers wanted parents to become involved in their children's education, and the administrators of the Sea Grant Program specifically wanted to encourage the children's interest in science and science-based careers.

In discussions of the above Phase I needs, an attempt was made to synthesize and distill the expressed needs into what was considered to be motivating and inspirational language. It was believed that the needs expressed by the city officials could be satisfied and that the population would benefit from the creation of an occupation-centered community. In the second example, the response to teachers and administrators was to create a parent-child program around the development of teams and team-building to focus on the academic progress of the child and, again, to go beyond to benefit the parent-child relationship in many other ways. Before conducting Phase II needs assessments, the concept of community was researched and translated into occupation-centered language. The meaning of the terms teams and team-building and what they might have to do with parenting was also explored.

The broad goal of the gardening program, then, might be to build community and the broad goal of the parent-child program might be to build teams. The broad goal of the homeless adolescent program discussed in the previous chapter might be to encourage self-efficacy and/or develop self-determination. You will recall that the Phase I need for the population of adolescents who are homeless was simply for "safe sex." Based on our community profile and our service profile, we believed that we could meet the expressed need to explore safe sex with this population, but our discussions prompted us to consider what safety might mean to these adolescents in

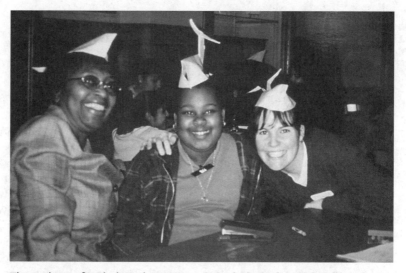

The making of "Whale Tail Party Hats" symbolizes the celebration of parent-child empowerment, awareness of our connection to the larger environment, and accomplishment of a fun and creative task.

the practice of their daily occupations. The issue seemed much larger than the Phase I expressed need. The issue seemed to be about self-efficacy and the components of what Ryan and Deci (2000) describe as self-determination (confidence, relatedness, and autonomy). Thus, our broad goal for this program was to encourage the development of self-efficacy and self-determination for the adolescents who participated.

In all of these examples, we are careful not to negate the Phase I need. In the discussions of that need, we develop a language for the Phase II assessment that offers more definition, explores the need(s) already identified, and perhaps offers a few additional options. Our Phase II focus group might include not only questions for discussion around what the adolescents themselves identify as sexual concerns (such as safety), but also other daily/weekly occupations where safety might be an issue (such as drugs, solicitation for prostitution, and so on). The questioning could include consideration of the factors involved in self-protection (for example, issues of confidence, information, and skills that impact self-esteem and self-efficacy). We then can develop objectives for occupation-centered programming that are closely aligned with both Phase I and Phase II needs, and in this way we continue to invite the support and cooperation of both groups. With this support, the program becomes a part of the community.

The above goals and others like them are empowering; they virtually invite investment and interaction of the participants. They excite us as well as those who may wish to fund our programs. As they stand now, however, they tell us very little. It is not possible to evaluate the goals of building community, or teams, or encouraging efficacy in such a way that one can measure effectiveness. Goals are not measurable as they are expressed; thus, we then couple these lofty, idealistic statements with clear, sound objectives that *are* measurable.

# Writing Measurable Objectives to Accompany Programming Goals

From our research and our dialogues, we develop one or perhaps two goals for occupation-centered community-based programs. Our goals are sufficiently global and comprehensive so that we will not need many to address the expressed needs for programming. Settling on appropriate goals takes some work, and in the process we must offer definitions and tease out meaning. When considering the previous examples, what does community mean? What about team-building, self-efficacy, or self-determination? As we grapple with the many ways we can translate the expressed needs into goals, we generate terms and phrases that will become our objectives.

DiLima and Schust (1997, p. 209) provide us with a list of characteristics for community programming objectives. They recommend that objectives must be performance, behavior, or action oriented. They must be clear and must state the level, condition, or standard of performance that is expected. They must be results-oriented and must have stated outcomes that are directly observable. They must have a specific time for completion, and, perhaps most importantly, they must be measurable.

To summarize, the objectives for community programs:

■ must be performance, behavior, or action oriented
■ must be expressed in clear language
■ must state the level, condition, or standard of performance that is expected
■ must be results-oriented
■ must have stated outcomes that are directly observable
■ must be oriented to time
■ must be measurable.

When we write objectives, we select from an assortment of verbs. Some examples include to learn, explore, promote, discuss, evaluate, identify, understand, determine, illustrate, recite, write, construct, define, demonstrate, challenge, accept, or support. Certainly there are many more from which to choose. With whatever we select, however, we must be able to determine when it has occurred; we must be able to **measure the outcome(s)**. Our choice of verbs indicates the action that will be performed. We will then follow the verb with a noun that will identify the expected outcome. We then finish with what level or condition we expect and when we expect it to occur. Note the following example:

The members will *demonstrate* their *commitment to the community* by *working in the community garden six hours each week* for the *twelve weeks of the program.*

You may have only one goal, but several objectives may be required for the participants of your program to be able to satisfy the goal. Your objectives offer the structure for your program. Keep them as simple and uncomplicated as possible, for you will have only a certain amount of time to accomplish them and everyone involved in the program—therapist, client, volunteer, and student—must be able to observe and recognize when the objectives have been accomplished.

For example, your goal for a day camp may be *to encourage movement and socialization through play.* You may enroll six children (or perhaps as many as twelve) for four five-hour days each week (or perhaps four two-hour days each week) for a period of two weeks; then you will have another group of children. Regardless of the number of children you decide to accommodate or the specific daily schedule, the objectives to meet the goal of encouraging movement and socialization through play must be accomplished in two weeks. Consider the following example of a measurable objective to meet this goal in the time specified.

> The children (or each child) will participate in *one group game each day* that will require *movement through a flexible crawl tube.*

Anyone working in the program described can observe and note when the objective has been satisfied; however, it would be virtually impossible for observers to consistently note the encouragement of movement and socialization through play. There are four terms—*encourage, movement, socialization,* and *play*—all open to broad, subjective interpretation; none is measurable without a specific objective. You might wish to practice defining these four terms for yourself; in the process, you will have begun to generate objectives for such a program.

# The Influence of "Mission" on Goals, Objectives, and Program Design

We cannot draft goals and objectives for programming without first having sufficient knowledge of the umbrella organization (that is, that organization that sponsors or supports the selected facility/agency) and the **mission** and *purpose* of that organization. Our Denver sanctuary, for example, might be sponsored by Catholic Charities; a similar program might be provided under the auspices of the Red Cross. The after-school, delinquency-prevention program we will be describing in Chapter 17 is provided under the multi-umbrellas of the Community Development Commission of the City Housing Authority, the University Extension Urban 4-H Club, and the City Parks and Recreation Department.

As we noted earlier, the mission of the sanctuary example was to provide free meals, shower, and bed in a safe environment. The need expressed by agency/facility administrators or other professionals working in that environment will reflect the mission and the purpose of the sponsoring organization, and that must be our first consideration in the design for programming. It may be an obvious oversimplification, but we would not expect to design a for-profit program to provide services for the homeless adolescent population frequenting the sanctuary. We also would not develop a "wellness" focus for a community-based program to serve the needs of a hospital whose mission is to serve the acutely ill; however, it might be appropriate if the hospital's mission also includes concern and protection for the health and welfare of the community it serves.

When you review the programming narratives described in Part V, you will see that almost all of the examples work from an early identification of the mission of the institution, agency, or organization. This is of significance when you are developing programming to support a particular community mission. Of course, if you are developing a freestanding program, then you will establish a mission of your own from which your programs will develop.

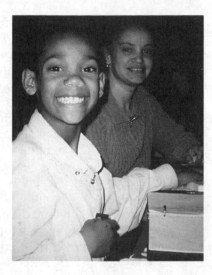

Meeting occupation-centered program goals can
be great fun for the planner and the participant!

The following example will demonstrate how the multiple missions of several
umbrella organizations and their combined needs can be translated and melded to
form an occupation-centered program. It also demonstrates how collaboration and
partnering may develop:

1. The Community Development Commission/Housing Authority expressed
   an original need to occupy the children who resided in housing authority
   projects during after-school hours until their parents returned home from
   work. Although not explicitly expressed, this need may have been prompted
   by recurring problems associated with graffiti, property damage, and gang
   violence.
2. Most of the children living in housing authority buildings attended a nearby
   public school. The teachers of the school supported the need for such a program and responded to this need with a structured way to encourage the
   children's after-school interest in education that would be engaging and fun.
   A science teacher at the school had heard a recent talk by primatologist Jane
   Goodall and wanted to sponsor a "Roots and Shoots" program for students.
3. The City Parks and Recreation Department sponsored the activities of a
   facility adjacent to the projects. They were interested in having the neighborhood children frequent their facility, particularly to encourage attendance at
   their weekend programming, but were understaffed in the afternoons when
   the housing authority needed programming. With the support of the school
   and the University Cooperative Extension, they had initiated an urban
   4-H Club chapter earlier in the year, and most of the chapter's activities
   were conducted on Saturday.

Granted, this is an extremely complex example, but it is likely that you will
have a number of missions to consider when you identify an opportunity to design

a program. In the above example, the missions did not appear to be competing with each other; they seemed, in fact, to be mutually supportive and the Phase I needs assessment confirmed these observations. There are recurring themes of community throughout these missions. The missions of the school and the Community Development Commission of the City Housing Authority were directed toward the education, protection, and development of children. The school's specific mission was to provide education to children in grades two through five. The Housing Authority not only provided housing to low-income families, but it also financially supported programming for the children in the community through the Community Development Commission. The city Parks and Recreation Department encouraged the health and fitness of children and adults through selected activity.

Two additional organizations were embedded in this mix. Through the sponsorship of the University Cooperative Extension, the 4-H Club's mission is "to enable youth to make wise choices and positive contributions to society throughout their lives." The club's mission is articulated through its motto: to "pledge my HEAD to clearer thinking, my HEART to greater loyalty, my HANDS to larger service and my HEALTH to better living" (4-H Clubs of America: http://www.4h-usa.org/). The science teacher brought another mission to the forefront through his interest in sponsoring programming developed around Goodall's *Roots and Shoots* projects for children around the world. Encompassed in the mission, the three major directives for this organization include a demonstration of care and concern for the community, the environment, and for animals (Goodall, 1978). This programming will be described in more detail in Chapter 17.

The enfolding of these missions provided an excellent opportunity to combine the interests and support of several organizations in the development of after-school occupation-centered programming for inner-city children. Skillful program design would be responsive to the socio-cultural development of the children through a structure of clubs rather than gangs. Goals and objectives would support community building, education, and perhaps a futures orientation. As occupation-centered practitioners, there are very few missions we encounter with which we are unable to relate. The previous example provides multiple opportunities for engagement in community-building while providing personal growth for each child involved in the program. The following is an example of a suggested goal for a program that will meet the Phase I needs and the combined missions.

Combined Missions: To *Build* Community.
Proposed goal: *To demonstrate* care and concern for the community through club projects that encourage *thinking, caring,* and *helping*.
A suggested objective to help us meet this goal might be: The children will cooperate to plan and carry out one neighborhood activity in the celebration of Earth Day.

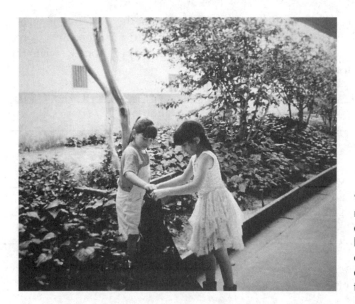

"Roots and Shoots" club members learn that cleaning up their neighborhood supports their club's goal to empower children to create change for positive global futures.

In this example, we have used caring and concern as indicators of investment in shared community, and cooperation has been defined as one measure of what we mean by community. Can you think of other ways to define community? Consider the above example. As it is expressed, does the goal capture all of the interests of those involved in providing mission statements? Does it capture all of the needs expressed in our brief description of Phase I assessment results? Does it generate excitement, interest, and spirit?

## Exercise 1

**Writing *Goals* and *Objectives* to Meet Multilevel Missions and Phase I Needs**

1.  Write below a goal for the combined missions example.

_____

_____

_____

_____

_____

Discuss your goal with classmates or colleagues. You might wish to reread the example, highlighting those portions that describe the collective missions and the needs.

2. Review the objective provided in the example. As the objective is written, you might suggest that it cannot be measured. How will you measure *to cooperate?* What might be a more measurable way to indicate cooperation? Rewrite the objective so that it is more measurable.

_____

_____

_____

_____

_____

3. Now write a measurable objective (or more than one) for the goal you wrote in step 1 of this exercise.

_____

_____

_____

_____

_____

_____

## Exercise 2

**Writing *Goals* and *Objectives* for Your Program**

Review all of the information you have collected as you have moved through the exercises to prepare you for this step. Consider the data gathered to develop your community and service profiles. If you have a sponsoring organization, review its mission and purpose. Reexamine the results of both the Phase I and Phase II assessments of need. Discuss how you will respond to the need(s). What do you want to accomplish for your targeted population? Will you provide prevention by offering programming to reduce the risks of illness, disability, or criminality? Will you provide remediation for the effects of illness and disability? Will you provide promotion and maintenance of health and wellness? Will you provide a combination of these things? You will want to revisit your early tentative ideas for goals and you might wish to return to some of the examples offered in this chapter. Write your ideas below.

1. Ideas for a program goal.

_____

_____

_____

_____

_____

Review the goal you wrote in the previous step. What does the goal mean to you? How will you define it for your community?

2. Develop several objectives that will permit your population to achieve the goal you have established. Write these objectives below.

_____

_____

_____

_____

_____

Review your objectives according to the criteria listed earlier in this chapter. Are your objectives written clearly? Are they measurable? Do you include the action that will occur, the outcome, the condition, and the time? Does each objective directly relate to the program goal? If an objective does not contribute to the satisfaction of the goal, then it must be rewritten or deleted. If more practice is needed, continue to work on these exercises until you have achieved the tight linking and clarity you will need to further develop the program. The quality of your goal statement and the accompanying objectives will establish the success of your program. There is sometimes a tendency to want to fold into your objective your rationale for selection of the objective (why) and (how) you will accomplish or meet the objective (your actual programming). The following is an example.

The students will learn to identify stress signals and to create a plan of action in order to decrease stress (thereby decreasing any guilt they may have felt when engaging in leisure).

We can understand what the programmers are trying to say, but the objective is confusing and difficult to measure in this format. If you find yourself writing such comprehensive and confusing objectives, consider practicing the following approach:

Objective: the students will learn to identify stress signals (in two weeks of programming).

Rationale: to decrease stress that may be prompted by guilt over engagement in leisure.

Programming: assisting the students in creating an 'action plan' to balance engagement in occupations.

It is now time to outline what sort of programming you will provide, on what kind of schedule, and for how long. Your goal and the accompanying objectives will provide the structure for this process. Your goal describes what you feel is most important to accomplish. Your objectives define, refine, and delimit the qualities that characterize your goal. The objectives describe not only what your population will do, but also when they will do it. Now your task is to develop the programming that will enable your population to meet the objectives that will satisfy the goal. It is a detailed and methodical process, and the links between actions and outcomes are equally as intricate.

## What Programming Will You Provide?

As you have accomplished the planning tasks in preparation for the work in this chapter, you have been developing the program you will ultimately provide. Many planners begin with the idea for a program and then seek to position and justify it through the steps of program development. As indicated earlier, this is likely the way that most experienced practitioners begin; the excitement generated by the idea springboards the work necessary to bring it to fruition.

We have all of our traditional options and more for how to practice in the community. Earlier we discussed several roles—including prevention, restoration, maintenance, and promotion—we might choose to develop a structure for our programs. These roles are not mutually exclusive; one program might, in fact, provide a goal and objectives to meet several of these directives. Regardless of the directive we select, there are some assumptions surrounding community-based practices. Practice in the community suggests that we become a part of our practice site—the community. Whether we reside there or not, we understand it and share in its problems and victories. There is an implicit expectation that we are responsive to the needs of the community, just as we are responsive to the needs of our client/patient/member. We understand that our client/patient/member is not only a member of the larger community, but of many other communities as well, and it is our task to encourage and enrich this person's contributions to all of these communities. We are aware of and responsive to what we might describe as the greater good. Although community-based programs need not always be charitable in structure, there is an expectation of charity in spirit. Occupation-centered community-based practitioners share in common a pervasive altruism.

In summary, the shared assumptions for community-based practitioners, then, include the following:

- We become *part* of our practice community.
- We are responsive to the needs of our community.
- We encourage and enrich the contributions to their many communities by our clients/patients/members.
- We share with other occupation-centered, community-based practitioners a pervasive altruism and a belief in the greater good.

These assumptions are directed toward strengthening community—and in the process strengthening its members. Alongside those who receive our services, we are community members. The assumptions listed in the previous paragraph could be described in the same way we have discussed goals; they are empowering and they help us feel connected to a greater purpose. Just as we have acknowledged with regard to goals, however, these assumptions do not structure what we will do, they only make us want to do! Where do we go from here?

# Theoretically Framing
# Your Community-Based Program

Practitioners develop organized ways of thinking about what they see, what they do, and how these things are interrelated. Reed (1998, p. 521) describes this as **theory**. She suggests that occupational therapy theory is concerned with occupational endeavor translated through four major concepts: the person, the environment, health, and occupation. From our discussions of occupation-centered community-based practice, it would seem that we are relying on occupational therapy theory not only to frame our discussions of this phenomenon, but also to guide our program design and development. In trying to understand and articulate the placement of occupation-centered intervention in the community, the author draws heavily on the theoretical orientation of occupational science (Clark, 1993; Clark, Parham, Carlson, Frank, Jackson, Pierce, et al., 1991; Clark, Wood, and Larson, 1998; Yerxa, Clark, Frank, Jackson, Parham, Pierce, et al., 1990). Larson, Wood, and Clark (2003) remind us that occupational science is an academic discipline. The formulating ideas for this discipline are extremely helpful as we think about the development of community-based programming; but we do not find the structure that is implicit in fully developed formal practice theories such as the Model of Human Occupation or Ecology of Human Performance. Crepeau and Schell (2003) distinguish between professional models (e.g. *Occupational Therapy Practice Framework*); formal theory (e.g. Model of Human

Occupation, Ecology of Human Performance, Occupational Adaptation, and Person-Environment Occupation Model); and a frame of reference (e.g. sensory integration) (p. 204). A **frame of reference**, then, would refer to a guide for a specific area of practice, as opposed to a formal theory that has more general application to practice. Theories may also inform **intervention strategies or approaches**. Two examples used a bit later in this discussion are Neurodevelopmental Theory and Learning Theory. Both of these theories provide fairly detailed guidelines for the application of these theories to practice, or intervention strategies and approaches. In addressing the questions stimulated by the interweaving of community, occupation, and intervention, we are searching for meaningful ways to integrate these concepts into a practice discipline appropriate for today and the future. In this process we may rely on all of the above examples.

Practitioners generally bring to the community one or more theoretical interventions that offer structure for the way he or she provides comprehensive services to patients/clients. In Mosey's definition, she suggests that frames of reference "provide a systematic description of and prescription for a practitioner's interaction with his domain of concern" (1981, p. 5). How do we select a theory, frame of reference, or intervention strategy that is the right one and the most comfortable one for us to employ in our practices? Selection of a theory or frame of reference (or more than one) for practice is first based on one's belief system; that is, it is based on what we believe about the world and what we believe about the people who occupy it. If we believe people define their own purposes in life and act on the world with intention, then we would seek an approach that offered respect for that belief and not one that might be antagonistic to it.

Occupational therapy practitioners commonly use the term occupation to describe how people act on or react to the world. The language of occupation is widely used today; however, there is still considerable variability in how this language is translated through the various theories and theoretical frames of reference. Perhaps this is how it should be; occupation unites us, but our choices of theories and frames of reference set us apart. This eclecticism will permit us to meet the wide variability of community-based need in many creative ways while remaining true to our foundations.

As mentioned in Chapter 2, we will also adopt larger, more comprehensive theories and models to umbrella our interventions that are most descriptive of the interactive community systems where our populations are served. Community models and occupation will provide the foundation for structures that will encapsulate other selected theories, theoretical frames or reference, and/or intervention strategies to guide individual intervention in the form of goal structures, objectives, and programming.

## Professional Models to Guide
## Our Program Development Processes

Although first based on our philosophical orientations, the next step in the selection of a theory, frame of reference, and/or intervention strategy supported by a theory or theories for practice may be quite pragmatic. There are three documents, specifically, that provide a comprehensive structure to assist the practitioner in developing a foundation for first understanding, and then implementing practice. Two of these documents: the American Occupational Therapy Association's official document **Occupational Therapy Practice Framework: Domain and Process**, 2002 and the World Health Organization's **International Classification of Functioning, Disability, and Health (ICF)**, first published in 2001, will be discussed briefly. These documents may be described as professional models helping to define the purview of our practices and, in the case of the *Framework*, the scope of practice. Both provide us with a way of thinking and understanding particularly suited to community practices. Such considerations as participation, health, and contextual factors are of utmost interest as we design community programs suited to adults and children. It is from a thorough understanding of these that practice theories may evolve to guide the practitioner.

## The Occupational Therapy Practice Framework: Domain and Process and the International Classification of Functioning, Disability, and Health (ICF)

Practice in the community can be facilitated through exploration of a common foundation and language for all occupational therapy practitioners, as well as others with whom we may wish to collaborate. The *Occupational Therapy Practice Framework: Domain and Process* and the *International Classification of Functioning, Disability, and Health* offer such a foundation and descriptive language.

The profession, through the volunteer sector of the American Occupational Therapy Association, specifically The Commission on Practice, provides us with guidelines and structures to assist our thinking, planning, and accomplishment of best practices in occupational therapy. One of the most recent of these documents to be adopted by the Representative Assembly of AOTA is the *Occupational Therapy Practice Framework: Domain and Process* (AOTA, 2002). The introduction to this document (referred to as the Framework) indicates that the intent is to "outline language and constructs that describe the profession's focus" (2002, p. 609). The document continues to hone the language of occupation and the accompanying concerns of activity. It describes engagement in occupation to support participation in life. Words wisely chosen to reflect the even more global interest in establishing a common language for all health care practitioners are outlined in the document *International Classification of Functioning, Disability, and Health (ICF)* (WHO 2000, 2001). The overall aim of this document is ". . . to provide a unified and standard language and framework for the description of health states" (2000a, 2). As in the Framework, the ICF uses the language of participation, activity, and context. The focus is on health as it is demonstrated (activities and participation) and as it is influenced by environmental and personal factors. The Framework outlines performance in areas of occupation (what we have historically termed work, rest, and play) to separate activities of daily living (ADL) from "instrumental" activities of daily living

(IADL). IADL's are thought to be descriptive of those activities that are oriented toward interacting with the environment and are, by nature, more complex (2002, p. 620). Because of the complexity found in the practice context of "the community," we may find that those activities of daily living described as "instrumental" are significant markers as we prepare to assist our community members to interface successfully with their environments. The Framework describes engagement as realized through performance skills and performance patterns. The individual acts (performance) on his or her environment (performance skills and patterns) through chosen or prescribed areas of occupation. Such performance is influenced by the context, the demands of the activity necessary for performance, and the specific factors (body structures and functions) demonstrated by the individual/client. The combination of these two documents, the Framework and the ICF, provides the practitioner with an appropriate and useful foundation to begin work in the multi-contextual environment of the community with a focus on health, ability, and access.

### Uniform Terminology for Occupational Therapy, 3rd Edition

The third document, *Uniform Terminology for Occupational Therapy, 3rd edition* has been rescinded as an official document of the American Occupational Therapy Association; however, it remains quite useful in helping us to develop a foundation for selecting goals and objectives and in establishing programming (American Occupational Therapy Association, 1994; Moyers, 1999). Although not necessarily intended for this purpose, through its organization and language the document provides us with practical guidelines for how to think about our service population. The contextual, temporal, and environmental characteristics of the population may prompt the choice of a theory, frame of reference, and/or intervention strategy that will provide the most useful way to view the patient/client/member. In addition, problems in function demonstrated in one or more of the performance areas may suggest component deficits (such as sensorimotor, psychosocial, and/or cognitive deficits), thus helping us to further define appropriate choices.

## Bringing Together Professional Models in the Selection of Theories and Frames of Reference to Inform Programming

Consider the following example using the three documents to inform our thinking as we continue the development of our programming ideas:

Our service population consists of children between the chronological ages of five to seven who have developmental ages of two to four *(Uniform Terminology)*. The children are experiencing problems performing in their primary areas of occupation that may include toilet hygiene, dressing, feeding and eating, functional mobility, socialization or social participation, and functional communication (*Uniform Terminology* and the *Framework*). Their problems may be in what the *Framework* defines as the performance skills defined as motor, process, and communication/interaction. Their immediate community consists of family and other children in the service environment. Context, then, is likely rich with cultural, physical, social, personal, and temporal parameters *(Framework)*. The *ICF* would describe these as environmental and personal contexts. Given this information, and more is available to us as we examine all of these documents, we might consider investigating two practice approaches—the sensory integration frame of reference (Baloueff, 2003; Parham and Mailloux, 2001; Mailloux and Burke, 1997) and the neurodevelopmental intervention approach (White, 2003)—that draw from developmental and neurological perspectives and theory to structure and guide our practice with these children. We might also wish to combine these with some aspects of a behavioral approach to intervention (Giles, 2003) drawn from learning theory or others that might be appropriate to meet the remediation, maintenance, and prevention needs of this service population and to ensure that they are fully engaged in the occupations of choice and need.

This example might also describe the ways we could structure our day camp program mentioned earlier. The goal for that program was to encourage movement and socialization through play. We could broaden the objectives for that program not only to address functional mobility and socialization, but functional communication, feeding, dressing, and toileting as well. We could attend to all of these "problem areas" through the medium of play guided by the theoretical frame of sensory integration, or we could combine sensory integration and neurodevelopmental theory and perhaps add others.

Whether your occupation-centered intervention is intended to help your population reduce risk and thus prevent illness, disability, or criminality; to intervene and remediate during the illness or disability process; or to maintain and encourage wellness and normal development, working from the structure and language of the *Framework*, the *ICF*, and *Uniform Terminology, 3rd edition*, and selecting one or more theories, theoretical frames of reference, and/or intervention strategies will provide the programming parameters for successful outcomes. There are several frames of reference and theoretical orientations informing intervention strategies described in Part V of this text to include the Model of Human Occupation, Occupational Adaptation, Ecology of Human Performance, Occupational Science, Social Learning Theory, and Self-Determination Theory. Following Exercise 3 is an account of how theories and models may be connected to goals and proposed programming. A model that is not described in programming examples, but is worthy of your further investigation is the Person-Environment-Occupation-Performance (PEOP) model that skillfully provides a bridge between professional models, occupation, and the community (Baum, Bass-Haugen, and Christiansen, 2005; Christiansen, Baum, and Bass-Haugen, 2005; Baum and Christiansen, 1997). If you would like to supplement your existing knowledge with regard to theoretical orientations and theoretical frames of reference used in occupational therapy intervention, review the extensive list of recommended readings at the close of this chapter.

Before we continue, we must revisit one more factor that was mentioned earlier in this chapter and one that contributes to the process of moving your patient/client/member from need to goal. This factor is clinical reasoning or what Schell refers to as "the basis of practice" (1998, p. 90). In many ways, clinical reasoning defines an occupational therapy practitioner's "way of being." Clinical reasoning describes the multifaceted process that encompasses all of the ways we utilize the information we have collected about a patient or client and the community—that is, through our theoretical orientations, our practice knowledge, and our experience. It also captures what has been described as more covert practice enmeshed in the "stories" that we and our patient/client utilize to develop and meet our goals (Fleming, 1994).

## Exercise 3

### Selecting Theories, Theoretical Frames of Reference, and Intervention Approaches to Guide Your Developing Program

1. Review the goal and the related objectives developed in Exercise 2. Discuss with your group and/or colleagues some potential theories, frames of reference, and/or intervention approaches and strategies that will support the concepts of occupation for the program you are developing.

Perhaps you are already using one or more theories or intervention strategies to guide your practice. Are they appropriate to structure the program you are proposing to meet the objectives and to satisfy your goal?

Note below one or more of your choices that are compatible with and supportive of your program goal and the accompanying objectives.

_____

_____

_____

_____

_____

2. Are you comfortable with your selection(s)? Is there agreement between these choices and your philosophical orientation? Your beliefs about people? Your

beliefs about occupation? Is there sufficient breadth and guidance to provide the structure for any assessment you might wish to do? Is there a good fit with your purpose of remediation, maintenance, or promotion and/or prevention? Make any notes with regard to these questions below; consider further investigation and research that might be useful.

_____

_____

_____

_____

The Model of Human Occupation was selected to guide several of the programs described in this text. Because the model addresses the motivation for engagement in occupation, how one elects to pattern engagement in occupation, the relationship between skills and performance, and the influence of context/environment on occupation, it is sufficiently broad to meet the needs of a wide range of program participants. It is also appropriate to structure programs targeting prevention and wellness as well as those targeting intervention (Kielhofner, 1995; Kielhofner and Barrett, 1998).

The adolescent sanctuary program mentioned earlier in Chapter 7 had as its goal "the development of self-efficacy." Objectives were developed to address the components of self-efficacy to include confidence, information, and skills. A review of the Model of Human Occupation provides us with language (such as volition, personal causation, values, interests, habits, and roles) to structure our program. An investigation into self-determination theory and the facilitation of intrinsic motivation, social development, and well-being further enhanced our understanding of self-efficacy.

In addition, the attention to the influence of environment on our population—within the context of urban homelessness—must be understood in the design of effective programming. This includes attention to what Dunn, McClain, Brown, and Youngstrom (1998) describe as ecology, or "the interaction between a person and the context" with resultant effects on behavior and task performance (1998, p. 531). In Chapter 7 we noted the multiple expressions of sexuality as adaptive responses to the potentially dangerous context of homelessness. Therefore, the theoretical construct of "adaptation" is significant to understanding our population's response to the community and to our programming. We might also find it useful to include Schkade's and Schultz's work on occupational adaptation (1998).

Clearly stated objectives guided by the selected theories, theoretical frame(s) of reference, and intervention strategies provide the framework for the design and development of programming that will enable our service population to satisfy needs and to meet the goal of services. The following equation summarizes this relationship.

Objective(s) + Theories, Frame(s) of Reference and Intervention Strategies = Programming = GOAL

Objective: Adolescents participating in the program will be provided with developmentally appropriate information and skills, which they can use to make informed choices about practiced sexual behaviors.

Theories/Frames of Reference/Intervention Strategies: These might include the Model of Human Occupation influenced by the theoretical underpinnings of the Ecology of Human Performance and Occupational Adaptation.

Programming: Modules might be developed to include the acquisition of information and the development of skills structured around the subsystems of volition, habituation, and mind/body performance.

GOAL: To advocate for oneself by effecting positive change in one's relationship with the environment (efficacy).

Finally, to complete our equation, we must add clinical reasoning:

Objective(s) + Theories, Frame(s) of Reference and Intervention Strategies + Clinical Reasoning = Programming = GOAL

## Exercise 4

### Designing Programming

1. Following your goal, your objectives, and the tenets of your selection of theories, frame or frames of reference, and intervention strategies what are your ideas for programming? (Refer to your textbooks, resources at the close of this chapter, and to Part V of this text for examples of programs if you need some help.) Note your ideas below.

_____

_____

_____

_____

Will your programming enable your service population to meet the established goal? The mechanics of what materials we will select or develop to provide programming and exactly how we will structure it (that is, weekly, daily, or monthly) will evolve as we continue to develop the program. For the beginner, developing programming in a step-by-step process is the best way to learn. For the experienced therapist, the process is less linear and problems are more easily anticipated and controlled during the planning process. But even experienced practitioners are often surprised and challenged by community practice environments and populations. Often it might appear to be more akin to chaos than order. There is always an element of trial and error even in the best of planning.

## Summary

Our earlier work in profiling our community and our service population and in gathering the results of the two phases of the assessment of needs has resulted in a goal for our program, which includes what we wish to accomplish for and with our service population. Our tentative goal and initial ideas for programming have been matched to evidence for successful similar practices and may have been scrutinized by "experts" practicing with a similar population within like contexts.

Goals provide us and our population with an attractive and empowering incentive that keeps us engaged in the process of moving forward. However, without objectives to help us define and then measure these goals, they are useless in helping us to design programs for the community. It is from these objectives that our day-to-day programming evolves.

In community practice, we approach the individual's need through the combined need of the population. However, we maintain our responsibility to the individual by adopting a way of thinking, or a theoretical approach, theoretical frame(s) of reference, and/or intervention strategies to guide our understanding and our choices of intervention. Our selected theories, frame(s) of reference, and intervention strategies can be compared to a pair of eyeglasses. When we put them on, we see the individual as an occupational being, but our use of occupation will be influenced by the theoretical orientation to practice that we have selected. Our selections provide us with ways to consider and to utilize occupation-centered thinking. The appearance of the actual program (the day-to-day activities) is a result of the goal, the objectives, and the theoretical frames and/or intervention strategies.

When you feel comfortable with your goal, objectives, your theories or frame(s) of reference, and/or your intervention strategies and when you have some ideas for programming that will move your population toward the expected outcomes, then you are ready to go on to the next step of establishing specific programming to include planning for staffing, space, equipment, and supplies. Who will do it? Where will it be done? What will you need to accomplish the programming and outcomes?

# References

American Occupational Therapy Association. (1994). Uniform terminology for occupational therapy, (3rd ed.). *American Journal of Occupational Therapy, 48,* 1,047–1,054.

American Occupational Therapy Association. (2002). *Occupational therapy practice framework: Domain and process.* Bethesda, MD: AOTA Press.

Azrin, S., & Goldman, H. (2005). Evidence-based practice emerges. In R. Drake, M. Merrens, & D. Lynde, (Eds.), *Evidence-based mental health practice.* (pp. 67–93). NY: Norton.

Baloueff, O. (2003). Sensory integration. In E. Crepeau, E. Cohn, & B. Schell, (Eds.), *Willard and Spackman's occupational therapy* (pp. 247–251). Philadelphia: Lippincott.

Baum, C., & Christiansen, C. (1997). The occupational therapy context: philosophy, principles, practice. In C. Christiansen, & C. Baum, (Eds.), *Occupational therapy enabling function and well-being* (pp. 28–43). Thorofare, NJ: Slack.

Baum, C., Bass-Haugen, J., & Christiansen, C. (2005). Person-environment-occupation-performance: A model for planning interventions for individuals and organizations. In C. H. Christiansen, C. M. Baum, & J. Bass-Haugen, (Eds.), *Occupational therapy: Performance, participation, and well-being* (3rd ed., pp. 373–385) Thorofare, NJ: Slack.

Charles, C., Gafu, A., & Whelan, T. (1999). Decision making in the professional patient encounter: Revisiting the shared decision making model. *Social Science in Medicine, 47,* 651–661.

Christiansen, C., Baum, C., & Bass-Haugen, J. (2005). Comparing the languages of: the ICF, the PEOP Model, and the AOTA Practice Framework. In C. Christiansen, C. Baum, & J. Bass-Haugen, (Eds.), *Occupational therapy: Performance, participation, and well-being,* (3rd ed.). (Appendix A). Thorofare, NJ: Slack.

Clark, F. (1993). Occupation embedded in a real life: Interweaving occupational science and occupational therapy. *American Journal of Occupational Therapy, 47,* 1,067–1,078.

Clark, F., Parham, D., Carlson, M., Frank, G., Jackson, J., Pierce, D., et al. (1991). Occupational science: Academic innovation in the service of occupational therapy's future. *American Journal of Occupational Therapy, 45,* 300–310.

Clark, F., Wood, W., & Larson, E. (1998). Occupational science: Occupational therapy's legacy for the 21st century. In M. Neistadt, & E. Crepeau, (Eds.), *Willard and Spackman's occupational therapy* (pp. 13–21). Philadelphia: Lippincott.

Crepeau, E. & Schell, B. (2003). Theory and practice in occupational therapy. In E. Crepeau, E. Cohn, & B. Schell, (Eds.), *Willard and Spackman's occupational therapy* (pp. 203–207). Philadelphia: Lippincott.

DiLima, S. N., & Schust, C. (1997). *Community health education and promotion: A guide to program design and evaluation* (p. 209). Gaithersburg, MD: The Aspen Reference Group.

Drake, R. E., & Goldman, H. (2003). *Evidence-based practices in mental health care.* Washington, DC: American Psychiatric Association.

Drake, R. E. (2005). The principles of evidence-based mental health treatment. In R. E. Drake, M. Merrens, & D. Lynde, (Eds.), *Evidence-based mental health practice* (pp. 15–32) NY: W. W. Norton and Co.

Dunn, W., McClain, L. H., Brown, C., & Youngstrom, M. J. (1998). The ecology of human performance. In M. Neistadt, & E. Crepeau, (Eds.), *Willard and Spackman's occupational therapy* (pp. 531–534). Philadelphia: Lippincott.

Fleming, M. H. (1994). Conditional reasoning: Creating meaningful experiences. In C. Mattingly, & M. H. Fleming, (Eds.), *Clinical reasoning: Forms of inquiry in a therapeutic practice* (pp. 197–235). Philadelphia: F. A. Davis.

Giles, G. (2003). Behaviorism. In E. Crepeau, E. Cohn, & B. Schell, (Eds.), *Willard and Spackman's occupational therapy* (pp. 257–259). Philadelphia: Lippincott.

Goodall, J. (1978). Institute for Wildlife Research, Education and Conservation. *Roots and shoots fact sheet*. Ridgefield, CT.

Guyatt, G., & Rennie, D. (2002).Users guides to the medical literature: A manual for evidence-based clinical practice. Chicago: American Medical Association.

Haynes, D., Devereaux, R., & Guyatt, G. (2002). Clinical experience in the era of evidence-based medicine and patient choice. *American College of Physicians Journal Club*, 136, AN.

Institute of Medicine. (2001). *Crossing the quality chasm: A new health system for the 21st century*. Washington, DC: National Academy Press.

Kellegrew, D. (2005). The evolution of evidence-based practice: Strategies and resources for busy practitioners. *OT Practice* (pp. 11–15). July 11.

Kielhofner, G. (1995). *A model of human occupation: Theory and application* (2nd ed.). Baltimore: Williams and Wilkins.

Kielhofner, G., & Barrett, L. (1998). The model of human occupation. In M. Neistadt, & E. Crepeau, (Eds.), *Willard and Spackman's occupational therapy* (pp. 527–529). Philadelphia: Lippincott.

Larson, E., Wood, W., & Clark, F. (2003). Occupational science: Building the science and practice of occupation through an academic discipline. In E. Crepeau, E. Cohn, & B. Schell, (Eds.), *Willard and Spackman's occupational therapy* (pp. 15–26). Philadelphia: Lippincott.

Law, M. (2002). *Evidence-based rehabilitation: A guide to practice*. Thorofare, NJ: Slack.

Law, M. (2005). Evidence-based practice: What can it mean for me? *Occupational Therapy Association of California Newsletter. Sept. 2005, 9*, Vol. 30, 15–16.

Mailloux, Z., & Burke, J. (1997). Play and the sensory integrative approach. In L. D. Parham, & L. Fazio, (Eds.), *Play in occupational therapy for children*. (pp. 112–125). St. Louis: Mosby.

Mattingly, C., & Fleming, M. (1994). *Clinical reasoning: Forms of inquiry in a therapeutic practice*. Philadelphia: F. A. Davis.

Mosey, A. C. (1981). *Three frames of reference for mental health*. New York: Raven.

Moyers, P. (1999, May/June). The guide to occupational therapy practice. *American Journal of Occupational Therapy, 53* (3), 247–322.

Parham, D. L., & Mailloux, Z. (2001). Sensory integration. In J. Case-Smith, (Ed.), *Occupational therapy for children* (pp. 329–379). St. Louis: Mosby.

Polkinghorne, D. (2004). *Practice and the human sciences: The case for a judgment-based practice of care.* Albany: State University of NY Press.

Reed, K. (1998). Theory and frame of reference. In M. Neistadt, & E. Crepeau, (Eds.), *Willard and Spackman's occupational therapy* (pp. 521–524). Philadelphia: Lippincott.

Relman, A. S. (1988). Assessment and accountability: The third revolution in medical care. *New England Journal of Medicine, 319,* 1220–1222.

Ryan, R., & Deci, E. (2000). Self-determination theory and the facilitation of intrinsic motivation, social development, and well-being. *American Psychologist*, Vol. 55, No. 1, 68–78.

Sackett, D., Rosenberg, W., Gray, J., Haynes, R., & Richardson, W. (1996). Evidence-based medicine: What it is and what it isn't. *British Medical Journal, 312,* 71–72.

Schell, B. (1998). Clinical reasoning: The basis of practice. In M. Neistadt, & E. Crepeau, (Eds.), *Willard and Spackman's occupational therapy* (pp. 90–100). Philadelphia: Lippincott.

Schkade, J. K., & Schultz, S. (1998). Occupational adaptation: An integrative frame of reference. In M. Neistadt, & E. Crepeau, (Eds.), *Willard and Spackman's occupational therapy* (pp. 529–531). Philadelphia: Lippincott.

White, B. (2003). Neurodevelopmental theory. In E. Crepeau, E. Cohn, & B. Schell, (Eds.), *Willard and Spackman's occupational therapy* (pp. 245–247). Philadelphia: Lippincott.

World Health Organization (2000, 2001). International classification of functioning, disability and health (ICF). Geneva, Switzerland, WHO.

Yerxa, E., Clark, F., Frank, G., Jackson, J., Parham, D., Pierce, D., et al. (1990). An introduction to occupational science: A foundation for occupational therapy in the 21st century. *Occupational Therapy in Health Care, 6,* 1–17.

## Related Internet Sites

4-H Clubs of America: http://www.4h-usa.org/

Jane Goodall: email: JANEGOODALL@wcsu.ctstateu.edu

Vast Spaces and Stone Walls: Overcoming Barriers to Postsecondary Education for Rural Students with Disabilities: http://www.tc.umn.edu/nlhome/g258/vitlink/heathl.html

Yahoo Online Index of Disability Web Sites: http://www.yahoo.com/yahoo/Society_and_Culture/Disabilities/

Jim Lubin's Disability Resource List: http://www.eskimo.com/~jlubin/disabled.html

Updated Versions of Disability Resources: http://otpt.ups.edu/Rehabilitation/Resources.html

O.T.Practice (www.aota.org)
American Journal of Occupational Therapy (www.aota.org)

## Internet Sites Related to Evidence-Based Practice

The Cochrane Collaboration (www.cochrane.org); also TRIP (Turning Research
    Into Practice) (www.tripdatabase.com)
ERIC Digests (www.eric.ed.gov)
The What Works Clearinghouse (www.whatworks.ed.gov/)
The Orlena Hawks Puckett Institute (www.puckett.org)
Center on the Social and Emotional Foundations for Early Learning (www.csefel.
    uiuc.edu)
National Guideline Clearinghouse Web Site (www.guideline.gov)
OT Seeker (free online database that contains systematic reviews and randomized
    controlled trials relevant to occupational therapy: (www.otseeker.com)
American Occupational Therapy Association's Evidence-Based Practice (EBP)
    Resource Directory: OT Search (aota.org)
OTD-BASE (20 occupational therapy journals) (http://www.otdbase.org)
PubMed (free public access to the MEDLINE database) (www.ncbi.nlm.nih.
    gov/entrez/)
Evidence Based Medicine Web Tutorial (http://www.usc.edu/hsc/nm/lis/
    tutorials/ebm.html)
Evidence Based Practice Centers (http://www.ahcpr.gov/clinic/epc/)
National Rehabilitation Information Center (NARIC) (www.naric.com); also
    RehabData
Collection of the Agency for Healthcare Research and Quality (www.ahrq.gov)
National Institute of Mental Health (NIMH) (www.nimh.nih.gov/)
*Substance Abuse and Mental Health Services Administration (SAMHSA)
    (www.samhsa.gov)
CINAHL (www.cinahl.com) (fee)
ACP Journal Club of the American College of Physicians (www.acpjc.org)
*The SAMHSA funded Implementing Evidence-Based Practices Project on DVD is
    a component of the Evaluation Edition of the Implementation Resource Kit.
    For purchase: Send a check for $15.00 made payable to Dartmouth College
    (to): Karen Dunn, NH, Dartmouth PRC, 2 Whipple Street, Suite 202, Lebanon,
    New Hampshire, 03766.

## Additional Recommended Reading

Allen, C. K., Earhart, C. A., & Blue, T. (1992). *Occupational therapy treatment goals
    for the physically and cognitively disabled*. Rockville, MD: American
    Occupational Therapy Association.
Ayres, A. J. (1979). *Sensory integration and the child*. Los Angeles: Western
    Psychological Associates.

Bly, L. (1991). A historical and current view of the basis of NDT. *Pediatric Physical Therapy, 3,* 131–135.

Christiansen, C., & Baum, C. (2005). (Eds.). *Occupational therapy performance, participation, and well-being.* Thorofare, NJ: Slack.

Coster, W., Tickle-Degnen, L., & Armenta, L. (1995). Therapist-child interaction during sensory integration treatment: Development and testing of a research tool. *Occupational Therapy Journal of Research, 15*(1), 17–35.

Dunn, W., Brown, C., McClain, L., & Westman, K. (1994). The ecology of human performance: A contextual perspective on human occupation. In C. B. Royeen, (Ed.), *AOTA self-study series: The practice of the future: Putting occupation back into therapy.* Rockville, MD: American Occupational Therapy Association.

Dunst, C. J., Trivette, C. M., & Deal, A. G. (1988). *Enabling and empowering families: Principles and guidelines for practice.* Cambridge, MA: Brookline Books.

Fisher, A. G., & Murray, E. A. (1991). Introduction to sensory integration theory. In A. G. Fisher, E. A. Murray, & A. C. Bundy, (Eds.), *Sensory integration theory and practice* (pp. 3–26). Philadelphia: F. A. Davis.

Hagedorn, R. (1992). *Occupational therapy: Foundations for practice. Models, frames of references, and core skills.* New York: Churchill Livingstone.

Kielhofner, G. (1992). *Conceptual foundations of occupational therapy.* Philadelphia: F. A. Davis.

Kimball, J. C. (1993). Sensory integrative frame of reference. In P. Kramer, & J. Hinojosa, (Eds.), *Frames of reference for pediatric occupational therapy* (pp. 87–175). Baltimore: Williams and Wilkins.

Mandel, D., Jackson, J., Zemke, R., Nelson, L., & Clark, F. (1999). *Lifestyle redesign: Implementing the well elderly study.* Rockville, MD: American Occupational Therapy Association.

Nelson, D. (1988). Occupation: Form and performance. *American Journal of Occupational Therapy, 42,* 633–641.

Parham, D. L., & Fazio, L. (Eds.). (1997). *Play in occupational therapy for children.* St. Louis, MO: Mosby.

Parham, D. L., & Mailloux, Z. (1995). Sensory integration. In J. Case-Smith, A. S. Allen, & P. N. Pratt, (Eds.), *Occupational therapy for children* (pp. 307–356). St. Louis, MO: Mosby.

Pedretti, L. W., & Pasquinelli, S. (1990). A frame of reference for occupational therapy in physical dysfunction. In L. W. Pedretti, & B. Zoltan, (Eds.), *Occupational therapy practice skills for physical dysfunction* (3rd ed.). Philadelphia: Mosby.

Reed, K. L. (1984). *Models of practice in occupational therapy.* Baltimore: Williams and Wilkins.

Roots and Shoots. (1998). *A curriculum packet to connect Los Angeles youth with their community, environment and wildlife.* Printed and distributed by the Los Angeles Zoo.

Scaffa, M. (2001). (Ed.). *Occupational therapy in community-based practice settings.* Philadelphia: F. A. Davis.

Schkade, J. K., & Schultz, S. (1992a). Occupational adaptation: Toward a holistic approach to contemporary practice. Part 1. *American Journal of Occupational Therapy, 46*, 829–837.

Schkade, J. K., & Schultz, S. (1992b). Occupational adaptation: Toward a holistic approach to contemporary practice. Part 2. *American Journal of Occupational Therapy, 46*, 917–925.

Schmidt, R. A., & Bjork, R. A. (1992). New conceptualizations of practice: Common principles in three paradigms suggest new concepts for training. *Psychological Science, 3*, 207–217.

Toglia, J. P. (1992). A dynamic interactional approach to cognitive rehabilitation. In N. Katz, (Ed.), *Cognitive rehabilitation: Models for intervention in occupational therapy* (pp. 1,041–1,043). Boston: Andover Medical Publishers.

Trombly, C. A. (1995). Theoretical foundations for practice. In C. A. Trombly, (Ed.), *Occupational therapy for physical dysfunction* (4th ed., pp. 15–27). Baltimore: Williams and Wilkins.

CHAPTER 9

# Staffing and Personnel

## Learning Objectives

1. To learn to connect the program goal and related objectives to staffing needs
2. To consider direct and indirect services required to meet the needs of the service population
3. To understand the relationship between the nature of services offered and the selection of staff to meet the needs of the program
4. To become familiar with the many potential roles of occupational therapy practitioners
5. To become familiar with the guidelines for supervision of occupational therapy personnel
6. To develop the job description for the occupational therapy practitioner(s) who will be hired for your program
7. To draft a sample advertisement to include the tasks to be performed (job description) and the credentials and experience desired for your proposed hirees

## Key Terms

1. Staff/Staffing Pattern/Personnel
2. Direct Services
3. Indirect Services
4. Occupational Therapist
5. Occupational Therapy Assistant
6. Activity Program Coordinator

7. Licensure/Credentialing
8. Registration/OTR; Certification/COTA
9. Supervisor/Supervision
10. Accrediting Agencies
11. Consultant
12. Entrepreneur
13. Advisory Board
14. Job Description

Will you be the primary staff member for your program? Certainly you might wish to start the program and perhaps stay directly involved indefinitely; but would your program better (and perhaps more economically) serve the needs of the community after start-up if you functioned as a consultant or as an on-site or off-site supervisor of other staff? Although you do not necessarily need to address these questions now, they are worth considering for your long-range planning. You might feel a bit overwhelmed with the demands of the initial planning process, but try to extend your thinking to first a one-year plan, then a two-year plan, and finally a three-year plan. Make your plans for controlled growth or perhaps for stability. While growth seems to be the "American way," you should always ask yourself why before you decide to grow. Decide if there is a need, and most importantly, consider what will be necessary to maintain quality if growth is in your long-range planning. Chaos planning in response to emergencies is not the way to operate a program or to ensure balance in the life of the programmer.

## Meeting the Needs of Your Patients/Clients/Members

The term **staffing** refers to the process of identifying, finding, and hiring those persons who will assist in providing the services to your population of choice. In some settings, these persons might be referred to as **personnel**, and in other settings they might be referred to as **staff**. Often in the language of the community, they are referred to simply as *the people who work here*. When anticipating your staffing needs, there are several considerations. First, what are the occupation-centered services you wish to provide? To answer this question, return to your initial planning. What is your purpose, your goal? What are your objectives for the program? In developing your goal and the accompanying objectives, you have carefully assessed the needs of the community and your population. Through this process, you have defined what services you will need.

You must also consider, however, the number of clients/patients/members you can accommodate while offering quality services. Several things will impact that decision. Certainly the funding for your program and the physical space where you will operate your program must be considered. It is possible that you will not have

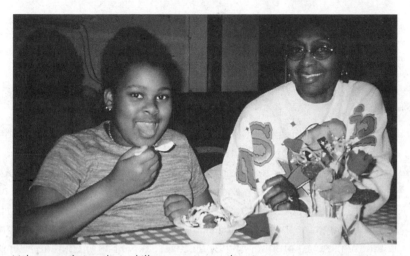

Volunteers bring their skills, expertise, and caring to many programs, which might be realized in the making and sharing of a banana split.

all the answers to funding and space when you begin; rather, you might focus on designing a program that is somewhat conservative, yet still responsive to the need. You might then seek funding and space with a strong and well-planned program design. When seeking grant funding, the initial "pilot" program is often purposefully small so that it can be well controlled to ensure that outcomes are met. An adequate funding amount can then be requested based on these early results.

We will want to know how services are offered to our population. We think of **direct services** as those services we provide that directly support the goal or goals of our clients/patients. These services might consist of assessment and/or intervention offered by a therapist. The term direct is more important when used to determine the costs of billing for professional services. **Indirect services** likely are less costly and include those services we provide through our programming that support our direct services. In the community programs described here, the distinguishing characteristics between these two kinds of services are not nearly as significant as they might be in a more traditional fee-for-service practice. You will want to identify the nature of the services you wish to offer because this will significantly impact who you hire and why. When considering staff to provide direct and indirect services, it will likely be the direct services that require specific and sometimes specialized knowledge and skills. While more indirect services may be designed and coordinated by a practitioner with specialized skills and knowledge (perhaps as a consultant), the day-to-day program may be conducted by someone with more generalized skills. As you make your decisions regarding the kinds of services needed to facilitate the goal achievement of your population, it will be helpful to review the description of the occupational therapy process provided by Rogers and Holm (1991) and Moyers (1999).

In addition to knowing how our services will be offered, we will also want to know when our population is available to receive services. This information was likely obtained in the Phase II needs assessment and must be considered now. The following example describes the reasoning that led to when this particular program was offered.

> When parents in the parent-child program were surveyed during the Phase II needs assessment, it became clear that all were working and would not attend a program that occurred immediately after school. Weekends were preferred for other things (such as shopping, laundry, and household chores). Early evening seemed the best time, although a potential conflict with dinner began to emerge. The solution was found through the inclusion of a shared meal as one aspect of the program that could then meet a number of the objectives, as well as encourage attendance.

Finally, we must decide on the configuration of our service delivery; that is, will we provide direct and indirect services to individuals or to groups? If you choose a group model, the size of the groups will be determined by whether your population consists of children or adults and the nature of their needs. (Malekoff, 1997; Howe and Schwartzberg, 2001).

For example, goal attainment for adolescents with behavior/conduct disorders requires the configuration of a smaller group size than might be successfully managed with a gardening group of individuals who are homeless. Likewise, a different level of staff expertise and supervision might be required for the two populations to meet their respective goals.

Direct group services to the adolescents in our example would likely require the education, skill, and experience of an intermediate or advanced practitioner (perhaps an entrepreneur). Although it would be designed and supervised by an intermediate or advanced practitioner/consultant, the gardening program could be conducted by an entry-level occupational therapist or by an intermediate occupational therapy assistant supervising occupational therapy aides, volunteers, and both occupational therapy and occupational therapy assistant students. Supervision requirements vary by practice setting and the needs of the client and, ultimately, are guided by the agency of employment and state requirements (*Guidelines for Supervision, Roles, and Responsibilities During the Delivery of Occupational Therapy Services*, AOTA, 2004).

Therefore, to anticipate staffing needs, you must determine the following:

- The needs and availability of the service population
- Potential funding sources and estimated funds available to support the program
- Physical space where the program is likely to be provided

- The nature of services needed—direct or indirect
- Configurations of service delivery—individual or groups.

When you have answered the above questions, you are well on your way to identifying a **staffing pattern**, or the configuration of staff assigned to the varying responsibilities for maintaining programming.

# Occupational Therapy Practitioners

## The Occupational Therapist

Our purpose is to design community-based programs that are occupation-centered, and at the center of all these programs will be one or more occupational therapy practitioners. Although they may not always be on-site, they will always be responsible for maintaining occupation as the central organizing theme of the program. Other personnel may be hired to support the multiple functions of the program, but occupational therapy practitioners are the gatekeepers of occupation and the ones to ensure that programs remain occupation-centered.

Our next task will be to consider what practice skills are required to provide quality services to our population and, further, what occupational therapy practitioners can best provide these services. At some level, the program will require the skills and knowledge of one or more occupational therapists, perhaps to design and develop the program, to provide direct or indirect services, or to supervise occupational therapy assistants or other personnel.

Generally, occupational therapists may be considered to be practicing along a continuum from entry level to intermediate level to advanced level based on their level of education, their experience, and their demonstrated practice skills. Whether your program will require the expertise of an entry-level, intermediate, or advanced practitioner will again depend on your goal and objectives and the services you wish to provide. You will want to review the *Guidelines for Supervision, Roles, and Responsibilities During the Delivery of Occupational Therapy Services* (AOTA, 2004) and, of particular importance, your state's practice act and regulatory agency standards and rules to match the service needs of your population to the skills and experience of the practitioner you wish to employ. In all matters of responsibility, including the concerns of staffing, the occupational therapy practitioner is first guided by the *Occupational Therapy Code of Ethics* (AOTA, 2004). This document reminds us of our responsibilities to the client/patient and to the profession we serve. Refer to Chapter 10 for an example of staff selection for a pediatric camp program.

To summarize, the program goal, objectives, and planned services determine:

- the necessary level of education;
- the level of experience; and
- the required skills and knowledge of the occupational therapy practitioner.

## The Occupational Therapy Assistant

The Occupational Therapy Assistant may also demonstrate the three categories of ability—entry level, intermediate, and advanced—based on the same considerations that were applied to the occupational therapist. Requirements for supervision are provided in the *Guidelines for Supervision, Roles, and Responsibilities During the Delivery of Occupational Therapy Services* (AOTA, 2004). As the levels of role performance increase (from entry to intermediate to advanced), the occupational therapy assistant requires less intense supervision. The *Guidelines* do not constitute a standard of supervision in any particular locality or place. Practitioners are expected to be aware of, and comply with state and federal regulations, as well as maintain workplace policies (AOTA, 2004; p. 159). Anderson (2005, p. 10) states that the "role of the occupational therapy assistant continues to expand, and it is each practitioner's responsibility to understand this role relative to the occupational therapist and state regulations." Both the occupational therapist and the occupational therapy assistant can serve as activity program coordinators. The **activity program coordinator** determines the activity needs and preferences of the clients, and identifies specific activity plans to achieve the client's goals. Programs vary greatly but most often are preventative, designed to maintain emotional, physical, cognitive, and social wellness. Adult day care programs and programs for the well elderly are examples of this type of programming.

## Credentialing

**Credentialing** is a process whereby one receives written evidence of qualifications to practice. Occupational therapists are credentialed and **registered** under the auspices of the National Board for Certification in Occupational Therapy, Inc. (NBCOT). In January, 2007, all persons who sit for the national examination must have received a Master's degree in occupational therapy and have completed the minimum of 24 weeks full-time Level II fieldwork. When the candidate has successfuly passed the examination, they may use the designation occupational therapist registered (**OTR**) following their name.

Credentialing by NBCOT is independent and separate from state regulation/**licensure**. Almost all states/jurisdictions, including the District of Columbia, Puerto Rico, and Guam, have some form of regulation of occupational therapy practitioners. Practitioners are encouraged to contact the appropriate state regulatory entity where they intend to practice. A list of occupational therapy regulatory bodies can be accessed on the NBCOT website (http://www.nbcot.org).

Occupational therapy assistants, as well, are credentialed, and **certified** under the National Board for Certification in Occupational Therapy, Inc. (NBCOT) Occupational therapy assistants must have completed a minimum of an Associate in Arts degree and 16 weeks' full-time Level II fieldwork to sit for the examination. When the candidate has successfully passed the examination they may use the designation certified occupational therapy assistant (**COTA**) following their name.

Occupational therapy assistants are regulated in some states and the state of employment should be contacted for any additional credentialing requirements.

## Supervision of Professional Personnel

Collaborative **supervision** of numerous levels of personnel is the key to operating a successful occupation-centered program. Of course, the continuum of supervision depends on the experience and skills of the supervisee; there is closer and more supervision for the entry-level practitioner (OTR, COTA, or Aide) and less supervision for the intermediate to advanced practitioner.

As noted earlier, AOTA Guidelines and state, federal, and workplace guidelines establish the specific requirements for supervision. In general, both the entry-level OTR and the entry-level COTA can supervise aides, technicians, care extenders, and volunteers. In addition, the entry-level occupational therapist may supervise all levels of occupational therapy assistants and Level 1 academic fieldwork students. Occupational therapists with one year of practice experience may supervise occupational therapy Level II fieldwork students; and occupational therapists or occupational therapy assistants with one year of practice experience may supervise occupational therapy assistant Level II fieldwork students. *Standards for an Accredited Educational Program for the Occupational Therapist* and *Standards for an Accredited Educational Program for the Occupational Therapy Assistant*; Accreditation Council for Occupational Therapy Education (ACOTE) (1998).

## Other Personnel

It is likely that you also will want to staff your program with other personnel to assist in the provision of direct and/or indirect services or to offer other support to the program. Office staff may be necessary, particularly in a for-profit venture where billing and receipt of payment for services is an integral part of the success of the program. The multiple roles of reception will also be important to many settings. Clients/patients must be greeted, phones must be answered, messages must be received, records must be updated, and so on. The decision to either employ these persons or to employ an external service will need to be made based on your mission and your volume of services. If your service is offered under the umbrella of another agency or agencies, they may provide these services. As your program develops, you might want to add opportunities for volunteers and/or interning students.

If you are designing and developing a community-based program as an experienced occupational therapy practitioner, you might want to contact the occupational therapy academic programs in your area to discuss their curricula and specific service learning/fieldwork/internship requirements. The costs of providing opportunities for students as opposed to the benefits has been a long-standing debate in the profession, particularly in recent "cost-crunching" times. However, in community-based programs, particularly those that are not-for-profit, students can learn while providing much-needed services. This is also true for volunteers. Volunteers offer a wealth of skill and experiences and are a valuable addition to a program. A program cannot expect to exist based on volunteer services or student services (volunteer, service learning, or interning) alone for two obvious reasons. First of all, both students and volunteers are time-limited. Since volunteers provide services because they want to, not because they have to, they often move on to other things, just as students do. Secondly, both groups are adjunctive, intended to enhance professional services, and both groups must be supervised. Although this second reason of supervision is not prohibitive, it must be considered. While there is always some cost involved in supervision, the richness of an educational environment added to the community mix far outweighs any dollar cost.

## Other Professional Personnel

Depending on your goal and your objectives, your program can also benefit from the services of other professionals, including speech therapists, physical therapists, special education teachers, and others. As with occupational therapy personnel, if you wish to involve the services of other therapy specialists, then you will need to carefully research their roles and requirements for supervision. The national and state organizations of other professions also publish documents describing service provision and supervisory requirements. If you plan to hire professional personnel in addition to occupational therapy practitioners, it will be necessary to contact these organizations.

Keep in mind, however, that the kind of programming that would require the consideration of multiple personnel at professional levels is more along the lines of a community-based, free-standing, or extended practice rather than much of the programming described in this text.

You will also need to become familiar with the credentialing of those personnel you intend to hire so that services are provided by properly credentialed and trained individuals. Academic standards for occupational therapy education are maintained by the Accreditation Council of the American Occupational Therapy Association according to the guidelines provided by the *Standards for an Accredited Educational Program for the Occupational Therapist* (ACOTE, 1998) and a separate but similar document for occupational therapy assistants titled *Standards for an Accredited Educational Program for the Occupational Therapy Assistant* (ACOTE, 1998).

## Accrediting Agencies

If there is to be further credentialing/accrediting of your organization/program, then you must become familiar with those agencies that provide this credentialing and you must know their requirements as well (not only for staff but also for other aspects of your program). Some examples of agencies that set standards for operations of health care provision include the Commission on Accreditation of

Rehabilitation Facilities (CARF) and the Joint Commission on Accreditation of Healthcare Organizations (JCAHO). Whether or not you will be required to meet the standards of these organizations or others will depend on the kinds of services you expect to provide and where they will be provided. You will need to explore this further when you initiate the early process of developing a program. If you are affiliating with another organization or agency, they can help you explore your role in any accreditation or credentialing procedures.

# The Consultant and the Entrepreneur

Let's consider two other roles, both appropriate to many kinds of community-based programs in terms of both required expertise and affordable costs, for the experienced occupational therapy practitioner. First, let's consider the role of the **consultant**. The consultant is one who provides consultation to individuals, groups, or organizations and does so within the systems related to practice, education, administration, or research. This role is not specific to occupational therapy nor is it restricted, within the profession, to occupational therapists. With consideration for state practice requirements and guidelines, the experienced occupational therapy assistant may also consult within his or her area(s) of expertise. Programming examples in this text span a broad arena of systems where a consultant with appropriate knowledge, experience, and expertise could first design and develop a program and then consult through the continuing phases. Epstein and Jaffe (2003) provide a comprehensive discussion of the various roles and responsibilities of the consultant under the rubric of "collaborative interventions for change."

Hanft and Place (1996) provide an example of the role of the consultant specific to the school system. They provide a model for consultation that includes the development of a strategy, which is followed by the development of a method according to the therapist's style (p. 77). This model is very appropriate for those who might wish to consult in other systems as well as the school system, and it is not unlike the process of community program development advocated in this text.

A consultant has the opportunity—and, we presume, the ability—to see the "whole picture." When entering an agreement with an organization, the consultant is obligated to provide the best advice/plan possible to assist the organization to meet the needs of its service population and the needs of the organization as expressed through its mission and philosophy. The consultant is able to do this without becoming enmeshed in the day-to-day operations of the organization; therefore, his or her vision for the organization can remain unclouded.

The consultant's practice and programming experience permits him or her to provide the very best strategies and methods to accomplish the goals of the organization. In fact, the consultant, along with the members of the organization, may have assisted in establishing the goals. In our discussions of program development, it is possible that the consultant would be hired to do all aspects of development described in this text, including the recommendations for the personnel to operate the program(s). The consultant might then stay on to consult at regular intervals. This role of consultant is not to be confused with the role of supervisor. In fact, the consultant might wish to supervise on-site professional personnel, but this would not be one of the expected roles of a consultant.

Hanft and Place (1996, p. 77) mention "style" as one of the elements in their consulting model. They suggest that style, or how you present yourself and your information to the organization, may include the following choices: "tell, sell, teach/advise; and encourage or support." When you function as a program planner/consultant in the community, you must engage in all of these behaviors and more. The skills and information drawn from your intellect, education, and experience must be matched with the strong qualities of leadership; you must have the ability to have a vision, to exude a sense of ethical responsibility (and as such, to merit trust), and to model a belief in the therapeutic and formative potential of occupation. And, perhaps most importantly, you must be convincing in the belief that community is integral to our professional strength and must be encouraged and protected as an ideal.

The role of the occupational therapy **entrepreneur** is also very appropriate to our discussions. Modestly, the name entrepreneur is given to the practitioner who is partially or fully self-employed in the provision of occupational therapy services. Of course, the consultant may fit this description as well, but we may think of the entrepreneur more as the independent contractor and private practice owner and/or operator. As an independent contractor, the entrepreneur offers services independently. As opposed to employees, independent contractors' work is task-driven; they often set their own hours, and they are paid by the job. They also supply their own resources to do the job, including any health insurance or benefits. These "resources" may also include employees.

Jesierski and Gauch (1996) and The Occupational Therapy Association of California (1999) offer suggestions for the entrepreneur to include the management of multiple employees. Foto (1999) discusses competence and the entrepreneur. Because of the growing numbers of practitioners assuming this role, she notes that the future stature of the profession may depend on the competency of these practitioners. In her view, competency of these independent practitioners will likely be judged by marketplace success (Foto, 1999; pp. 765–769). As a private practice owner and operator, the entrepreneur may select from a number of business options. He or she may choose to enter into a partnership, group practice, corporate organization, joint venture, or may operate a sole proprietorship (Richmond, 2004). A partnership simply means that you are going into business with at least one other person and likely more than one. Ryan, Ray, and Hiduke (1999, pp. 196–198) describe the arrangement as "psychologically comforting," while legally it is little more than an accounting entity. Joint venture means somewhat the same thing, but is less a business term than one to describe a shared "adventure." A sole proprietorship, of course, is the opposite of these. You start the business on your own, without partners. A group practice likely means that you will be practicing fairly independently in the company of other professionals. Most often, support services (that is, billing, supplies, equipment, reception, and so on) are shared by the group, along with cost. You may elect to incorporate your business. Corporations are often a way that a small business can limit liability, channel heavy expenses, guarantee continuity, improve the tax circumstances, upgrade the business's image, and perhaps offer employees internal incentives (Ryan, Ray, and

Hiduke, 1999; pp. 201–202). It is certainly recommended that none of the above enterprises be entered into without first completing some substantial research, consulting a business attorney, and consulting a certified public accountant.

# The Advisory Board

The one other category of persons we should consider in the process of program development is the **advisory board**. Karsh and Fox (2003, p. 287) describe the advisory board or committee as a "panel of representatives from all interested organizations and groups in the community who are concerned with a particular program and will help design, support, and oversee it." They go on to describe how important a good advisory board is to the funding process.

An astute programmer will recognize the advantages of appointing a group of persons from the surrounding community to assist in providing expertise and in offering "links" to those in the community who may be of assistance as we develop and market our program to include program participants, shareholders, and stakeholders. This group generally consists of professionals from occupational therapy or other disciplines, laypersons, consumers, and/or caregivers. It is unusual that they are paid; however, travel expenses may be reimbursed if they must come from some distance for meetings, and as a courtesy, a meal is often provided along with the meeting. Experienced members of this group may also provide mentoring to the programmer, which is particularly useful if the programmer does not share in the culture of the community.

## Exercise 1

**Developing Your Staffing Plan**

In the exercises presented in previous chapters, you developed the goal and objectives for your community-based service population, you selected a theoretical orientation and/or frame of reference to guide the selection and provision of services, and you began to develop your ideas for programming that would enable your population to meet the goals. Continue to develop your program by answering the following questions and noting your responses in the space provided.

1. What, if any, direct service(s) will your program provide?

_____

_____

_____

_____

_____

2. If you intend to provide direct services, what level of occupational therapy practitioner will you require?

_____

_____

_____

_____

3. What, if any, indirect service(s) will your program provide?

_____

_____

_____

_____

_____

4. If you are providing indirect service(s), who can best provide these?

_____

_____

_____

_____

_____

Although we will more carefully develop the volume of services and anticipated service configuration when we consider costs, these things will impact staffing in a number of ways, and you might wish to consider them now. For example, offering services in less traditional time slots such as evenings and weekends might appeal to many patients/clients/members as well as staff who wish to work full-time during the days at another facility (perhaps another facility where benefits are paid). Such a schedule might also appeal to fieldwork students who seek part-time or nontraditional options. Weekend or evening time slots might also relieve concerns for space, since many occupational therapy clinics and facilities offer programming primarily in weekday formats. Leasing space for evening and weekend programming might benefit everyone concerned.

If you intend to supplement your program with volunteers, the day and time services are offered will likely affect the age and experience of your volunteers. Retired adults may wish to volunteer during weekdays; students, on the other hand, might prefer to help after school and on weekends.

A combined volunteer model is recommended to supplement services for our earlier community gardening program example. In the gardening program described, retired gardeners preferred the early morning hours for working in the gardens, as did some of the members. Other members, some retired volunteers, some working adult volunteers, and younger (working or in school) volunteers preferred the late afternoon and early evening. Still others were available on weekends. Service-learning students balanced out the options. On the surface, this might seem problematic, but with a continuous thread of direction and supervision, these options invite creativity and flexibility with tasks such as tilling, planting, weeding, and watering in the early mornings; picking, cleaning, preparing, and socializing under the trees in the afternoons; and viewing seed and equipment catalogues, researching options (such as a "taco" garden and an "early Native American" garden), building benches and ponds, and attending community meetings in the evening or on the weekend.

The community garden was restricted by the fact that gardening space was at a premium. In order to involve as many members as possible, it was necessary to operate on a broad seven-day schedule. The garden also dictated this kind of attention. Thus, a wide array of personnel over a broad programming schedule was required. The two important requirements for the occupational therapy practitioners were 1) advanced supervisory skills and experience; and 2) skills and experience in program management and coordination. There were other requirements, but the preceding were of most importance. For example, interest and experience in psychosocial practice and an interest in gardening were advantages but were not critical.

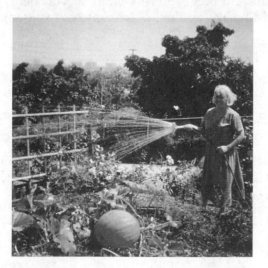

Watering a garden project in the early morning hours is enjoyed by a garden club volunteer.

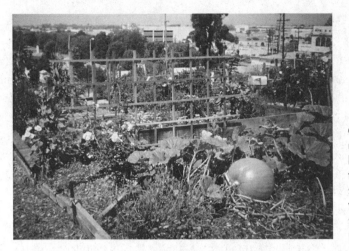

Overlooking the city, an urban pocket garden can bring many pleasures to all involved–members, staff, students and volunteers–while achieving significant goals for the participants.

5.  Considering the gardening example, what is your present planning with regard to how and when you will provide services? How will these plans dictate the paid and perhaps volunteer staff that you will require?

_____

_____

_____

_____

_____

6.  Consider what you will want your occupational therapy practitioner(s) to do. Make a list of the tasks that will make up the job (separately, if you anticipate hiring more than one).

Some examples for the occupational therapy manager of the community garden program include the following:

- Management of the gardening program to include staff, supplies, materials, equipment, scheduling, and budgeting
- Hiring, training, and supervision of staff

- Training and development of volunteers
- Supervision of students to include service-learning, level 1, and level 2 fieldwork students
- Monitoring program objectives and revising and updating as needed
- Monitoring all aspects of program evaluation
- Preparing statistics, documentation, and proposals for funding reapplication or for new funding

While in other kinds of programs, expertise and experience with a particular service population might be the most important factor, in this example it was not.

Make your list of tasks below.

_____

_____

_____

_____

_____

    In the development of the above list, you have created the **job description** for the occupational therapy practitioner or practitioners that will provide services for your program. If you are the one who will do this, can you do the job that is required? From the job description, you can identify the credentials and experience that will be required to perform the job, and an advertisement can be written. You may wish to review examples of employment/job listings in the American Occupational Therapy Association's *OT Practice* (otpractice@aota.org). You may also wish to review newsletters and websites of your state organization.

7. Following your review of examples in professional sources, try writing a draft advertisement for the position you described above (the advertisement also markets your program, so you will want to describe it in the most accurate and positive way).

_____

_____

_____

You might choose to place your advertisement in national sources, local sources, or sometimes both. This choice is substantially influenced by cost and by what you believe to be the local/regional availability of qualified therapists. If you already anticipate that funds will be limited, you might circulate a job description and advertisement in the form of a flyer to academic programs (for recently certi- fied practitioners) or to State Association Chapter Newsletters for more experi- enced practitioners. A well-designed, strategically placed flyer is also a good way to attract volunteers.

## Summary

Finding well-prepared, ethical, and creative staff may be one of the most complex challenges to developing new programs. Once you have developed the goal, objec- tives, and ideas for the program, it is usually not difficult to write a job description for the occupational therapy practitioner(s) and other staff. The next task is to mar- ket your program to potential staff through carefully placed and well-written advertising. When considering the staffing of a new or extended program, you must consider the match between the needs of the service population and the expertise and experience of the practitioner. If supervision of other personnel or students will be expected, then the experience and practice credentials of the occu- pational therapy practitioner must be carefully considered. A thorough review of the *Reference Manual of the Official Documents of the American Occupational Therapy Association* will provide the foundation for first advertising for and then selecting the appropriate practitioner or practitioners to provide the program. Chapter 11 will offer additional discussion of considerations for hiring and retaining staff.

## References

American Occupational Therapy Association. (2004). *Reference manual of the official documents of the American occupational therapy association, Inc.* (10th ed.). Bethesda, MD: AOTA.

American Occupational Therapy Association. (2004). Guidelines for supervision, roles, and responsibilities during the delivery of occupational therapy services (10th ed., pp. 159–167). *Reference manual of the official documents of the American occupational therapy association, Inc.* Bethesda, MD: AOTA.

American Occupational Therapy Association (2004). Ethics (10th ed., pp. 115–141). *Reference manual of the official documents of the American occupational therapy association, Inc.* Bethesda, MD: AOTA

American Occupational Therapy Association (1998). *Standards for an accredited educational program for the occupational therapist; standards for an accredited educational program for the occupational therapy assistant.* Bethesda, MD: AOTA

Anderson, D. (2005). The OTA role . . . It depends on who you ask. *OT Practice.* Aug. 8, Vol. 10, Issue 14.

Epstein, C., & Jaffe, E. (2003). Consultation: Collaborative interventions for change. In G. McCormack, E. Jaffe, & M. Goodman-Lavey, (Eds.), *The occupational therapy manager* (pp. 257–286), Bethesda, MD: AOTA Press.

Foto, M. (1999). Competence and the occupational therapy entrepreneur. *American Journal of Occupational Therapy, 52*(9), 765–769.

Hanft, B. E., & Placc, P. A. (1996). *The consulting therapist: A guide for OTs and PTs in schools.* San Antonio, TX: Therapy Skill Builders.

Howe, M., & Schwartzberg, S. (2001). *A functional approach to group work in occupational therapy.* Philadelphia: Lippincott.

Jesierski, R., & Gauch, P. (Eds.). (1996). *On your own: An introduction to private practice and self-employment.* Ottawa, Ontario: The Canadian Association of Occupational Therapists.

Karsh, E., & Fox, A. (2003). *The only grant-writing book you'll ever need.* New York: Carroll and Graf Publishers.

Malekoff, A. (1997). *Group work with adolescents.* NY: Guilford Press.

Moyers, P. (1999). The guide to occupational therapy practice. *American Journal of Occupational Therapy, 53,* 247–322.

Occupational Therapy Association of California (Sponsors). (1999). Growing in size: Employment law, employee retention, and employee records. *Branching out: Private practice and beyond.* Sacramento, CA: Author.

Richmond, T. (2004). Business Structure. In T. Richmond, & D. Powers, (Eds.), *Business Fundamentals for the Rehabilitation Professional* (pp. 25–48). Thorofare, NJ: Slack.

Rogers, J. C., & Holm, M. B. (1991). Occupational therapy diagnostic reasoning: A component of clinical reasoning. *American Journal of Occupational Therapy, 45,* 1,045–1,053.

Ryan, J. D., Ray, R. J., & Hiduke, G. (1999). *Small business: An entrepreneur's plan* (5th ed.). Fort Worth, TX: The Dryden Press.

## Related Internet Sites and Telephone Numbers

*OT Practice* otpractice@aota.org
NBCOT: http://www.nbcot.org
Occupational Therapy Products: http://www.aota.org
AOTA Educational Standards: http://www.aota.org/students/standot.html
Developing a Small Business: www.lectlaw.com; www.awsource.com;
    www.hg.org; www.cnnfn.com/smbusiness
U.S. Small Business Administration: www.sba.gov; (1-800-U-ASK-SBA)
EEOC Guide: Reasonable Accomodation and Undue Hardship Under the ADA:
    www.eeoc.gov/docs/accommodation.html; (1-800-669-3362)
Equal Employment Opportunity Commission: (1-202-663-4900)
Pacific Disability and Business Technical Assistance Center:
    http://www. pacdbtac.org; (ADA Hotline: 1-800-949-4232)
The Job Accommodations Network:(1-800-526-7234)

# CHAPTER 10

# Space; Furnishings, Equipment, and Supplies

## Learning Objectives

1. To understand the distinction between *space* and *environment*
2. To learn to project space/environment needs from program goal(s) and objectives
3. To determine square footage needed to provide intervention and support services to meet program objectives
4. To determine the need for utilities, plumbing, and safety to support the objectives of the program
5. To compare the characteristics of service provision to the characteristics of available space to determine where negotiations may occur without compromising program goals
6. To understand the relationship between the program goal, the nature and volume of services to be provided, and the furnishings, equipment, and supplies that will be required to operate the program
7. To distinguish between furnishings, equipment, and supplies
8. To understand the distinction between capital and noncapital equipment
9. To identify the characteristics that determine the categories of expendable and nonexpendable supplies
10. To develop a list of furnishings, equipment, and supplies needed for your anticipated program along with accompanying suppliers, quantities, and costs
11. To develop a short-term and long-term cost projection for the furnishings, equipment, and supplies needed to support the goal(s) of your program

## Key Terms

1. Space/Dedicated Space
2. Environment
3. Safety/Ergonomics
4. Volume of Services
5. Furnishings
6. Capital and Noncapital Equipment
7. Supplies (Expendable and Nonexpendable)
8. Cost Projections
9. Direct and Indirect Costs; Overhead

You now have taken your early idea, and either alone or with your classmates, colleagues, or partners you have developed a brief profile of the agency, the community, and the population. You have assessed the need for services both from those in the agency and/or the community and from the population to be served. You have reviewed developing trends that may impact this program (issues of societal concern such as stress, violence, growing populations of homeless mothers and children, poor, underserved elderly, and so on). From the results of this work, you have selected a goal or goals and supporting objectives for the program.

Considering these goal(s) and the objectives, you have identified specific directions for programming that will meet the needs of the agency or organization, the community, and the service population. You have determined your staffing needs, including the levels of skill, knowledge, and expertise that will be required to satisfy your goal(s). You also know what levels of supervision will be needed. To review, you have accomplished the following:

- Profiled the agency, community, and service population
- Assessed the need from the community and/or agency and the service population
- Reviewed trends that might impact your program
- Selected a goal or goals for your program
- Selected objectives to support your goal or goals
- Designed programming to meet the objectives of your service population
- Identified the staff that will be needed to support the range, volume, and nature of programming required to satisfy the goal(s).

You are now ready to identify the remaining resources needed to conduct the program according to your design and plan.

# Planning the Utilization of Existing Space: Environments and Context

Let's consider space. Actually, that statement is a bit vague; what we are really doing is not just considering space but analyzing, designing, and engineering environments. **Space** happens to be where we complete these activities; it defines our parameters. Before you begin this process, think about **environments** and how they impact outcomes. Space denotes emptiness; think of it as a blank canvas on which we paint images. Just as you transform a blank canvas, you can transform the space designated for your program into a positive environment with color, light, and contours.

The same space can invite entirely different outcomes when the environment is created with the needs of the population in mind. For example, consider the choice of classical music and stimulating color for an older adult population or cartoon favorites and subdued color for a population of potentially hyperactive children (or perhaps the reverse depending on the theoretical framework selected by the planner).

Now let's return to the tracing of our progress. If you have initiated planning at the invitation of an agency or organization, it is likely that the agency or organization has identified some space it thinks would be suitable for the proposed programming. While this offered space may be small and less than ideal, it is usually adequate to begin. Remember that the space, in part, will structure the volume and design of service offering. Initially, you should be conservative until you have matched your objectives to outcomes, so a small space is not necessarily restrictive.

If space is offered by the facility, it probably is not presently in priority use; for example, it might be a storeroom (to be emptied); a garage (to be cleaned out); a partially covered patio; or the sharing of a dining room or a classroom. It may be an occupational therapy clinic space that is available evenings and on weekends. If you will have **dedicated space** (used for your purposes exclusively), you will have much more flexibility in programming; if not, you will need to negotiate the sharing of space around other programming that may already exist. Occasionally part of the negotiation process includes the need to revisit your objectives and the structure of your program as well as the volume of services you wish to provide. You might not be able to realistically meet the needs of either the facility, community, or the service population as they originally were assessed. If you are an inexperienced planner, this is an extremely challenging juncture, for you want to meet all of the need. It is likely that if your program evaluation results indicate that you were successful with a smaller component of the population, you can negotiate for more (and maybe more desirable) space. If your initial work was accurate, then your goal or goals do not change, regardless of what negotiations you must make along the way.

Before you begin to actually identify and acquire space, revisit the work you have already accomplished, including your goal(s), your objectives, the nature of

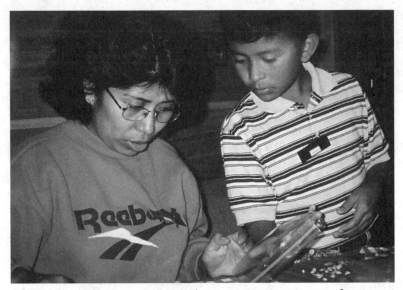

Often a classroom environment is the most appropriate space for programs centered around the occupations of the "student."

services you wish to provide, and the volume of services that you will provide to meet the identified needs. You cannot negotiate until you know what you want—the best-case scenario.

Worthy of mention in our discussion of space and environments is the *Occupational Therapy Practice Framework*'s guidelines for context (2002, p. 613). Context, as well, defines programming "space" but requires us to stretch our conceptualization of "space" just a bit. Context, where and how intervention may occur, according to the *Framework*, includes not only physical concerns, but also cultural, social, personal, spiritual, temporal, and virtual. All of these conditions are interrelated and occur within and surrounding the client, and they all influence performance. As we consider all of the factors that may influence our decisions about choosing the most persuasive and appropriate environment for programming, we will remain cognizant of these interrelated contexts.

## Exercise 1

**Identifying the Required Space to Meet the Needs of Your Program Design: Square Footage**

Consider the space/square footage required for each participant served (that is, an area that is a 2-foot square will contain 4 square feet). Remember that many service models can be considered, including rotating groups or individuals and weekday, weekend, or evening scheduling.

The earlier example of the day camp to promote movement and socialization through play could be offered in a number of different ways to accommodate the needs of the community. For example, you could offer two groups a day, each for one-half day; four groups a day for shorter periods; groups that rotate on one or two-week schedules; or after-school groups. Depending on space and staffing, perhaps concurrent groups could be accommodated. Neville-Jan, Fazio, Kennedy, and Snyder (1997, pp. 144–157) describe an elementary to middle school occupation-centered transition program that utilized scheduling concurrently with the children's academic day.

1. Note below your anticipated program schedule and the square-footage space needs (both indoor and outdoor as required by your program).

_____

_____

_____

_____

_____

Consider the space/square footage for any equipment your goal(s) and objectives require.

The planner of the day camp, for example, intended to access the objectives and goal primarily through the sensory-integrative frame of reference. Both indoor and outdoor space was considered in accommodating equipment such as the flexible crawl tube and a ball-crawl for a program providing service to six children between the ages of four and five.

The parent-child program, first introduced in Chapters 8 and 9, blended integrated community sites with classroom-style table-and-chair work space for both a parent and a child of middle-school age that took into consideration the varying heights and weights of the participants.

2.  Note below your anticipated space needs for equipment.

_____

_____

_____

_____

_____

3.  Will your program require space for files, office equipment, and office supplies? Note below what will be needed and the approximate square footage required.

_____

_____

_____

_____

_____

Consider any additional equipment/supplies for your program (including what was noted above) such as assessments, arts and crafts, and so on. What kind of storage will be required? Also consider office supplies. Will your supplies/equipment require secured (locked) storage? If you need to move supplies from place to place (programming in more than one location), do you need storage for supply carts?

For example, the space for the community garden was dictated by the size of the ground plots available to the program (later negotiation permitted the acquisition of additional space). The acquisition of a secured storage shed for equipment/tools and supplies, however, was not negotiable.

4.  Note below your anticipated storage needs.

_____

_____

_____

_____

_____

## Exercise 2

**Utilities and Plumbing**

Again consider the design of your program and the anticipated nature and volume of services to be offered. Consider the toilets, sinks that you will need, and the location. What will be the needs of your population for adaptations, for accessibility, and for structural changes to the fixtures? Do you need a bathroom in the intervention area, or will one dual-purpose bathroom serve both the intervention area and perhaps reception? Does the bathroom need to be large enough for diaper/clothing changes? Will you need a tub and/or a shower?

1. Note below your needs for bathrooms.

_____

_____

_____

_____

Will you require water sources and/or sinks in the intervention areas? Will you need a water source/sink for arts and crafts? Will you have specialized needs such as over-sized sinks for paper making with the addition of a clay trap in the sink drain? Will you include orthotics or other treatment procedures requiring plumbing? An outdoor faucet is a necessity for filling inflated swimming pools and for cleaning up children after a day camp activity.

2. Note below your additional needs for water/sinks.

_____

_____

_____

_____

Consider your needs for dedicated telephone lines, computer access (for intervention and/or staff needs), and utilities. Will you require heavy-duty electrical wiring for equipment? Specialized lighting? Wall and/or floor outlets? Outside outlets?

3. Note what you will require below.

_____

_____

_____

_____

_____

## Exercise 3

### Safety/Ergonomics

Consider any special requirements to ensure the safety of your service population and your staff. Will you require security for the building and/or the parking lot? If you are working with a facility, you might not be able to control this; but it is certainly a question to ask, particularly if your staff will be working evening or weekend hours when other employees might not be present. Will outside areas require security walls or fences (for example, are you servicing potential "runaways")?

**Ergonomics** is defined as the "science of fitting the task to the worker and not the worker to the task" (Fenton and Gagnon, 2003). Ergonomics structures the interaction of the worker with the equipment, work process, and workstation design. Not only is the worker's well-being protected but the company/business has far fewer injuries and days lost on the job. What are the ergonomic needs of your clients/employees? Are computer workstations at appropriate heights? Is lighting appropriate? Consider equipment and tasks to ensure safe lifting.

1. Note below your needs with regard to the above considerations.

_____

_____

_____

_____

Do you anticipate facility-specific safety requirements with regard to space design (such as codes or restrictions)? If so, what might be the potential impact on your program? When you survey the existing space, make note of any safety concerns you may want to have addressed.

2.  Note your responses below either now or after you have surveyed the proposed space.

_____

_____

_____

_____

_____

## Exercise 4

**Space and Environment**

What kind of environment do you wish to create? Will your intervention require individualized space that is free from distractions? A large space for group intervention that might include games, exercises, and maybe dancing? A patio area? A room for parent/family conferences? A waiting area for clients/patients/families? A formal reception area?

Consider color, furnishings, windows for natural lighting or more subdued artificial lighting, sound (such as distracting noise), and privacy.

1.  Note below your needs with regard to the creation of an environment that will facilitate the achievement of objectives.

_____

_____

_____

_____

_____

## Exercise 5

**Considering Additional "Contexts"**

Thus far, in this chapter, our work has been primarily within the physical context. It may seem a quantum leap to go from defining the square footage of a room/environment, the concerns of physical space, to such considerations as how culture, social, personal, and perhaps spiritual and virtual concerns will impact performance. It is likely you've been considering these factors all along, but may not have categorized them. How have these dimensions of "environment" influenced your choices in programming?

_____

_____

_____

_____

_____

# Taking a First Look and Then Another

If you have not already done so, it is time to take a critical walk-through of the space where you will be providing your program. Before this visit, carefully consider your responses to the exercises you just completed with regard to the space requirements deemed necessary to meet the objectives of your program. If necessary, make a second visit; walk the space and determine the exact square footage that is available to you for intervention and storage. Compare these figures with the results of your earlier exercises. Spend time envisioning how the space will be laid out and how people will get in and out of it. While you are there draw a rough floor plan and note the details of the space, including placement of doors/exits, windows, closets, electrical outlets, lighting, telephone lines, and anything else that presently exists in the designated space. For exact square footage, use graph paper to scale (for example 1/4" = 1 foot). See Figure 10–1 for an example of a floor/space drawing for a pediatric intervention program.

## Exercise 6

**Comparing Your Rough Space Drawing to Your Original Plan**

Carefully compare your drawing of the available space with the results of the previous exercises. Discuss any discrepancies you might find. On another sheet of graph paper, note any additions or alterations that meeting your program goal will require. What compromises are you willing to make? Remember that you might be willing to negotiate the mode of service delivery and you might also reconsider your objectives, but you cannot alter your goal and still meet the needs of your service population and the community.

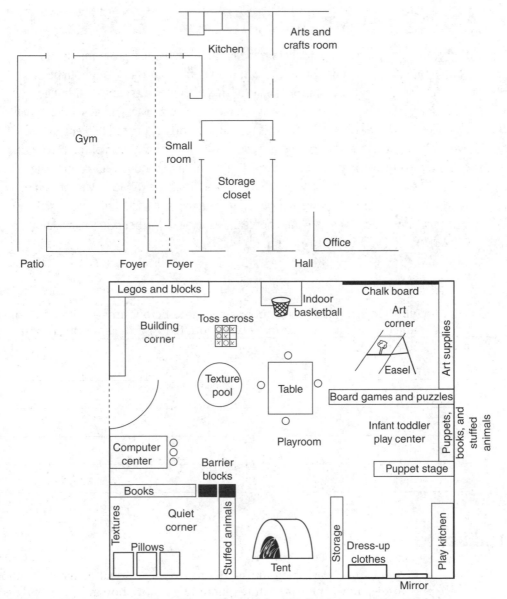

**FIGURE 10–1** Example of a Floor/Space Drawing for a Pediatric Intervention Program

In the planning of the elementary to middle school transition program mentioned earlier, the most desirable space (one without distraction) was thought to be a small classroom or meeting room adjacent to the regular classroom. Although it was added later when the program was expanded, such a space initially was not available. The format for programming was redesigned and negotiated to blend and flow with actual classroom and playground activities during the course of the daily round of activities supporting the occupation of "just going to school"/education. The goal of the program accurately reflected the need; thus, negotiation was possible. Without such preliminary work in assessing the need, the assistance of the school administrators and teachers would not likely have been forthcoming (Neville-Jan, Fazio, Kennedy, and Snyder, 1997; pp. 144–157).

1. After you have made your comparisons, note below any additions or alterations in the existing space that must be negotiated in order for your program to meet the goal(s).

_____

_____

_____

_____

_____

## Ideal Space

You might want to draft what could be described as an ideal or most desirable space plan to keep in your file for future planning; for now, however, you will need to negotiate from what you require to meet your goal(s), not necessarily from what might be ideal. Space is a desirable and scarce commodity for most agencies and organizations, particularly if they are not-for-profit. However, if you have followed through on the previous exercises and have an accurate and detailed assessment of needs, then you will have an informed position from which you can negotiate. Do not settle for less than what you require to satisfy your goal(s). If you must negotiate for less space (reduced square footage) or less desirable space than you intended (inadequate storage, no windows, and so on), then you may need to alter your objectives and the volume of services you can offer. You will need to be clear about this in your negotiations. Also consider your bottom line for negotiation. There is always a point from which you might decide that you cannot meet the expected need or cannot do so while offering quality services. Negotiation does not mean compromising ethics, integrity, or quality. If it comes to this, you know to step away and perhaps broker your plan elsewhere in the community.

## Designing New, Remodeled, or Renovated Space for a Private Practice

If you are designing space for a private for-profit practice, you can be more creative in the expression of your needs. However, even if you have substantial freedom in space design, it is critical that you always be realistic in what you must have to meet your goal(s) and objectives. If you are successful as you initiate programming and if your outcome measures demonstrate this success, then you will be in a position to negotiate for additional and perhaps more desirable space.

Assuming careful planning and good business savvy (or advice), it is likely that private practices will soon outgrow their space and will find the need to expand into other existing space. It would be advisable to keep this in mind if you anticipate leasing space for a freestanding practice. Consider a business building that is zoned appropriately for your practice, with easy access, elevators to upper floors, adequate parking, and with potential to lease adjoining space when the practice grows. This will help in the future to avoid the time, potential client loss, and expense of having to move everything to a new address.

If you are starting a private practice, then the space plan must be detailed, accurate, and comprehensive. This is also true if you are "shopping" for existing space to remodel or if you are able to design your space as a building is being constructed. As a culture, occupational therapy practitioners have a good sense of space, environment, and design; however, the design of a practice space from the ground up requires the services of an architect and perhaps other design professionals. Certainly you must carefully collaborate from your area of expertise, which is knowledge about the characteristics and needs of the community, the service needs of your population, attention to multiple contexts, and the characteristics of adapted environments.

There are a few other points to consider if you intend to design and plan a private practice. Just as we discussed previously, conduct all steps of the programming process, including the needs assessment, trends analysis, and the community profile. Although you might believe that you know the community, it is likely that you only know it from your own perspective (that is, the environment that supports your chosen occupations). Of course, place your practice within the community you wish to serve, with consideration for the round of activities that your targeted client/patient population engages in daily and weekly. If your program's targeted population includes children with learning and/or emotional disorders who are seen after school or on Saturdays, consider the daily occupations of the parents and families, and place your practice close to areas such as schools, athletic fields, and shopping.

If a mother or father is able to first drop off one child for soccer practice, another for an after-school music lesson, and another for therapy then shop for dinner, your practice will be more successful than one that is located outside of (his or) her round of daily activity. Convenience is also a factor for adults who come for therapy before or after work or during their lunch hours. "Mapping" your community and the daily occupations of your targeted population and their families and using this "map" to locate your practice and develop your programming hours will be a long-standing advantage to you. While it might seem to be common sense, placing your practice convenient to the occupational routines of your client/patient population is also a sophisticated marketing strategy.

The above considerations also hold true for the planning of day camps for differently abled children. Again, parents may have to balance the needs of other children, their own work schedules, and the needs of a differently abled child. In the case of a day camp, offering low-cost transportation is a real plus, but sometimes simply offering a small space for parents and caregivers to have a cup of coffee, chat with others, and relax is enough to get children there when otherwise they might not have been included. Anticipating and addressing the needs of a caregiver while providing intervention to the client/patient/camper permits the planner to meet several objectives. In addition, if our camp example also includes the siblings of the service population, several needs may be satisfied. Additional programming for these caregivers through focused "help" sessions while their children are receiving services might be a wise marketing tool or, in some cases, another point of potentially profitable service.

The wise utilization of space—whether a room, a building, or a location within a community—is often key to the success of a program. As stated by Ryan, Ray, and Hiduke (1999, p. 119), "one of the most important decisions an entrepreneur has to make is where to locate his or her business . . . location, location, location."

## Furnishings, Equipment, and Supplies

Now that you have accomplished your preliminary planning and have identified your space/programming environment, it is time to furnish it. Again, revisit your goal(s) and objectives. It seems redundant by now, but your well-crafted and informed goal(s) and objectives structure every plan and every decision that you make as you develop your program. We have all witnessed programs where there is an apparent lack of planning, direction, and structure. Consider, for example, treatment rooms filled with laundry lists of supplies and equipment because they were assumed to be important to an occupational therapy practice. This particularly happens when a planner solicits donated items without a clear sense of the program's direction. To avoid making a generic list of, for example, twelve reachers or five boxes of raffia or five inflatable swimming pools or four computers with cognitive retraining software, let's begin by defining exactly what we want to accomplish.

goal/objectives + target population + theoretical orientation/frame(s) of reference + staff + space + service volume = furnishings, equipment and supplies.

As we have already noted, our first considerations include our programming goal, our accompanying objectives, and our population to be served. In Chapter 8 you developed the theoretical orientation that you would use to structure your intervention. The **volume of services**—or how many clients/patients/members you would see in the course of a day, week, or month—was established as you considered the needs of your population and the number of staff, their qualifications, and their skills. These considerations also helped you select and plan the space where the program would take place. As summarized in the above equation, all of these considerations form the pieces of a puzzle that will lead you to the furnishings, equipment, and supplies that you will need to operate the program.

Let's examine how all of these considerations come together to result in our recommended inventory of furnishings, equipment, and supplies. You will recall that earlier we reviewed the space needs for a day camp example.

The goal of the day camp was to promote movement and socialization through play, and the sensory-integrative frame of reference was selected to facilitate the objectives designed to accomplish the goal. The available space could easily accommodate the program design to offer services for six children between the ages of four and five, four days a week from 10:00 A.M. to 3:00 P.M., for two weeks. This service model was then repeated for new groups of children. Children require attention both to facilitate the achievement of intervention objectives and to guarantee safety. For the six children, there were two occupational therapists, one occupational therapy assistant, and two student volunteers. In addition to direct service, administrative tasks and marketing/promotion were shared by the two occupational therapists.

The program was conducted both indoors and out-of-doors. The out-of-doors area combined a large sand strip with a grassy area for sensory-integrative games and activities. An awning covered four picnic tables for lunch, snacks, and arts and crafts. A smaller indoor area was available for the occasional rainy day and was used primarily for storage.

This service-delivery model could be expanded if the children came to camp for only half-days or if two camps were run simultaneously. Such decisions would require that the planners revisit their objectives and their goal. Could the campers meet their objectives in only half-day visits? How would this decision affect the staffing pattern? What would happen if two camps were run simultaneously? Would more space be required? More supplies and equipment? How would this decision impact the staffing pattern? Could the objectives continue to be satisfied? Would new objectives be required to meet the goal? Would these potential changes in the service-delivery model continue to meet the needs as expressed by referring community therapists, teachers, and parents? (See Figure 10–2 for a partial supply list for this program.)

This example demonstrates several things. The equation we have offered to take us to our decision of what equipment and supplies we will need to provide the program is certainly not linear. With each option we might consider, there are pros and cons. It is our developing clinical reasoning that permits us to integrate all of these potential choices into a best-case scenario for the child/camper. Certainly adding more children to the camp while hiring fewer staff and not increasing supplies or equipment has the potential to "make more money." Or, does it? Can we consider that offering the very best services (that through our evaluation process we can guarantee are effective) may be more lucrative over time?

## How Do You Find What You Need?

We have mentioned several service items in our day camp example that will have to be purchased, including picnic tables, games and activities, and arts and crafts supplies. The picnic tables and perhaps the games will be a one-time purchase, but the supplies for arts and crafts will require continuous replacement. If you are a practicing therapist, choosing the furnishings, equipment, and supplies for your program will not be difficult. On the other hand, if you are a student, you will first need to peruse the catalogues of suppliers that occupational therapy practitioners use to furnish their practices. Although some of the supplies and equipment surround you in your classrooms, until now you may not have been aware of how and where they were obtained or how much they cost. (See the partial list at the end of this chapter for companies that provide equipment and supplies.)

The issue of cost brings us to another important consideration: we have not yet established a budget for our program (that will come in the next chapter). Depending on how you have become accustomed to handling your personal budget, you might be a little confused about designing a program without knowing what you can afford. If you are a student, you should use what might be described as *optimistic budgeting*, or designing the best-case scenario of what the program *should* be. When you know what you want and what it will cost, then you target the funding. If you

---

**FIGURE 10–2  Sample Cost Sheet for a Day Camp**

This particular day camp program is a variation of the one described in earlier chapters. It is an extension of a pediatric not-for-profit practice, but it also welcomes the siblings of clients. It is staffed by full-time employees of the practice during the three summer months. The following is the service provision formula: two four-day weeks (=) one camp session (×) 3 summer months (=) six sessions (×) ten day campers each session (=) a total of 60 children serviced. The following is a partial cost sheet for the program. *Items marked with an asterisk (\*) indicate a partial list.*

1. **STAFFING**

   a. Full-time camp: occupational therapist (OTR) entry-level
      Yearly gross salary (=) $46,000
   b. Part-time camp, part-time practice: occupational therapist (OTR), six years experience, sensory-integration certification
      Yearly gross salary (=) $62,000
   c. Part-time camp, part-time practice: certified occupational therapy assistant (COTA), one year experience
      Yearly gross salary (=) $28,000
      Total yearly professional salaries (=) $136,000
      Approximate combined benefit packages (×) 20% (=) $27,200
      Total professional employee cost to company (=) $163,200
   d. Part-time camp, part-time practice: office assistant
      Yearly gross salary (=) $19,200
      Approximate benefit package (×) 20% (=) $3,840
      Total administrative staff cost to company (=) $23,040

2. **MARKETING**

   a. Computer-generated flyers hand-distributed by practice professional staff to parents of children already being seen in the practice and to Regional Center offices. Approximately 200 flyers distributed at a cost of $.02 per flyer (=) $4.
      Sixty registrations and deposits were received, and a waiting list was quickly generated that exceeded the capacity of the camp. Thus, no further marketing to obtain campers was required.
   b. Personal marketing to local businesses and companies to obtain donated equipment and supplies and tuition scholarships was part of the responsibility of the therapists who were 100% camp time. An end-of-summer "thank you" picnic lunch for donors and full-time campers was donated by a local caterer.

**FIGURE 10–2 Sample Cost Sheet for a Day Camp—continued**

### 3. OVERHEAD

    a. Utilities: Water and trash pickup were the only requirements and were at an approximate cost of $52 for the summer (absorbed into the larger practice bills).

    b. Van rental (1 × each week of camp) (=) 12 (×) $17 (=) $204

### 4. EQUIPMENT (Capital)

    None Required

### 5. EQUIPMENT*(noncapital): Purchased locally, so no shipping charges.

    a. 4 picnic tables with attached benches (ea. $210) (=) $840

    b. 4 large inflatable wading pools (ea. $42) (=) $168

    c. 3 kinder chutes (ea. $49.95) (=) $149.85

    d. 3 soft ring toss games (ea. $18) (=) $54

    e. 1 parachute (=) $215

    f. 15 beach balls (ea. $1.99) (=) $29.85

       Total cost of equipment if purchased*: $1456.70

       Items 1, 2, and 5 Were Donated: −1223.00

       Actual cost of equipment to company: $ 233.70

### 6. NONEXPENDABLE SUPPLIES* (purchased for full summer)

    a. 1 class-pack scissors—included 36, left and right handed (ea. $32) (=) $32

    b. 1 class-pack paint brushes—100 assorted (ea. $28) (=) $28

    c. 3 packs printmaking sponges—35 assorted shapes (ea. $15) (=) $45

       Total cost of nonexpendable supplies for summer*: $105

### 7. EXPENDABLE SUPPLIES* (figured for one two-week session (×) 6 sessions)

    a. 10 1.7 fl. oz. nontoxic, nonflammable glue sticks (×) .99 ea. (=) $9.90 (×) 6 sessions (=) $59.94 (Note: bulk of 100 glue sticks at a cost of $.52 ea. offered a savings of $.47 per stick (=) total cost of $52.00.)

    b. 2 class-pack assorted construction paper—500 sheets (×) $4.72 ea. (=) $9.44 (bulk savings of approximately $.03 per sheet over smaller pkg.)

    c. Crayola washable paints nine colors: 1 gallon each (×) $15.95 gal. (=) $143.55

    d. 500 paper paint pans (=) $9

Total cost of expendable supplies for summer* (six sessions) (=) $213.99
Total cost of expendable supplies for summer * (divided by six sessions) (=) $35.67
approximate supply cost for each session (divided by 10 children per session) (=)
$3.57 approximate supply cost per child.

## Considerations for Establishing Fees and Funding Camp Tuitions

If we had generated a complete list of equipment and supplies for this example (as
you will for the program you are designing), we would be able to closely figure the
cost of the program for each participant. Knowing this exact figure will help us
establish tuition costs for each camper in this program and would also help us
estimate the costs of adding more sessions or more children per session. For
programs such as this, some planners/managers also figure a breakdown of
salary/equipment/overhead charges per client along with supplies in order to arrive
at a per-person cost.

   If the campers require extremely close attention for effective intervention and for
safety (for example, children with behavior disorders or other special problems), then
we might need to hire more staff and perhaps additional time of specialized
professional staff. The cost of higher levels of staff expertise and more personal
attention are generally figured into the client's costs. We might also consider training
volunteers for the program or adding students. Both volunteers and students require
professional time for supervision, and these costs must be included in the financial
mix but are not generally included in the client's costs.

   Funding options for a camp such as the one described in this example include
the following:

1. Private pay (may be considered day care for tax purposes)
2. Regional centers or other avenues of pay already established for the child's
   therapy
3. Donated "scholarships" based on financial need

are unable to acquire enough financing to run the program exactly the way you
want, you can make reductions in a number of areas (such as volume of services,
staff, equipment, and supplies) before start-up and during the first year, while still
meeting your needs/goal(s). As you become a more experienced planner, you will
always have a funding source and a "ballpark" figure for funding in mind. You then
will match each step of the process to the anticipated source and potential amount
for funding.

## Furnishing Your Program

The term **furnishing** refers to the furniture we will need to provide the program that will help our clients/patients/members meet their objectives and the goal, or goals of the program. What will be required to furnish a welcoming environment? Will you require work tables, chairs, lamps, a television, VCR, a DVD player, a radio, a sofa, a bed, and so on? Many of the programs described in this text have operated on little more than the above list. Most have required minimal supplies, and a few have required some equipment; however, equipment for therapeutic purposes has seldom been included. From our examples, you might think that community-based programs are always low-budget, "shoe-string" ventures that seldom, if ever, require expensive furnishings or equipment. However, keep in mind that the furnishings, equipment, and supplies are dictated by your goal or goals, your objectives, and the needs of your target population, not by their placement in the community. While not intended to be therapeutic, a riding garden tiller that would permit several of the community gardeners in our earlier example with physical limitations to be central to the development of new garden space was a fairly high-end expense.

If you are designing a private practice, the way you furnish it will be extremely important to how you market and promote your practice to your selected population. While the primary aim in some of our community examples was a comfortable, inviting, and safe environment, the private practice will certainly provide all of these things and more. A well-appointed reception area and intervention environment, for example, contribute more than comfort to a practice setting. The setting must appeal to the senses of the consumer, and will enhance the quality of the intervention. Think about what you have learned about the multiple "contexts" that influence outcomes of intervention. Consider, also, how much the environment and furnishings contribute to your acceptance of practicing professionals (such as your doctor, dentist, counselor, or therapist), assuming that the quality of services is equal.

## Exercise 7

### How Will You Furnish Your Program?

1. Consider what furnishings you will require to meet the set objectives and goal(s) of your program. Consider the volume of services and the age and differing abilities of your target population (for example, will adaptations be required in furnishings?). List below the furnishings you will need along with costs from your catalogue sources (such as Sears, J.C. Penny, or others of your choice).

| Furnishings | Source | Anticipated Cost |
| --- | --- | --- |
| _____ | _____ | _____ |
| _____ | _____ | _____ |
| _____ | _____ | _____ |

_____     _____     _____

_____     _____     _____

_____     _____     _____

## Equipment

Equipment is categorized in terms of cost and useful life (the length of time the equipment is expected to be in service—usually two years or longer). Although the category of equipment may vary from one agency or institution to another and may be specified by granting/funding sources, for our purposes we will consider any equipment needed to support the programming at a cost of $1,000 or more to be in the category of **capital equipment**. Equipment may be intended exclusively for therapeutic purposes (such as adaptive playground equipment or work hardening equipment), but our garden tiller is also equipment that would fall into this category, even though its intended purpose is not to provide therapy. Standard playground equipment and many kitchen appliances would also be considered as capital equipment (unless the umbrella agency or funding source places such things in the category of *furnishings*, which is something you will determine when you actually do your budget). We consider most equipment to be nonexpendable; that is, we will expect to use it many times and for many clients/patients/members. Of course, eventually the equipment will wear out and will need to be repaired and/or replaced and such replacement costs will be anticipated in our long-range budget planning, as will service contracts for repairs. Any equipment below the cost of $1,000 is considered **noncapital equipment** and is also included in the category of nonexpendable.

## Exercise 8

**Selecting Equipment for Your Program**

1. List below all of the equipment you will need for your program (if you will not need equipment, simply indicate *none*).

_____

_____

_____

_____

_____

_____

2. When you have completed your equipment list, refer to the catalogues and determine the source and the cost of each piece of desired equipment. Note these items below, and place an asterisk beside the equipment that is in excess of $1,000 (capital equipment).

Equipment                 Source                 Anticipated Cost

_____          _____          _____

_____          _____          _____

_____          _____          _____

_____          _____          _____

_____          _____          _____

_____          _____          _____

3. You can now make two lists of equipment—one for capital equipment and one for noncapital equipment.

Capital Equipment                    Noncapital Equipment

_____          _____

_____          _____

_____          _____

_____          _____

_____          _____

_____          _____

In fact, you might not have to purchase all or any of the furnishings or equipment for your program. If the agency is providing a space, it might also provide the loan of furnishings and equipment. In many of our examples, the tables, chairs, computers, and kitchens of the facility/agency were used. However, it is always good to know all of the costs should you wish to recreate the program elsewhere. Some facilities/agencies will also expect that you replace any equipment that is stolen or damaged because of negligence or misuse by you or your clients/members. Although we would expect that this would not occur, knowing the cost sometimes helps programmers to be more aware of security and maintenance.

## Supplies

Now consider **supplies** needed to support the services provided by your program (such as computer software, arts and crafts, paper, pencils, toys, garden seeds, cooking ingredients, and so on). Consider supplies needed per client/patient/member on a daily/weekly basis. Also consider what supplies are **expendable** (such as masking tape or plant fertilizer, which must be replaced when they are used) or **nonexpendable** (such as scissors, gardening forks, or inflatable wading pools, which can be used several times without replacement). If you have used wading pools in your practice, you know that they are a good example of an item that could be considered either expendable or nonexpendable. They are, in fact, listed as a nonexpendable supply item, but if you purchase the cheap ones, they are extremely vulnerable to rips and punctures and might not last the course of one day. Over the long haul, spending a little more for equipment and nonexpendable supplies is very wise. Again, make your lists from what you want, and decide later where you can cut some corners without jeopardizing your goal(s) and the quality of your program.

Assessments/screening instruments also generally are listed under nonexpendable supplies (except for paper forms, of course). These will be considered in Chapter 11 and will be included in the combined supplies selected to support your client/patient/member services in the development of the total budget.

## Exercise 9

### Selecting Supplies for Your Program

1. Consider now what *nonexpendable* supplies you will need to begin your program. To determine the number of items needed, consider the number of clients/patients/members that you will service, the daily or weekly time schedule, and the specific supplies required to provide the program. Consider the following examples:

Six campers serviced daily (=) six pairs of right-handed scissors and (to be prepared) three pairs of left-handed scissors.

Six campers serviced daily (=) two "quality" inflatable wading pools (three children to each pool with no hard edges to encourage safe movement as well as socialization).

Twelve community gardener/members attending daily (=) twelve pairs of gardening gloves.

Twelve community gardener/members attending daily (=) four spading forks, four long-handled hoes, and four short-handled hoes.

Using the above formula to help determine quantity, note below the *nonexpendable* supplies you will need for your program, the source, amount, and anticipated cost (remember that if you have sufficient storage, sometimes it is substantially cheaper to order in bulk even though it may be more than you require at the present time). Write your formulas below.

| Nonexpendable Supplies | Source | Quantity | Anticipated Cost |
|---|---|---|---|
| _____ | _____ | _____ | _____ |
| _____ | _____ | _____ | _____ |
| _____ | _____ | _____ | _____ |
| _____ | _____ | _____ | _____ |

2. Decide now what _expendable_ supplies you will need to start your program and to operate it for one cycle of clients/patients/members. Consider the following examples:

Two four-day weeks (=) eight one-hour arts and crafts sessions (×) six day campers (=) 12 (1.7 fl. oz) nontoxic, nonflammable glue sticks (estimated that gluing would be involved in 1/3 of the arts and crafts activities, assumed one stick would be used per child per week, and anticipated little waste and better product with the glue stick as opposed to a bottle of less expensive glue).

The community garden is supplied with expendables in gardening "cycles" to include planting, maintaining, harvesting, and clearing.

Planting cycle (=) area of garden (×) twelve gardeners/members (=) 72 packets of assorted seeds, twelve spools of row-marking string, 100 row-marker sticks, and five large bags of fertilizer (estimated planting of some individual and some group choices, including annual flowers, herbs, and vegetables for future saleability; assumed that row-marking string and sticks are cheaper in quantity and are easily stored; and assumed that supplies are donated or purchased locally).

Using the examples as guidelines, note your formula below for determining the expendable supplies that you will need.

_____

_____

_____

_____

_____

List below the *expendable* supplies you will need to provide your program for one cycle.

| Expendable Supplies | Source | Quantity | Anticipated Cost |
|---|---|---|---|
| _____ | _____ | _____ | _____ |
| _____ | _____ | _____ | _____ |
| _____ | _____ | _____ | _____ |
| _____ | _____ | _____ | _____ |
| _____ | _____ | _____ | _____ |
| _____ | _____ | _____ | _____ |

## Exercise 10

### Long-Term Budgeting

Most budgets will be based on three-month, six-month, one-year, and three-year cycles. This may be referred to as short-term budgeting (what you require to operate one cycle of your program) and long-term budgeting (what you require for several cycles of your program, usually up to three years). Long-term budgeting requires that you make **cost projections**, including a percentage increase for inflation. For our purposes in this chapter, we are only considering the costs associated with furnishings, equipment, and supplies. We will consider other costs in the chapter to follow.

Consider the equipment noted in the previous exercise. Will any of it require replacement over the course of a three-year period? When we figure the final budget later, we will include **indirect costs** such as the costs of service and maintenance contracts and **overhead** (electricity, telephone, Internet, and so on). For now, however, we are only considering some of our **direct costs**, or those costs for equipment and supplies that will directly support the client/patient/member services.

1. Note below any equipment (capital or noncapital) that you anticipate may need to be replaced during the first three years of your program.

| Replacement of Capital Equipment | Anticipated Cost (consider inflation) |
|---|---|
| _____ | _____ |
| _____ | _____ |
| _____ | _____ |
| _____ | _____ |

| Replacement of Noncapital Equipment | Anticipated Cost (consider inflation) |
| --- | --- |
| _____ | _____ |
| _____ | _____ |
| _____ | _____ |
| _____ | _____ |

2. Now consider your *nonexpendable* supply list. How often will you need to replace these supplies?

For our earlier example, the gardening gloves and the wading pools probably would be the most vulnerable to "short lives." For example, a good pair of gardening gloves with rubber or leather palms would be expected to last the home gardener for perhaps a year or more with proper care. Twelve pairs of such gloves would cost about $30 each, or $360 out of a 12-month budget. It is not likely that all of our gardeners/members will wear out gloves equally, so we could cut some corners and spend $7 for a pair of good (but not the best) gloves and anticipate that they would probably last a year for some of our less enthusiastic gardeners and six months or three months for others. We could then anticipate glove replacement in increments over three months, six months, and a year. In reality, gloves are items that gardening-supply stores might donate, but we want to know what they cost in the event that we must pay for them.

A durable, inflatable wading pool might last through a summer of two-week camper rotations or approximately six eight-day cycles (with each of two pools meeting the needs of three children each and with the combined pools sheltering some 288 small bodies over the course of a summer). Although it is possible that these pools will last all summer, it is likely that at least one will require replacement at a cost of around $42 to $45 during the three-month interval.

Make your calculations and note below what *nonexpendable* supplies you anticipate replacing, how often, and the anticipated (plus inflation) costs.

| Nonexpendable Supplies | Replacement Cycle | Anticipated Costs |
|---|---|---|
| _____ | _____ | _____ |
| _____ | _____ | _____ |
| _____ | _____ | _____ |
| _____ | _____ | _____ |
| _____ | _____ | _____ |
| _____ | _____ | _____ |

3. What will be your replacement cycle for *expendable* supplies? Will you bring in new groups every two weeks like our day camp example? Will your cycle be every month, three months, or six months? Will you have new members/patients/clients cycling through your program all the time? Will your expendable supplies be exhausted in cycles like the community garden example?

For the community garden, the most expensive season of the year was the first one—the planting season. Seventy-two packets of seeds cost from $.50 to $2.10 per packet depending on the quantity of seeds per packet (100–8,000) and how exotic the potential plants were considered to be. The hemp twine for row marking sold for $8.95 per 200-foot ball, and the wooden markers were $5.00 for 100. The program later received a donation of nonexpendable metal row markers that would have cost $22.95 per 50 if purchased and ten flats of live seedlings that would have cost approximately $15.00 per flat.

Although starting up the garden each season appeared to be expensive, for most of the year, costs were substantially reduced. Therefore, the budget for the year was heavily inflluenced by the planting season and was less influenced by the maintenance (fertilizer and mulch) and the harvest and clean-up. The garden was organic so there were no chemical pesticides to purchase; this also enhanced marketing for produce and floral sales; however, the task of maintenance and removing pests required more attention on a daily basis.

Note below your anticipated *expendable* supplies and when you will anticipate replacement along with your projections of cost (consider that inflation will also impact your expendable supplies).

| Expendable Supplies | Replacement Cycle | Anticipated Costs |
|---|---|---|
| _____ | _____ | _____ |
| _____ | _____ | _____ |
| _____ | _____ | _____ |
| _____ | _____ | _____ |
| _____ | _____ | _____ |
| _____ | _____ | _____ |

## *Summary*

First, anticipating space needs by matching them closely to program goal(s) and objectives will place the planner in an excellent position to prepare for the necessary negotiation that will take place in the process of locating, or sometimes being assigned, space for program operations. A detailed analysis of the size and nature of space required for intervention, the plumbing and utilities needed, and considerations for safety and ergonomics place the planner in a good position to review available space with a careful eye toward what negotiations may be made without compromising the goal(s) of the program. Although somewhat different than the space considerations of the planner working in cooperation with an agency/facility, the space needs of those who anticipate initiating a freestanding practice continue to be based on the community and service profiles, the comprehensive assessment of needs, and on-going reviews of trends that might impact the success of the program.

In preparing to initiate a program, you will need to obtain (and likely purchase) a number of items to facilitate the achievement of objectives and, ultimately, the goal(s) of the program. These items fall under the categories of furnishings, capital and noncapital equipment, and expendable and nonexpendable supplies. Furnishings are those things that we would describe in our households as "furniture," including tables, chairs, sofas, lamps, beds, and dressers. They may be considered part of our indirect services in some cases (such as providing a comfortable reception area) and direct services in others (such as tables and chairs for activities or perhaps a bed for activities of daily living practice). In program design and development, many of these items are intended to add comfort and style to the space where we will carry out our intervention rather than to directly support the intervention itself.

Equipment may be intended for therapeutic purposes such as playground equipment designed specifically to facilitate the sensory-integration aspects of a child's development. On the other hand, it may be used to encourage participation such as the riding tiller or tractor for the community garden. In most settings, equipment is categorized by cost. Although the amount may differ depending on the setting, generally those items over $1,000 are considered to be capital equipment, and those under this purchase amount are considered to be noncapital equipment.

Supplies are also categorized but not usually by cost. They may fall into the category of expendable, or those things that are "used up" by participants in the course of their direct-service program. Items that have a longer life, or are not "used up" in the process of intervention, are termed nonexpendable items. All of these items cost the program money, and they are considered to be a substantial part of the budget process—both short-term and long-term. Of course, there are other indirect and direct costs to programming, which will be considered in detail in Chapter 11. In this chapter, we will consider all of the costs to operate our program and, in the chapter to follow, how we will pay these costs.

## Selected Companies That Provide Equipment and Supplies Appropriate for Occupation-Centered Programming

- Attainment Company, Inc.
  P.O. Box 930160
  Verona, WI 53593-0160
  800-327-4269
  *multiple options/supplies for children and adults with special needs

- Best Priced Products, Inc.
  P.O. Box 1174
  White Plains, NY 10602
  800-824-2939
  *rehabilitation supplies and equipment for adults and children

- Childswork/Childsplay
  P.O. Box 1604
  Secaucus, NJ 07096-1604
  800-962-1141
  Email: care@GenesisDirect.com
  *social and emotional needs of children and adolescents

- Communication Skill Builders
  3830 E. Bellevue
  P.O. Box 42050-CS4

Tucson, AZ 85733
602-323-7500
*communication supplies for adults and children

■   Communication/Therapy Skill Builders
(A Division of the Psychological Corporation)
555 Academic Court
San Antonio, TX 78204-9941
800-211-8378
*pediatric and adult assesssment and intervention

■   Dick Blick Art Materials
P.O. Box 1267
Galesburg, IL 61402-1267
800-828-4548
www.dickblick.com
*arts and crafts supplies for the artist and teacher

■   Discount School Supply
Box 60000
San Francisco, CA 94160-3847
800-627-2829
www.DiscountSchoolSupply.com
*arts and craft supplies, manipulatives, toys, books, language/science; social
awareness; active play/dramatic play; furniture for children

■   Eastman
Northwest District Headquarters: Denver
303-576-1000
Southwest District: Phoenix
602-269-3131
*office furniture and products

■   Enrichments (for Better Living)
P.O. Box 579
145 Tower Drive
Hinsdale, IL 60521
800-323-5547
*adult and pediatric rehabilitation supplies and equipment

■   Flaghouse
601 Flaghouse Drive
Hasbrouck Heights, NJ 07604-3116
800-793-7900

www.flaghouse.com
*adult and pediatric rehabilitation supplies and equipment; physical education and recreation supplies and equipment . . . for school, office, institutions, and health care facilities

- Imaginart
  307 Arizona Street
  Bisbee, AZ 85603
  800-828-1376
  Email: imaginart@aol.com
  *therapy supplies for pediatrics, physical rehabilitation, and mental health

- K.Log, Inc.
  P.O. Box 5
  Zion, IL 6009-0005
  800-872-6611
  K-log.com
  *furnishings for offices, classrooms, and multipurpose environments

- Lilypons Water Gardens
  6800 Lilypons Road
  P.O. Box 10
  Buckeystown, MD 21717-0010
  800-723-7667
  www.lilypons.com
  *supplies, equipment, plants for water gardening, fish, snails, and frogs

- NorthCoast Medical, Inc.
  187 Stauffer Blvd.
  San Jose, CA 95125-1042
  800-821-9319
  *adult rehabilitation and fitness supplies; hand therapy supplies

- PCI Educational Publishing
  2800 NE Loop 410 Suite 105
  San Antonio, TX 78218-1525
  800-594-4263
  *supplies for cognitive and emotional independence

- Sammons Preston Rolyan
  P.O. Box 5071
  Bolingbrook, IL 60440-5071

800-323-5547
www.sammonsprestonrolyan.com
*supplies and equipment for adult rehabilitation

■   S & S Opportunities
P.O. Box 513
Colchester, CT 06415-0517
800-937-3482
*adult and pediatric rehabilitation equipment, supplies, and
furniture

■   S & S Healthcare
P.O. Box 513
Colchester, CT 06415-0517
800-243-9232
www.snswwide.com
*arts, crafts, games, and exercise for therapy and rehabilitation

■   Sears Home Health Care
20 Presidential Drive
Roselle, IL 60172
800-326-1750
*adult rehabilitation equipment

■   Shepherd's Garden Seeds
30 Irene Street
Torrington, CT 06790-6658
860-482-3638
www.shepherdseeds.com
*garden seeds—ordinary to the exotic—and gardening supplies

■   Smith and Nephew, Inc
One Quality Drive
P.O. Box 1005
Germantown, WI 53022-8205
800-558-8633
*adult rehabilitation supplies

■   Tandy Leather Crafts
TLC Direct
1400 Everman Parkway
Fort Worth, TX 76140-5089
888-890-1611
www.tandyleather.com
*leathercraft kits, Indian Lore; leather hides and tools for the craftsperson
and hobbyist

- Wellness Reproductions, Inc.
  23945 Mercantile Road, Suite KM
  Beachwood, OH 44122-5924
  800-669-9208
  *supplies and resources for mental health facilitators and educators

- Whole Person Associates
  210 W. Michigan
  Duluth, MN 55802-1908
  800-247-6789
  www.wholeperson.com
  *stress management, wellness-promotion, and emotional self-care
  resources

# References

American Occupational Therapy Association (2003). *Occupational therapy practice framework: Domain and Process*. Bethesda, MD: American Occupational Therapy Association.

Fenton, S., & Gagnon, P. (2003) Work activities. In E. Crepeau, E. Cohn, & B. Schell, (Eds.), *Willard and Spackman's occupational therapy* (pp. 342–346). Philadelphia: Lippincott.

Neville-Jan, A., Fazio, L. S., Kennedy, B., & Snyder, C. (1997). Elementary to middle school transition: Using multicultural play activities to develop life skills. In D. Parham, & L. S. Fazio, (Eds.), *Play in occupational therapy for children* (pp. 144–157). St. Louis, MO: Mosby-Yearbook.

Ryan, J. D., Ray, R., & Hiduke, G. (1999). *Small business: An entrepreneur's plan* (5th ed.). Fort Worth, TX: The Dryden Press.

# CHAPTER 11

# Costs and Projected Funding Needs

## Learning Objectives

1. To recognize the important features of program evaluation and cost determination in maintaining program viability
2. To appreciate the importance of maintaining occupation and quality of life in the outcome measures of programs while managing costs
3. To understand the various cost structures for programs to include those that are for-profit and those that are intended to be not-for-profit
4. To become aware of the multiple considerations when hiring and retaining an employee, to include financial implications
5. To learn to figure costs for your program and anticipate funding needs
6. To become comfortable with the budget terms and descriptions utilized in funding proposals

## Key Terms

1. Budget
2. Budget Line/Budget Narrative/Budget Justification
3. Revenue
4. For Profit/Not for Profit or Non-Profit
5. Fee for Service
6. Indirect Costs/Overhead
7. Direct Costs

8. In-kind
9. Insurance
10. Malpractice/Professional Liability
11. Benefits
12. Hiring/Retention
13. Outsourcing

There are two critical dimensions of the community programming proposal. While they are no more or less important than other aspects of the proposal, when it comes to anticipating long-term success of the program, *carefully determining the cost and evaluating the effectiveness of the program* make the difference in its staying power and its funding. Frequently the programmer least favors developing these two areas, but they are the areas that separate the daydreamer from the true proactive planner.

If we could maintain our excitement and momentum through the processes of budgeting and evaluation-planning, then we would find evidence of many more successful and long-running programs. Sadly, many programming efforts are like sparklers on the 4th of July; on July 5 they have disappeared into the landfill. The idea that will last, on the other hand, is supported by sound money management and careful evaluation of outcomes. How do we deal with our budgetary concerns? What will this program cost? How will it be funded? What does it mean to manage the finances of a program?

Smith (1996) outlined the key categories that an occupational therapy financial manager must be alert to in light of the external environment within which health care organizations function. Her discussions describe the multiple levels of financial accounting and management known to most occupational therapy managers. Focusing largely on service billing, her categories included such tasks as establishing prices and pricing policies and the negotiation of reimbursement contracts with third-party payers and individual payers (Smith, 1996; pp. 63–100). Although Smith's information may be more suited to what we might describe as a clinic or hospital-based, treatment focused practice, her words also ring true for many freestanding practices. Jabri (2003) discusses financial planning and management with an eye for service quality. Focusing on strategic planning to establish a sound financial plan, she alerts the reader to the power of effectively managing a budget in order to manage the service quality of the department, or one's business (Jabri, 2003; p. 147). Smith shares with Jabri considerations of certain aspects of cost accounting such as strategic planning and monitoring productivity and efficiency as critical to all programming, whether it be treatment-based intervention, wellness promotion, or prevention. These considerations apply whether the administrative structure is a for-profit private practice or a not-for-profit program operated under the umbrella of another agency or agencies.

Liebler and McConnell (2004), Jabri, 2003, Thomas (1996), and Logigian (1994) discuss cost management as well as additional roles of the financial manager. Accountability is the key word in financial management, whether it is in health care or the business sector. In terms of accountability in occupation-centered, community-based programs, the linkages between occupation, quality improvement, and program evaluation must be supported and encouraged alongside the present-day concerns for efficiency and cost-effectiveness. We cannot afford to let the current payment systems restrict our creativity, diminish our goals, or compromise our ethics.

Edwards (1997) supports the measurement of quality of life that goes beyond our usual parameters for quality improvement and medical measures of outcome. Certainly meaning and life quality are outcome measures to be pursued in our programming efforts, even in the face of cost reductions and downsizing. Although difficult to accomplish, we should not minimize the need to consistently and accurately define and measure these characteristics of carefully planned and truly occupation-centered programming as we work to anticipate and manage costs.

## Costs and Budgets

Figuring costs, budgeting, and anticipating resources can be a challenge. Some program planners prefer to set lofty goals, plan big, and be prepared to scale back; other planners like to start small and expand their thinking later. Starting with a "big" plan is a way of encouraging excitement and creativity, and in many ways it widens the scope of opportunity. However, the "big" plan is seldom obtainable in the early efforts. As long as the planner is prepared for this and is willing to grow in increments (postponing the larger version for some time later on the three-year time line), planning can progress smoothly. Thus, good management ensures the reality, and for both the conservative and the aggressive approach, a long-range plan is critical.

Regardless of the nature of the intervention, all programs have expenses that must be funded. In previous chapters, you began the process of outlining your programming costs to include furnishings, supplies, equipment, space, and personnel. These items begin to form lines in your budget. In its simplest form, a **budget** is a fiscal plan for a program that includes an itemized list of anticipated income (revenues) and expenses. Karsh and Fox caution us that for a grant funding proposal, the budget must reflect as closely as possible the activities and staffing described in the narrative (Jabri, 2003; p. 289). In other words, the budget must be closely tied to goals, objectives, and programming and it must be specific and accurate. They go on to define a **budget line** as an item (line) in a budget; for example, one occupational therapist at a specified salary, or supplies and equipment (see Figure 11–1 for an example of budget lines).

For most funding applications, a **budget narrative and budget justification** is required (Karsh and Fox, 2003; Smith and Tremore, 2003; Browning, 2001). A **budget narrative** is a verbal description of each line item in the budget, describing how the amount was calculated and how the item relates to the program **(justification)**. For example, in the staff line item: occupational therapist (full time @ $54,000 per year), our narrative justification might be: *A full-time occupational therapist is required to conduct programming and supervise the occupational therapy student program; salary is comparable to what occupational therapists with pediatric and supervisory experience make*

| Line Item | Cost |
|---|---|
| **Staffing** | |
| Occupational Therapist (full-time @ $54,000 per year) | $54,000 |

| Line Item | Cost |
|---|---|
| **Operational Expenses** | |
| Postage | $2,700 |

**FIGURE 11–1**   Examples of Line Item Budgeting

*in this geographical region*. Although the formats may differ, all funding organizations expect to see clearly how the budget costs relate to the activities to be provided.

For our initial learning experience, we will approach the budget process by first drafting a list of all of our anticipated expenses and then making a projection of our needed income from these expenditures. This needed income may come from a number of sources, including **revenues** generated by payment for services, revenues from program-generated products or services, or what we will describe as general funding (comprehensive funds for programming from an agency or foundation). For those who are anticipating initiating a private practice, this list of costs first becomes part of your start-up worksheet and then your business plan.

Before we begin to draft such a cost sheet in the initiation of our budget, however, there are some additional categories of expense that we have not yet considered, including overhead, insurance, and benefits for employees. Whether or not you are responsible for these expenses will depend on what kind of program you are planning. In all of the areas of financial management, our level of responsibilities and specific tasks will fall along a continuum depending on the nature of the program. There are obviously fewer fiscal (money-related) management responsibilities for the planner/manager who works under the umbrella of another agency or agencies than there would be for the planner who is establishing a business/private practice. Of course, someone must assume the responsibilities— and perhaps liabilities—of financial management, but in many cases, it will be someone other than you. Whether you are responsible or not, it is important that you thoroughly understand the process so that you can anticipate what will be required to ensure the financial success of the program.

# The Nature of Your Program

Occupation-centered practitioners may offer their services under many different administrative structures. It is important to distinguish between those kinds of practices we are describing as independent and private versus those programs that are established under the administrative umbrella of another agency or facility. If you are an employee, then the contents of this chapter are generally the concern of your employer (the agency/facility). Of course, you would be expected to maintain a budget for your program and generally provide administrative services, but it is not likely that you would be responsible for funding the collective costs of your program, although you might be expected to write grants and seek to obtain funding.

Although it does not have to be, a private practice is usually **for-profit**; in other words, it expects to have money left over after expenses are paid. These practices are much different from those that are **not-for-profit or non-profit**. Not-for-profit programs intend to pay expenses, but they do not intend to make money. Not-for-profit programs may be eligible for numerous grants and gifts that a for-profit program would not be; this is discussed in more detail in Chapter 12. Although both kinds of programs may charge their patients/clients fees, the intent to make a profit over expenses, or not to, is the difference. Whether a program is for-profit or not-for-profit does not necessarily impact the salaries of employees. In fact, salaries may be higher in not-for-profit programs than those in for-profit programs, and benefits may be better. Many of the programs described in this text, for example, are not-for-profit and do not charge a **fee for service** (that is, the clients/members are not charged for the therapist's services). In fact, many of these programs are supported through grant funding and indirectly through student tuition for *service learning* or *fieldwork*. In these ways, a preceptor can be paid, any needed equipment and supplies can be purchased, and overhead is paid. In some cases, there is some revenue generated (for example, through the sale of garden produce or hand-made craft products); however, these monies are funneled back into the program for the purchase of supplies, or to the members. Sometimes these programs require a trial period—several months or maybe longer—in order for the program staff and participants to establish a firm rapport with the community and to evaluate the effectiveness of the program. A small start-up grant or gift may be appropriate during this "pilot" period of becoming established; however, more funds would likely be available if applied for after the program has been evaluated for effectiveness. Even though a program is not-for-profit, it is important to remember that no program is "free." Someone pays, but how much and in what way can be very convoluted.

If you are a student, just beginning to learn about programming and funding, it is important to remember that everything is accounted for in your program cost sheet and budget, from the needs of your employees to each piece of paper and pencil that you may use to provide your program. Whether you have assured funding before you begin, perhaps from your collaborators/agencies, or you intend to seek it as part of the planning process, nothing will happen unless you know exactly how much money will be required. See Chapter 10 for a sample cost sheet developed for a variation of our earlier day camp example.

# Overhead, Direct Costs, Indirect Costs, and In-kind

**Indirect costs** (often called **overhead**) refer to cost items such as utilities (electric, gas, water, telephone, and Internet access), rent payments, maintenance costs, and sometimes insurance premiums that collectively support your program. If you are starting a private practice, overhead has to be carefully accounted for and usually begins immediately when you obtain space. When you apply for grant funding to support a not-for-profit program, overhead costs generally are grouped and included as a percentage of costs in the amount prescribed by the particular granting agency. You would be able to obtain this information from the granting agency and the prospectus for the specific grant. There may be other expenses to consider associated with licensing, certification, or accreditation, depending on the nature of your services.

**Direct costs** are those expenses for services and products that you need for the program and are not otherwise available at your facility/organization. You may or may not see this term in funding application packages, which is also true for the term indirect costs. The **In-kind** budget line is a term associated with grant funding applications and is where you list any financial contributions that your agency/organization will make available to the grant-funded program. In-kind support or contributions may include such things as staff time, space and utilities, and possibly volunteer hours. You would, then, not include these things in your funding request.

## Reducing Risks: Insurance

For occupation-centered community-based programs, at least three kinds of **insurance** must be considered. The private-practice planner generally will be responsible for all of these. The first is the insurance for your practice or company. Insurance, which is always about managing risk, can protect your practice from loss due to fire, public liability, and crime, among other things. When considering insurance for your company, you must first decide on the type of insurance you will need, and then you must decide on the amount of coverage. As a general rule, do not risk more than you can afford to lose. You should also talk to several insurance agents who are accustomed to offering policies to similar practices.

The second type of insurance is **malpractice** or **professional liability** insurance. Malpractice insurance covers against claims from clients/patients who suffer damages as a result of services you or your employees perform. You may wish to offer employees this insurance coverage as part of their employee **benefit** package, although many companies require that employees provide their own malpractice insurance. Students are already familiar with malpractice or professional liability insurance since all receive this coverage when they enter their occupational therapy clinical program. Some people mistakenly believe that malpractice insurance is only appropriate when you are "learning" to be a practitioner and that when you actually become a practitioner, you no longer require it. However, the reality is that in today's litigious climate, the more you know, the more you acquire responsibilities—and the more malpractice coverage you require!

The third category of insurance is also the responsibility of the private practitioners or those who will be responsible for employees. There are three categories of insurances that help employees manage risk and therefore help employers maintain their businesses. Providing *health insurance* for yourself and for your employees may seem to be a big expense when you are establishing your business plan, but consider how much work might be lost if you do not provide it. You can always offer a better insurance package than your employees could find on their own, and they may choose not to provide their own. In order to keep their employees healthy and to help them balance life at home with life at work, many small businesses offer incentives such as limited child care, exercise programs, and weight management/substance abuse programs. Occupation-centered practitioners who own businesses should be the first to consider these benefits for their employees.

You will also want to include *disability insurance, life insurance,* and *worker's compensation* insurance. If you are the owner of the business, disability insurance is critical, and you may also wish to offer it to employees. Ryan, Ray, and Hiduke (1999) suggest that disability for a business owner is a much greater risk than death. While life insurance may not offer a direct advantage to the owner of a practice, it is a service to the employee and the employee's family, and it is generally not as costly as the other insurances. Worker's compensation protects employees if they are injured while on the job. As mentioned previously, occupational therapy practitioners must be aware of ergonomics and should ensure that the workplace does not provide risks to the safety and well-being of employees.

## The Potential Costs of Employees

There are several questions that come to mind when we hire employees to assist with our program. In Chapter 9 we discussed the various roles of the professional and nonprofessional staff you might wish to hire to support the services of your program. We also discussed how to develop a job description and an advertisement to initiate the employee search. This was the easy part. The **hiring** and **retention** of employees make up a large part of your anticipated labor and budget. We have already discussed the insurances and other benefits you may wish to provide, but there are additional considerations that will impact your finances as an owner of a practice.

First you must decide when you will hire your employees. Will you hire them before your first client or concurrently? If they are hired concurrently with the arrival of clients, how will the preparation and final planning be accomplished? Will you do it? Perhaps you can hire some temporary or part-time employees. In this case, you are able to delay paying benefits during the preparation phase. Although the percentages vary, many employers provide certain benefits only to employees who work more than 80% of a full-time work schedule. However, consider that you might require a high level of professional experience and expertise to assist with the final preparations—perhaps expertise that you do not have. In this case, you will want to offer all of the potential options you can to attract the person you need. If you are starting a for-profit practice, you may wish to offer this first employee stock options or profit sharing as an incentive to help with the final preparations. Hiring and then keeping (retaining) good employees is the key to a successful private practice. All of these questions must be considered before you run your ad. In addition, you must budget the cost of placing employment advertisements and any costs that may be incurred for recruitment. Not only is this true in the beginning, but it must be anticipated as the program begins to grow. Of course, salary must be considered, as well as employment taxes (social security, unemployment, and Medicare) and additional benefits such as retirement, vacation, sick leave, and family leave.

The best way to determine professional salaries is to talk to other managers in your area to obtain a range for the kinds of services you wish to provide. This is another reason to network and to belong to your professional organizations. The professional organizations may also be able to provide you with salary ranges, but will not likely be as current as your colleagues. For other staff, you can find salary comparison data on the Internet at http://recruitmentextra.com/salarysurveys.html and at www.wageweb.com. When you have decided exactly what kind of employees you want and when you wish to hire them, it is time to place the advertisement and to begin the screening and interview process.

## Pre-Employee Screening, Interviews, and Hiring: Maintaining Compliance

As with many of the planning tasks we have discussed, this is yet another area where you may have differing levels of responsibility depending on whether you are starting your own practice or assisting the company you work for in the employee hiring process. Screening may include a number of measures to verify that your potential employee has provided you with truthful information. A careful review of the resume initiates the process, which is followed by contacting references and verifying state and national certifications and licenses. The next steps can include pre-employment medical examinations, finger printing, and perhaps drug screenings. One or more in-person interviews are employed, and in addition to standard interview questions, role-playing of intervention scenarios particular to your program might be appropriate.

If hiring is your responsibility, you should review legal and illegal pre-employment inquiries before you schedule an interview. You can obtain these from http://www.nolo.com. Also contact the civil rights office for your state and the Department of Industrial Relations for guidelines they may provide. Refer to the list at the close of this chapter for other sources that may be helpful.

When you have completed the interview process and are prepared to make an offer, you should check to see that your new employee can legally work in the United States and have that person complete an Employment and Eligibility Verification Form (I-9); you must also be familiar with the requirements for complying with the Americans with Disabilities Act (ADA). As occupational therapy practitioners you should be familiar with the *ADA Title I: Employment provision* and may, in fact, have encountered it in the workplace. As an employer, your responsibilities are even greater. Refer to the ADA and also to Regulations to Implement the Equal Employment Provisions of the Americans with Disabilities Act. Since the *9–11* incident threatening national security, and the resulting *Homeland Security Act*, foreign trained therapists are more stringently monitored. Contact the NBCOT website for updates if considering the services of a foreign trained therapist.

As the owner of a practice, you must also be compliant with all labor laws and all tax laws with regard to employees. It is recommended that you become familiar with the U.S. Department of Labor Statutes, the Fair Labor Standards Act, the Immigration and Nationality Act, the Occupational Safety and Health Act (OSHA), and the Employee Retirement Income Security Act (ERISA). (See the references at the close of this chapter for more information.)

If you find it necessary to dismiss an employee, it may be equally problematic. Consider the above resources should firing become necessary, and spell out all procedures at the first day of hire in an employee handbook or manual.

## Employee Records

If you are the owner or soon-to-be owner of a practice, you must maintain records for all employees. These include all of the basic information (such as name, address, social security number, and so on) as well as the original application and the results of any pre-hire inquiries. As the employee continues with your company, you add performance reviews, continuing education, and notations of any disciplinary action. Your state Fair Employment Office can provide you with additional information for what must be maintained in an employee's file and for how long. Human resource files are considered legal documents and may be requested in any malpractice suit or other legal action, so it is best to be proactive by being sure that they are complete. For non-profits, employee files, including updated resumes, will make the process of grant application and reporting more efficient.

## Summing Up Costs

Now that we have considered expenses related to employees, we have covered the standard cost items. As you think of other items that are indirectly or directly related to client/patient services, remember to consider all associated costs. For instance, perhaps you anticipate the need to lease a van for transportation. Remember that if you transport clients/patients, you will need additional insurance coverage and an appropriate driver's license. An occasional trip might be accommodated less expensively by hiring outside vans or buses (**outsourcing** transportation).

Once you have listed your start-up costs and the costs for one cycle of your program, you can project these for extended periods of time. These extensions of time, from one year up to three or five years, will include areas where you wish to grow (such as more or different staff, perhaps more space, or additional equipment).

The next chapter is intended to provide you with some direction for how your services might be paid for or how to seek funding. It is not intended to provide you with specific directions for who and how to bill for services or exact resources where you might find loans for a private practice or a grant to initiate a program, but enough information is provided to guide you to the specific information and resources that you will need to make these decisions. If you are a student, you will have (or have had) coursework complementary to this text. This coursework will guide you in the specifics of such management responsibilities as determining costs for services, anticipating and projecting revenue, developing an actual bill, and determining how to interface your interventions with appropriate payment services.

## Exercise 1

**What Kind of Program Do You Have?**

1. Discuss with your classmates, colleagues, or partners whether your program is free-standing or is under the management umbrella of another agency or agencies. Is your program intended to be for-profit, not-for-profit, or a service-learning component of an academic program or community agency?

To help you define your responsibilities, you must decide if you will be the planner and manager of a program as an employee of an agency or institution or if you will be owner and manager.

Note below what kind of program you have and why you believe this to be the case.

_____

_____

_____

_____

2. With regard to the characteristics of your program as noted above, write below what your responsibilities will likely be with regard to selection, hiring, and retention of employees; purchase and maintenance of furnishings, equipment, and supplies; the marketing of the program; and management of the budget.

Selection, hiring, and retention of employees.

_____

_____

_____

Purchase and maintenance of furnishings, equipment, and supplies.

_____

_____

_____

_____

Marketing of the program (to the community and potential consumers).

_____

_____

_____

_____

Managing the budget for the program.

_____

_____

_____

_____

## Exercise 2

### Developing a Cost Sheet for Start-Up, One Year, and Three Years of the Program

You have already accomplished a large part of the task of developing a cost sheet in the exercises you completed for Chapter 9 and Chapter 10. When you have completed Chapter 12, you will have all of the projected costs for the program. You may wish to revisit Chapter 10 for a cost sheet example.

Return to your lists of furnishings, equipment, and supplies and your staffing requirements. Using the structure provided by the example, define your costs in the following exercises.

### Start-Up, One-Month, and Yearly Costs

Our first consideration will be the professional and nonprofessional staff that you will require to run the day-to-day programming. Revisit the discussion in Chapter 9. To first determine your staffing needs, you must consider the needs and availability of the service population, the physical space where the program will be offered, the nature of the services you expect to provide, and the configuration of service delivery. Because professional staff can be expensive, you should also begin to give some attention to your anticipated budget and your potential funding, although you must first consider your program goal and the needs of your target population. You must be able to justify your costs; however, it is always important that you do not jeopardize the quality of your program by seeking to reduce costs too soon.

1.  Consider your costs for staffing (including the cost of advertising, salary, and benefits for full-time employees). For company-paid benefits, you can estimate approximately 20 percent of the salary figure, but realize that this can vary substantially.

Staff Position          % of time          Monthly/Yearly Gross Salary          Benefits

_____

_____

_____

_____

Total cost of staff salaries and benefits.

For one month _____ For one year _____

Total costs of start-up hiring _____

Total staff associated costs (advertising positions, salaries, and estimated benefits):

_____

2.  Return to the exercises in Chapter 10 for your estimated cost lists for furnishings, equipment, and supplies. Finalize all estimated costs (including shipping) for start-up and for one cycle of your program (for example, one month, three months, and so on); note below your total costs for each of these categories

Total cost of capital equipment for start-up _____

Total cost of noncapital equipment for start-up _____

Note any replacement of equipment that may be required over a three-year period and anticipated cost.

_____

_____

_____

Total cost of furnishings for start-up _____

Note any replacement of furnishings that may be required over a three-year period and anticipated cost.

_____

_____

_____

Total cost of nonexpendable supplies for start-up _____

(Remember to include any assessment materials here or in the question that follows.) Note any replacement of nonexpendable supplies and the estimated cost (what are the anticipated cycles for replacement—six months? one year? more?).

_____

_____

_____

Total cost of expendable supplies for one programming cycle _____

What is the anticipated cycle for replacement of supplies? _____

What is the resulting 3-month, 6-month, and/or yearly total costs of supplies

_____

3. Note below your estimated overhead for one month and for one year (carefully consider how you will operate your program, seasonal changes, anticipated fluctuations in service volume, and how this may impact overhead) Utilities (gas, electric, water, trash disposal, other).

Monthly Estimate                              Yearly Estimate

_____

_____

_____

Other overhead costs you may anticipate (such as equipment maintenance contracts, security, transportation, and so on).

_____

_____

_____

Total estimates of overhead for          One month _____

                                        One year _____

4. A detailed marketing plan will be developed in Chapter 13, and you will wish to return to this exercise to record specific costs. For now provide a rough estimate of what you may wish to spend for such things as brochures, business cards, telephone "yellow page" ads, and so on. You can finalize the costs later. Record your estimates below.

Marketing Methods                Cost for Start-Up          Yearly Cost

_____

_____

_____

_____

_____

5. Carefully review your developing program proposal for any anticipated costs that you may have forgotten to include. If you find additional costs, record them in the appropriate categories.

6. Add all of the above totals to determine an estimated figure of operating costs for your program for one year and for three years.

Total operating costs for one year:

_____

Total operating costs for three years (remember that this figure will reflect inflation and will not necessarily include all of the categories in your start-up and one-year costs).

_____

## Summary

The strength of your program evaluation plan and the accuracy of your cost sheet are critical to the funding success of your program. Through this process of planning program evaluation and anticipating costs and later, funding, you must maintain the importance of occupation and the more qualitative aspects of meaning in your program design and plan. In the potentially restrictive environments of today's health care, it is important to not lose sight of the goal and purpose of your program.

This chapter has proposed numerous resources for you to explore as you develop your budget and your financial plan. You have completed a brief review of your plan, and you have decided exactly what you hope to accomplish and how you aim to do it. Your careful analysis of what will be needed to operate your program in previous chapter exercises has now resulted in the combined estimated costs of your program. In the chapter to follow you will choose the direction you wish to go and identify your proposed funding source(s).

## *References*

Browning, B. (2001). *Grant Writing for Dummies.* New York, NY: Wiley Publishing, Inc.

Edwards, D. (1997). The effect of occupational therapy on function and well-being. In C. Christiansen, & C. Baum, (Eds.), *Occupational Therapy enabling function and well-being* (pp. 557–572). Thorofare, NJ: Slack.

Jabri, J. (2003). Financial Planning and Management. In G. McCormack, E. Jaffe, & M. Goodman-Lavey, (Eds.), *The Occupational Therapy Manager* (pp. 147–176). Bethesda, MD: AOTA.

Karsh, E., & Fox, A. (2003). *The only grant-writing book you'll ever need.* New York: Carroll and Graf Publishers.

Liebler, J., & McConnell, C. (2004). *Management principles for health professionals* (pp. 293–326). Sudbury, MA: Jones and Bartlett.

Logigian, M. (1994). Cost management. In K. Jacobs, & M. Logigian, (Eds.), *Functions of a manager in occupational therapy* (pp. 99–121). Thorofare, NJ: Slack.

Smith, N. (1996). Financial management. In M. Johnson, (Ed.), *The occupational therapy manager* (pp. 63–100). Bethesda, MD: American Occupational Therapy Association.

Smith, N., & Tremore, J. (2003). *The Everything Grant Writing Book.* Avon, MA: Adams Media.

Thomas, V. (1996). Evolving healthcare systems: Payment for occupational therapy services. In M. Johnson, (Ed.), *The occupational therapy manager* (pp. 577–602). Bethesda, MD: American Occupational Therapy Association.

## Recommended Readings

American Occupational Therapy Association, Inc. (1996). *Managed care: An occupational therapy sourcebook.* Bethesda, MD: Author.

Jackson, L. (1998). Idea 97. *O.T. Practice.* Bethesda, MD: American Occupational
    Therapy Association.
Kannenberg, K., Fine, S., & Lang, S. (1996). Reimbursement guidelines. In
    M. Brinson, & K. Kannenberg, (Eds.), *Mental health service delivery guidelines*
    (pp. 63–74). Bethesda, MD: American Occupational Therapy Association.
Occupational Therapy Association of California. (1999). *Branching out: Private
    practice and beyond.* Sacramento, CA: Author.
Regulations to implement the equal employment provisions of the Americans
    with Disabilities Act (1998). 29 CFR 1630.2(5). Washington, DC: U.S.
    Government Printing Office.

## Internet Sources

Legal and Illegal Pre-Employment Inquiries: http://www.nolo.com
National Association of Women Business Owners (NAWBO): www.nfwbo.org
General Business Salary Comparisons:
Recruitment Extra!: http://recruitmentextra.com/salarysurveys.html
    Wage Web: www.wageweb.com
Occupational Safety and Health Administration (OSHA): www.osha.gov
Equal Employment Opportunity Commission (EEOC) (202-663-4900):
    www.eeoc.gov/smallbus.html
Department of Labor: www.dol.gov
Internal Revenue Service (IRS): www.irs.gov
U.S.Department of Justice, Americans with Disabilities (800-514-0301;
    202-514-0301): www.usdoj.gov/crt/ada
Immigration and Naturalization Service:
    www.ins.usdoj.gov/employer/index.html
The American Occupational Therapy Association (FAX-on-request) 800-701-7735
The National Board for Certification of Occupational Therapy (NBCOT):
    http://www.nbcot.org

# CHAPTER 12.

# Funding Your Program

## Learning Objectives

1. To investigate the multiple ways to fund community practices
2. To explore the nature of ones' practice appropriate to funding sources
3. To learn the vocabulary of "funding"
4. To understand the process of grant preparation and application
5. To distinguish the structure and function of the various funding agencies

## Key Terms

1. Public and Private Funding Sources
2. Private Payer/Pay Out-Of-Pocket
3. Gift Tuitions/Matched Funding
4. Collection Agency
5. Cash Flow
6. Sliding Scale
7. Proposal
8. Grant
9. 501(c)(3)/Determination Letter
10. RAG, RFP, RFA
11. Foundation
12. LOI (Letter of Inquiry/Letter of Intent)
13. Cover Letter/Abstract/Executive Summary
14. Capital
15. Business Plan

# What Kinds of Funding Are Appropriate for Community-Based Programs, and What Kinds of Funding Are Appropriate for "My" Program?

In order for you to answer this question you must first consider who you are, as a service entity, and just what it is that you want to do. This was where we started the program development process. What is the *problem* that you (and/or your organization) want to solve, what do you need to do to *solve* it, and what will it *cost?* Cost may be one of the last things considered; but in this chapter, it's the *motivator*. Answers to these questions and others as you develop your proposal will help you determine what kind of funding you'll need to operate your program, and what preparation you'll need to make to find and obtain that funding.

As noted in the previous chapter, and depending on the services you wish to provide, you may rely on private and public insurers for individual clients and patients. You may also look toward federal legislation for persons with disabilities, both adults and children. Occupational therapy practitioners must remain abreast of past and current legislation that will benefit their particular clients. There is federal funding for programs that are designed to help disabled persons successfully integrate into the community through education, vocational training, social skills, medical services, and independent living skills. Reed (1992) provides a classic historical account of federal legislation beginning with World War I and encourages all practitioners to be alert to legislation (past, present and future) that will benefit his or her clients. It is also necessary that practitioners advocate for client/patient access to present legislation through knowledge of public laws, as well as assume advocacy roles for needed future legislation.

Most of the programs described in this text are designed to promote health and well-being and prevent illness or injury for the individual and/or for the larger community. Programming of this nature requires the occupational therapy practitioner to constantly explore and expand differing and varied funding sources. In a 1998 special issue of *The American Journal of Occupational Therapy* devoted to community health, Brownson (1998) noted that we are looking at health from an ecological perspective and health care as a continuum from health promotion to tertiary prevention . . . expansion of occupational therapy roles in this way will require the exploration of new and different sources of funding (Brownson, 1998; p. 64).

As you ask yourself the above questions you may determine that you will require grant funding of some kind; but discovering the need for grant funding is not enough. "The most successful programs are mission driven, not grant driven" (Karsh and Fox, 2003; p. 13). According to these authors, you don't develop your program simply to obtain funding; but, if you need funding you'll likely find a granting organization interested in your program.

# Potential Funding Sources

## Public and Private Funding Sources

At the close of the previous chapter, and this one, you will find a number of resources that can help you make your way through the potentially confusing maze of anticipating and covering your costs. While these resources describe structurally sound systems, specifics are usually a bit behind what is actually happening in the rapidly changing world of today's health care. Always seek out the most current information.

What might be described as **public funding** for occupational therapy services includes both insurance and grant-based programs. Federal and state insurance programs such as Medicare, Medicaid, and worker's compensation require constant attention to updated policies and procedures. Membership in your professional organizations can greatly facilitate this process, such as the American Occupational Therapy Associations' *One-Minute-Update* and other electronic venues for maintaining currency. Examples of grant-based public funding programs include the Individuals with Disabilities Education Act (1990) and the Older Americans Act (1965). We also must remain attentive to the policies of **private funding** sources; insurance benefit programs such as Blue Cross/Blue Shield, managed care organizations, and other commercial insurers. If you plan to bill Medicare or private insurances as an independent practitioner, it is recommended that you work as an employee within a system that receives some of their compensation from these agencies before you try it on your own; or perhaps hire a consultant early on to assist with the provider applications and advanced preparation. Once you understand the systems and know the correct coding for billing required by the particular carrier or agency to facilitate payment, you can likely do it on your own. You can also access the Web sites of your particular carriers for the latest updates. The American Occupational Therapy Association's *Fax-on-Demand* provides updates regarding the latest summaries of frequently utilized CPT codes and Medicare fee schedules (the AOTA web-site and *Fax-on-Demand* number is listed at the close of this chapter).

Even though substantial preparation is required to receive payment for services through public and private insurances, many occupational therapy practitioners who engage in community programming wish to fit their services into the more conventional payment models just described. However, there are many ways to access funding options. Being responsive to trends will also assist the programmer in utilizing the appropriate language and descriptions to better position him or herself for funding. The clinical psychologist Vega (1998) provides one example when he describes a developing trend in the middle 1990's toward interest in behavioral disease management, which is also an area of interest to occupation-centered practitioners. He encourages psychology practitioners who wish to engage in this kind of programming to go directly to local hospitals with their well-developed educational programs targeting the facility's wellness programs and cardiac units. There is a message for occupation-centered practitioners here as well, for we also promote education/skills-based wellness programming. Vega (1998) goes on to propose that disease management, whether somatic or behavioral, will target those diseases that have high cost, high frequency, and high chronicity. As a nation we remain concerned about cancer, diabetes, heart disease, asthma, and obesity. Cost savings for purchasers of insurance coverage is the key to the future. Avoiding stress injuries in the workplace through the practice of ergonomics is a current example, responsive to trend, and is rich with opportunity for occupational therapy practitioners; as is multi-contextual programming promoting safety for all ages. Building on Vega's suggestions (1998, p. 3) consider the following strategies:

1. Managing a population via capitated or subcapitated contracts;
2. Be flexible in the way you offer programming; be able to *match* the need;
3. Propose what you think (*know*) you can do, based on what you've done (*programming effectiveness, yours or that of others before you . . . published evidence*);
4. Be willing to *partner, collaborate* and work as part of a team (*author's emphasis*).

If these ideas match your interests as an occupation-centered program planner, you can tailor the development of your proposal(s) toward these ends. Although licensure laws attempt to, and do for some payment systems, "carve out" territories for practitioners, few of the caregiving professions really "own" anything today. The market share goes to those who have the skills and information to do the job cost-effectively and to those who demonstrate that they can do what they claim. None of the health/wellness-oriented professions have a secure foothold in today's market and they all are searching for opportunities.

## Private Payers

If you anticipate operating a practice as a for-profit business, the first professional relationships you must establish are with an attorney and/or a tax advisor. The next and most lasting relationship is with an accountant/bookkeeper. You will likely need help in setting up monthly profit and loss statements and certainly to keep track of accounts payable and receivable. There are computer software programs (such as *QuickBooks*) to help you if you decide to handle your own finances, which you may want to consider, at least in the early stages before your business grows. How will you know whether you can make it on your own? Consider the size of your start-up practice, and look at how you manage your personal finances; these two things will help you make the choice of whether to try to manage the "business" side of your practice or to hire someone to assist you. Remember, as well, that "on your own" doesn't necessarily mean alone; working with partners, establishing collaborations, utilizing personal resources are the keys to successful programs and practices.

This brings us to another form of payment for services in which the client/patient, or **private payer**, pays **"out-of-pocket."** In many of the developing community-based practices, it is not uncommon that clients/patients/parents pay directly for the services that are provided. Many parents are accustomed to paying for special classes, music lessons, sports, and camp fees; paying for occupation-centered intervention for their children is seen as being of little difference. Older clients are accustomed to paying for classes, sports club memberships, and prevention programs (such as *Weight Watchers*). Many occupation-centered wellness and prevention programs are similar in structure. Oftentimes, such as in a camp program, there may be many forms of payment, including private pay for those who can, donation-based **gift tuitions** for those who cannot, and public and private funding for those who are eligible. Donated "gift tuitions" or "scholarships" for children who can not afford a camp fee may be obtained from local Fire Departments, Police Departments, or other community service providers and businesses. Seeking such funding from professional sports organizations and larger companies is also a good idea. Some organizations/businesses will provide **matched funding** for programs. For every dollar (or tuition/programming fee) that you raise through small funding activities such as bake sales, garage sales, car washes, etc., they will match with a like donation/gift of their own. Remember that the tax advantage for these organizations or individuals is to restrict their "gifts" to not-for-profit organizations.

If you anticipate receiving out-of-pocket payment for services you may require the assistance of a **collection agency**. For a fee, these agencies will help you retrieve payment from clients who are past due in their accounts. For a specified time, your bookkeeper will follow those who are delinquent (usually 30 days), then the bill is turned over to a collection agency. Sometimes insurance companies take a period of time to pay for a service, but usually you can anticipate receiving payment; that may not be the case with private payers. Depending on the volume of services you offer, this could present a substantial problem for your **cash flow**. Cash flow is the actual money you have on hand to operate your business. Remember that you can be turning a profit in a private practice but still have no money on hand—perhaps another reason to hire an accountant. For programs/businesses that rely on out-of-pocket payment, it is strongly recommended that a receptionist (not the therapist) collect the fee from the client before intervention. Although there is an associated cost, making the arrangements to accept credit card payments will facilitate the payment process; however, it also means that a client may have to be turned away. Most therapists are reluctant to refuse treatment, particularly for children, so a **sliding scale** fee structure may help. This means that fees are set based on the income and ability to pay of the client/parent. The top of the fee scale is for those who can pay more, with adjusted increments for those with fewer resources. Remember, though, that for a private practice there is always a "bottom-line;" an amount of revenue that you must generate to keep your business solvent and, ultimately, profitable.

## Public and Private *Grant* Funding

According to Karsh and Fox (2003, p. ix), seasoned grant writers, "Grant writing is one of those seemingly benign terms that tap into about every neurosis imaginable." Can I get *one*? Do I know enough? If I get *one*, what will I do with it? And, by the way, as Karsh and Fox (2003), and others remind us, we don't "write grants," we write **proposals** in order to *win* **grants** (Karsh and Fox, 2003; Smith and Tremore, 2003; Brown and Brown, 2001). This is exactly what you're doing if you've followed the process in this text; you are creating a proposal. In order to seek grant funding, some tweaking and perhaps additional development will be necessary, but you will have done some work in all of the areas of program design that a granting/funding agency is interested in.

Perhaps a few additional cautions are required. Although writing grant proposals is the primary fund-raising tool for organizations that provide essential services to a community, the process is extremely competitive. People use the phrase "to win a grant" because that's how it works. Not everyone "wins." Regardless of the granting agency, however, to even be in the competition, you must have a proposal of extremely high-quality. The elements of a proposal are basically the same no matter who the grant-maker is or how much money the grant provides. The proposal will convince the grant-maker of your capacity to identify, and then implement and sustain a quality program. Most experienced grant-writers would agree that submitting a poorly thought out, poorly developed, poorly written proposal is sometimes the most damaging thing you can do to your long-term prospects. The message is, if you're not ready, don't submit a proposal. Smith and Tremore (2003) emphasize the need for "good writing." They offer some general hints: 1) use everyday language; 2) avoid jargon; 3) be politically correct; 4) avoid sexist language; 5) explain acronyms and terms; 6) use strong, active verbs; and 7) speak with authority. Whatever you do, don't adopt the tone that "we can only do this . . . *if* you give us the money." If the work is important you'll figure out a way to do it (Smith and Tremore 2003; pp. 185–191). You're giving the agency the *opportunity* to fund your program; you're not begging.

Who am I? What do I want to do? This question was asked earlier in this chapter and the answers are of particular importance now that we're considering applying for grant funding. Knowing who you are and what you want to do determines where you go for your money. Organizations who seek funding fall into three or four general categories. According to Karsh and Fox (2003), these are: 1) grassroots organizations; 2) social service agencies and other service providers; 3) advocacy groups; and 4) individuals. Grassroots organizations may range from neighborhood-improvement groups (managing graffiti) to obtaining uniforms for the little-league baseball team. Advocacy groups are interested in specific issues such as funding for special schools, or trying to raise awareness for various sociopolitical forums such as rights for individuals with disability (two of many examples). Individuals may seek grants to fund their projects. Artists, writers, film-makers, and scholars make up this group. Of primary importance to most of us, as occupation-centered practitioners, is the second category of organizations, that of social service agencies and other service providers.

## Social Service Agencies and Other Service Providers

These organizations are either not-for-profit (also called nonprofit) organizations or local government agencies set up to address the needs of groups of people of all ages and types: children's day care, after-school programs, violence prevention, pregnancy and substance-use prevention for teenagers, immigration counseling, domestic-violence prevention for families, health, sanitation and perhaps housing needs of a community, and many other similar examples (Karsh and Fox, 2003; Barbato and Furlich, 2000). It is likely that your developing proposal targets one of the above populations. Not-for-profit social-service organizations may operate one small program; perhaps providing services for a small group of children; larger nonprofits and government agencies may run large numbers of programs for all ages and needs. Funding needs may run from a few hundred dollars to a few million and funding sources may include individual donors, private foundations, corporations, and government funding agencies.

If service providers are nonprofit, as opposed to government agencies, they are usually incorporated under state laws and receive tax-exempt status from the Internal Revenue Service. The term **501(c)(3)** refers to the section of the Internal Revenue Code that authorizes this type of organization, or the term **determination letter**, indicating the document from the IRS stating that your organization is tax exempt. Karsh and Fox (2003) describe the process of using state incorporation papers or an IRS determination letter to prove you're a not-for-profit, because most foundations and government funders only give to such organizations (Karsh and Fox, 2003; p. 6). The term not-for-profit as opposed to nonprofit is the technical term in the law and recognizes that the *purpose* of an organization is "not for profit" and that, although the organization could show a budget surplus, it is not likely. As an aside, if you are a "for-profit" practice and show a deficit, it doesn't automatically make you a "not-for-profit" organization.

Contributions to 501(c)(3)s are tax deductible, so individual donors as well as foundations and government entities are more inclined to fund this type of organization. If you are not already working under the umbrella of a not-for-profit agency (and you need to know this) then the process will involve a lawyer and substantial paperwork to form the nonprofit corporation. In some communities, a private attorney may provide this service at low cost or for free, "pro bono." It will take several months to prepare the paperwork and to wait for the IRS to review the documentation. Allow sufficient time on your *time-line* before you prepare to seek funding.

Even though you receive a nonprofit status, it may take time to win grant funding. Although some foundations are interested in brand-new organizations, most funding agencies expect to see a significant track record of service with some funding, a committed board of directors, sound fiscal health, good leadership, a clear vision/mission, the proven capacity to implement programs, and the ability to sustain projects, activities, staff, and programs (Barbato and Furlich, 2000; Brown and Brown, 2001; Knowles, 2002; Karsh and Fox, 2003). In most cases, a substantial amount of work has to be done before you seek a grant.

## The Funders, Who Are They?

The federal government gives grants. State and local governments give grant-like funding in the form of contracts. Private foundations, corporations, and individuals (through a fund or trust) give grants. In some parts of the country, a regional association of grant-makers (**RAG**) may publish a standard or common application form that grant seekers can use for all participating foundations in that area. Some RAGs also publish a common report form.

Government grants are generally announced through *requests for proposals* (**RFPs**). These may also be called *requests for applications*, or **RFAs**. These communications tell the applicant the nature and cost of the program that must be proposed. They include guidelines, due dates, and other information. For examples of RFPs you might wish to view the Foundation Center's weekly *RFP Bulletin*. The *Bulletin* is a free e-mail subscription, arriving weekly and containing over a dozen weekly grant announcements with links to the relevant Web sites. The Web sites contain guidelines, application forms, and other announcements. Brown and Brown (2001, pp. 77–93) provides substantial information about funders, generating leads, foundation resources, guides to funding periodicals and funding opportunities on the internet.

## Foundations

**Foundations** range in size from very small family foundations (grant decisions made by family members) and small budgets under $100,000 to enormous organizations that have many staff members and give away millions of dollars each year. Examples of such large foundations are: Robert Wood Johnson Foundation, the Carnegie Corporation, the Kellogg Foundation, the Kresge Foundation, and the Ford Foundation. Large foundations publish requirements that are as specific as the RFP for government grants but smaller foundations are far less prescriptive.

In general, *family foundations* have specific and narrowly focused giving patterns based on the intentions of the donor or the interests of current family members who are the officers or trustees. *Independent private foundations* will usually have at least a small professional staff, and often began as family foundations but are no longer controlled by the original donor or the donor's family. Even though there may be a separation from the origin of the foundation, Karsh and Fox (2003, p. 16) tell us that private foundations remain ethically, and in most cases, legally bound to follow the donor's intent. If the original endowment or bequest said the money was to be used for the protection of Siamese cats or the training of potential opera singers (female, age 9–15), then that's what it's used for. In most cases, though, the parameters are broader; for example "health services for children of poverty-level families."

United Way is an example of a *federated fund*. Federated funds were created to benefit the community by pooling donations from individuals and businesses and using those funds to support nonprofit organizations. Unlike most other foundations, federated funds devote a large portion of their resources to ongoing fundraising efforts.

*Corporate foundations*, or *company sponsored foundations* are independent foundations created by large corporations with funds from the business itself. In most cases the foundation functions like other foundations, receiving proposals and making grants, but giving may be tied to the corporation's own goals.

*Community foundations*, or *community trusts* occupy a place in every state and Puerto Rico; usually there are several of these local foundations. Karsh and Fox (2003, Appendix V) provide an extensive list by state. Three random examples are: Cesar E. Chavez Community Development Fund in Keene, California; the New York Community Trust at Two Park Avenue, NY; and Community Foundation of the Texas Hill Country, Kerrville, TX. Community foundations have been set up to administer individual trust funds or pools of funds from individual donors who don't want to create a new foundation but do want to benefit their community in some way. To determine if there is a community foundation in your area, go to your local library (perhaps even your phone book), or go to a listing at the Foundation Center's Web site (see Web site addresses at end of chapter).

*Financial institutions* have always administered charitable trusts set up according to a donor's instructions. Proposals to a trust held by a financial institution are much the same as proposals to other foundations.

## How Do You Find Foundations?

The *Foundation Center* is a national organization that provides support to foundations and information to the potential grant seeker. There are Foundation Center Libraries in five cities across the United States: New York, Atlanta, Cleveland, Washington, DC, and San Francisco. In many other locations, a public library or nonprofit organization is designated as a Foundation Center Cooperating Collection. (See Web site address at the end of the chapter for more information.)

*The Foundation Directory* is perhaps the most important resource for potential grant seekers, but there are many other directories that describe foundations and corporations by location, program interests, size of grants given, and many other characteristics. *The Foundation Directory* reports on foundations with assets in excess of $2 million or annual giving of at least $200,000. Other versions of the Directory provide information for those private and community foundations in the United States holding assets from $1 million to $2 million or with annual granting programs from $50,000 to $200,000. A companion document, *Guide to U.S. Foundations, Their Trustees, Officers, and Donors*, provides brief data on foundations with assets below $1 million and giving programs of less than $50,000 annually. The Foundation Center Libraries also maintain foundation annual reports. The foundation annual reports will provide helpful clues to the kinds of activities the foundation prefers to fund, the dollar amounts offered, and other characteristics of eligibility. *The Foundation Directory Online* can be subscribed to, but first check your library; they may already subscribe.

Before submitting a proposal to a foundation, you would be wise to call or write (or access their Web site) for their annual report, grant application form or guidelines (some may not offer guidelines), descriptions of programs funded, and any other information that you can get. The more information you have the better your chance of submitting an acceptable proposal. Generally, your application/proposal will be rejected outright if it doesn't meet the recipient's guidelines. Another source of information about a particular foundation is their tax return (referred to as *990s*).

These tax returns almost always include a list of organizations funded and the amount of money given to each. Some may indicate the particular program funded. The 990s are usually available through an internet Web site called *GrantSmart* (see end of chapter for Web address).

*Corporations* and *local businesses* may fulfill their civic responsibilities through grants and sponsorships to nonprofit organizations. As an example of a private funding organization, the Pfizer pharmaceutical company's corporate philanthropy includes, among many other agendas, maternal and child health programs to help low-income, high-risk parents get prenatal and well-baby care and information. Occupation-centered community nonprofit programs such as those targeting skills for teen mothers, those designed to encourage nurturing mother-baby shared occupations, or those providing screening for developmental milestones in infants and children would be appropriate for this organization (Children and Youth Funding Report, 1998; pp. 10–11).

Business donors or sponsors are often the best place for a small organization to begin to seek funding and to establish a successful track record in using these gifts. Start with your local bank, or perhaps a retail store. Ask the manager if they provide assistance to groups like yours and what you have to do to apply for it. Ask if he or she would look at your proposal and give you an opportunity to talk about it. Wherever your community is located, urban or rural, it is likely that a Wal-Mart retail store is somewhere at the heart of it. If you are looking for a small amount of matching money (up to $2,000 to double what you already have) for your children and youth program, consider this organization. *Civic* associations in which local business people participate, like the Chamber of Commerce, Lions Club, Rotary, and Kiwanis, often have giving programs or provide sponsorships for local organizations or programs. Each association will have its own priorities and most gifts will be small, but it's a way to partially fund your pilot program in preparation for seeking larger amounts of funding. It might be all you need.

## Federal Grants

The federal government awards many billions of dollars in grant funds each year. A federal grant is an award of federal money made to accomplish some general public purpose (Karsh and Fox, 2003; p. 22). The nature of the grant, who is eligible, how the award is given, and the terms and conditions are specified in the legislation that creates each grant program and in detailed regulations (*regs*). The legislation provides the structure for any restrictions or limitations and for the extensive reporting requirements that are generally required.

Just as the *Foundation Directory* provides information about foundation funding; the *Federal Register* does the same thing for federal granting monies. The *Federal Register* is a daily publication that reports on official federal actions, including all federal funding opportunities. Announcements for grant programs, often with the whole application package, appear in the *Federal Register*. Occasionally, the announcement will appear as part of a department's grant-making plans for the year, which provides substantial lead time for your application. It is more likely, though, that notification will allow 30 to 90 days for an application response. Without access to the *Federal Register* you won't be able to make competitive federal applications for funding. As with other funding announcement documents mentioned earlier, you can likely find a copy at your library, or obtain internet access. Karsh and Fox (2003) provide a "guide" to searching *The Federal Register Online* (Karsh and Fox, 2003; p. 29). Many federal agencies have their own Web sites where they publish grant information. You'll want to access these sites as well. Some examples of interest to occupation-centered practitioners are: *Department of Health and Human Services* (related sites: *Administration for Children and Families, National Institutes of Health,* and *Substance Abuse and Mental Health Administration*) and the *Department of Education.* (See end of chapter for Web sites.)

In general, federal (also state and local) grant proposals are complex and time consuming to prepare. It is virtually impossible to develop and write a comprehensive, technical grant application in the short window of time that most federal programs offer between announcement and due date. This is one of the reasons it's important to develop your proposal far in advance. Brown and Brown (2001) suggest that the grant seeker develop a system of year-round grant seeking. These authors propose that one can *demystify* grant seeking by "organizing your office and practicing the right work habits so you can get more and better grant proposals out the door and more money coming in, *without suffering* (Brown and Brown, 2001; p. xix). Many organizations devote key personnel to the year-round process of seeking funding. According to Brown and Brown (2001) there is a "grant-seeking" cycle that first involves the meticulously prepared proposal with comprehensive files containing all of the collected information for each component of the proposal, from goals and objectives for programming to the results of outcome evaluations, to staff job descriptions and resumes. When you prepare a grant, regardless of the agency, you have everything they could possibly ask for.

## Dealing With the Application

Many first-time grant seekers skim or speed-read the application. They are generally interested in how much money they can get, the questions that must be answered in the proposal, and the absolute midnight deadline the grant has to be driven to the local Fed-Ex! In fact, if you hope to be successful, the whole package must be read carefully and more than once.

Successful grant writers (Knowles, 2002; Barbato and Furlich, 2000; Smith and Tremore, 2003; Karsh and Fox, 2003) suggest that, as you become familiar with the application (and they don't all look the same), you should ask yourself these questions:

1. Am I, or is my organization even eligible to apply for the grant described in the package?
2. Does my idea for a grant mesh with the grant-maker's?
3. What kinds of projects has the grant-maker funded recently?

4. How much money is the grant for, and will it cover my expenses? Most grant applications stipulate the approximate amount of funding that will be awarded. Some only tell you what the total amount will be and approximately how many grants will be given. Others give a maximum possible award or an average.

5. Do I really have to answer *all* of the questions? Yes! Most grant applications include a list of questions or topics that you must address in a specific number of pages; some may restrict the number of words per question. You must answer all of the questions or address every topic that is included in the application and with the number of pages/words specified.

6. What if there are no real questions? Foundations, particularly, may simply describe what they want you to tell them without asking specific questions, or they may suggest what they'd like to see in the proposal. They may say something like this: *"we are interested in learning as much as possible about the applicant . . . this includes budget (past, current, projected), audited financial statements, an IRS letter explaining tax status, and examples of past accomplishments . . . the main body of the application should not exceed 15 pages"* (Karsh and Fox, 2001; p. 290).

7. What if I don't find any guidelines, instructions, or specific questions? In this case, you may wish to write a **letter of inquiry (LOI)**. Something like an abstract, discussed a bit later, this letter is a brief summary of your organization, its purpose, the need you wish to address, your program to address the need, the cost of your program, and the amount you're requesting. You will also want to include why you selected this particular funder and how your program will fit their overall interests. Follow this with a telephone call. The LOI refers to both *letter of inquiry* and **letter of intent**.

8. A *letter of intent* is requested by some funders to determine approximately how many applicants they may expect to receive applications from.

9. What information/documents am I likely to need? You can review the chapters in this text for much of the information you'll need: mission/goals, objectives, programming, staff, floor plan, associated trends, the community and population profiles, needs assessments and evaluations, budget, and current funding sources. In addition, you may need personnel policies and procedures, staff resumes, job descriptions, organizational charts, names of board members, evidence of collaboration/partnering with other individuals/disciplines/ organizations, certificate of incorporation as a not-for-profit organization, and proof of tax-exempt status. Of more importance all of the time is the question of *"how you will sustain your program when the grant runs out?"* In all cases, read the application carefully so that you don't leave anything out and generally, don't put in things that aren't asked for.

## The Grant Proposal

It's important for you to appreciate that grantsmanship refers to the *process* of collecting information, developing your ideas, and writing. It is a process that you initiated with

Chapter 1 in this text. It is much more than just answering a series of questions. Certainly you may need to answer questions, but you will do so from information collected during the process of developing your program. Knowing yourself and your community will help you establish the context for your work—what you want to accomplish, and it will help you find the best grant-maker for your purposes. It is essential that you get the funder to believe in your ideas and to trust that you, as the leader, know what you're doing and have the sense of purpose to do it. The basis for this "trust" is established alongside the development of your program.

In most cases, the actual "pieces" needed to accompany your proposal for funding will include:

1. the cover letter;
2. the cover sheet;
3. the abstract, or executive summary;
4. the table of contents; and
5. appendices (attachments).

You know from the development of your community programming proposal what a table of contents, a cover or title sheet, and appendices include, but you may not be familiar with the **cover letter**, and/or the **abstract/executive summary**.

A **cover letter** is an introduction and is the first document in a grant application. Most often it is used on foundation and corporate requests, not in applications for federal or state funding but, again, read the directions to be sure. The letter should be reflective, sincere, and provide only a taste of what's to come in the grant request. It is generally best to do the cover letter last, after you've completed the entire grant application. Remember, though, it isn't simply a summary. The cover letter must be persuasive and it's likely the only appropriate place in a funding proposal to get personal. Barbato and Furlich (2000), in their book *Writing for a Good Cause*, outline the process of crafting proposals and what they describe as 'other persuasive pieces for nonprofits.' The cover letter is the first line of *persuasion*; it tells the reader right away whether the proposal is worth reading. Mary Bellor, president of the Philip L. Graham Fund in Washington, D.C. is quoted in Barbato and Furlich as saying "I read the cover letter first; I want to see who you are, what you do, who benefits, and why it matters . . . I want a preview of what I'm going to find in the proposal, I don't want a summary" (Barbato and Furlich, 2000; p. 86).

The **abstract** or **executive summary** is a brief, one-page overview of what the grant reviewer will find in the full grant application. It is written (or assembled) after the grant application narrative has been entirely written. It should be one-page only and Barbato and Furlich (2000, p. 23) recommend even less than that. Browning (2001, pp. 119–120) recommends lifting key sentences from the following areas of the proposal, keeping them in the same order as they are in the narrative:

■ your proposed initiative,
■ program design/plan of action,

- problem statement/statement of need,
- goals,
- measurable objectives, and
- impact on problem.

Other grant writers (Barbato and Furlich, 2000; pp. 92–93) recommend an even more succinct version that includes:

- the problem you want to address;
- your proposed solution; and
- how much your proposal requests.

## Banks and Lending Institutions

If you are planning a for-profit program/practice, then some of your funding needs may fall into the category of a loan. It is generally expected, however, that you have your own **capital**. If you have other sources of income and collateral (home equity, stocks, or bonds), you might be in a position to borrow funds in addition to your own. Of course, there's always some risk that must be considered if the practice struggles. A solid **business plan** with good projections and supporting data is a prerequisite to requesting a start-up loan. Ryan, Ray, and Hiduke (1999, p. 6) suggest the following outline for developing a business plan appropriate for seeking funds from a lending agency (you will recognize in their suggested plan many of the components you have already prepared during your planning process):

1. Cover sheet
2. Statement of purpose
3. Table of contents

- The Business

    a. Description of business
    b. Marketing
    c. Competition
    d. Operating procedures
    e. Personnel
    f. Business insurance
    g. Financial data

- Financial Data

    a. Loan application
    b. Capital equipment and supply list
    c. Balance sheet
    d. Break-even analysis
    e. Proforma income projections (profit and loss statements)

Three-year summary
Detail by month, first year
Detail by quarters, second and third years
Assumptions upon which projections were based
f. Proforma cash flow
Follow guidelines for letter E

- Supporting Documents

Tax returns of principals for last three years
Personal financial statement (forms supplied by lender)
If franchised, a copy of the contract
Copy of proposed lease or purchase agreement for space
Copy of licenses and other legal documents
Copy of resumes of all principals
Copy of letters of intent from suppliers, etc.

These authors also suggest the following Web site to assist in the preparation of this plan: www.sba.gov/starting/indexbusplans.html. Clearly, this route is not for the "faint of heart," and you should still seek the services of an accountant. It should be comforting to know, however, that the planning you have already accomplished is the foundation upon which you can attach the additional pieces.

## What Happens Next?

You place your completed application in the mail, and you wait. You will generally know when the selections will be made, and when you can expect notification. You may not hear if you're not selected, so a phone call may be acceptable if the granting date has passed and you've heard nothing.

When the applications arrive at the granting agency (never accepted after the deadline) they are evaluated and points are attached to each section of the proposal/application indicating strength/weakness. Generally, in the application information, you'll be informed how the evaluation will be determined. The irony is that sometimes you'll receive a high score, but receive no funding. Only a few of the best scores can be funded. However, you should note your scores and be pleased with your high scores. You have learned something valuable for the next application. If you have low scores, do better the next time.

If you receive notice that your application has been funded, most often for three to five years, your work begins. You can't abandon your program, take the money and go to Tahiti. You have an unrelenting responsibility to meet the terms of your proposal. Are there strings attached to the grant award? You can be sure of it. All granting organizations expect reporting on a regular basis. They will want to know that your program is making a difference (evaluation results) and they will want to know that their money is well-spent. Read carefully what kind of reporting is expected, what documents may be needed, and what the reporting deadlines are.

Even for small amounts of money, there are expectations that require reporting procedures.

## Exercises

*If you are a student likely this portion of your work will be for learning purposes only and even though you may make a mock grant application you won't submit it to an agency. That will come later when you can devote the necessary time and effort to actually implement and run a program.*

### What Kind of Program Do You Have?

1. Refer to Exercise 1 in the previous chapter. Is your program *not-for-profit*, or is the intention to be *for-profit*?

_____

_____

_____

_____

   If you are *not-for-profit*, review what you would need to do to seek 501(c)(3) status. Remember if you are working under the umbrella of a not-for-profit agency . . . this work will have already been accomplished. Either way, for the purposes of learning review the process and information you will need and note below.

_____

_____

_____

_____

2. Refer to Exercise 2 in the previous chapter. Carefully evaluate your costs. It is unlikely for the purposes of your student exercises that you have a budget accurate enough for a grant application; however, you should have all the pieces and can make a fairly accurate estimate of the sum you will need to operate your program for.

Start-Up _____

One Year _____

Three Years _____

In what lines of the budget do you think you'll need to do additional work to be prepared to make a funding application? Note any areas below.

_____

_____

_____

### Identifying Potential Funding Sources?

3. Review the potential funding sources noted in this chapter compared to the goal and purpose of your program. If you are working under the umbrella of another not-for-profit organization, ask if they already have grant funded programs and the nature of them (perhaps they receive a portion of their funding from *United Way* or other similar organizations).

Will you bill insurances? Will you establish a sliding fee scale and accept out-of-pocket pay? Will you consider a private foundation? Will you wish to seek a federal grant? If you intend to be a for-profit, you may wish to consider a small business loan.

Discuss funding options with your classmates, colleagues, or partners to determine which ones seem most appropriate for your program. Note your choices below.

_____

_____

_____

_____

### Learning as Much as Possible About Your Selected Funding Source:

4. You're now ready to go to the library, the Web sites, and the directories to learn as much as you can about your selected funding source. Find the best *fit* with your purpose, your goal and your program. Note below what sources you will use.

_____

_____

_____

_____

Obtain a grant application package from the agency you've selected and become familiar with it. Evaluate the requested application information compared to what you have in your proposal. Where will you need to do more work? Some funding sources (such as federal and private organizations and lending agencies) require a fairly lengthy application process. Revisit your time line and be sure to include the funding process.

_____

_____

_____

_____

_____

## Summary

This chapter has provided you with a general outline of funding sources as you anticipate how you will initiate and maintain your program. You have examined the characteristics of your program and come to decisions about potential funding sources. If your venture calls for external funding either through grants or a loan, then you must anticipate that early in your planning. It was not the purpose of this chapter, or this text, to tell you everything you need to know to acquire funding for your program. It provides an overview and some guidance. There are many excellent resources listed in the reference portion at the end of the chapter; use them to fill in any gaps you might find. Select the direction you wish to go, make a plan, utilize the resources and move ahead.

## References

Barbato, J., & Furlich, D. (2000). *Writing for a good cause*. New York: Simon and Schuster Publishers.

Brown, L. G., & Brown, M. J. (2001). *Demystifying grant seeking*. San Francisco, CA: Jossey-Bass Publishers.

Browning, B. (2001). *Grant writing for dummies*. New York: Wiley Publishing.

Brownson, C. (1998). Funding community practice: Stage I. *The American Journal Of Occupational Therapy* 52(1), 60–64.

Children and youth funding report. (1998, November 4). Silver Spring, MD: CD Publications.

Karsh, E., & Fox, A. (2003). *The only grant-writing book you'll ever need*. New York: Carroll and Graf Publishers.

Knowles, C. (2002). *The first-time grantwriter's guide to success*. Thousand Oaks, CA: Corwin Press Publishers.

Reed, K. (1992). History of federal legislation for persons with disabilities. *The American Journal of Occupational Therapy 46*(5), 397–408.

Ryan, J. D., Ray, R., & Hiduke, G. (1999). *Small business: An entrepreneur's plan*. Philadelphia: The Dryden Press.

Smith, N., & Tremore, J. (2003). *The everything grant writing book*. Avon, MA: F + W Publications.

Vega, P. (1998, October). Industry trends. In *Practice strategies, A business guide for behavioral healthcare providers*. Washington, DC: American Association for Marriage and Family Therapy.

## Internet Resources

Administration for Children and Families:
    http://www.acf.hhs.gov/grants.html
Business Plans: www.sba.gov/starting/indexbusplans.html
Department of Education: http://www.edu.gov
    http://www.ed.gov/topics/topics.jsp?&top=Grants+%26+Contracts
Department of Health and Human Services:
    http://www.hhs.gov/agencies/grants.html
Health Resources and Service Administration:
    http://www.hrsa.gov/grants.htm
National Institutes of Health: http://www.nih.gov/grants/guide/index.html
Substance Abuse and Mental Health Administration:
    http://www.ssamhsa.gov/grants/grants.html
Federal Register: http://www.access.gpo.gov/su_docs/aces/aces!40.html
The Foundation Center: http://www.foundation.center.org
http://fdncenter.org/funders/grantsmart/index.html
http://fdncenter.org/funders/grantmaker/gws_corp/corpl.html
http://fdncenter.org/funders/cga/index.html
http://gtionline.fdncenter.org
National Institute of Health: http://www.nih.gov/grants/guide/index.html
National Association of Women Business Owners (NAWBO): www.nfwbo.org
U.S. Department of Justice, Americans with Disabilities
    (800-514-0301; 202-514-0301): www.usdoj.gov/crt/ada;
    http://www.usdoj.gov/10grants/index.html
The American Occupational Therapy Association (FAX-on-request) 800-701-7735
The Grantsmanship Center: http://www.tgci.com
Grantwriting Resources: http://www.fundsnetservices.com/grantwri.htm

Publications and Services of the Foundation Center, 79 Fifth Avenue, New York,
    10003-3076 (800-424-9836); Foundation Center's World Wide Web site:
    http://fdncenter.org
U.S. Census Bureau: http://www.census.gov
After-School Program Information: http://www.afterschool.gov

## General Research Directories

The following are published by the Foundation Center, New York:

*The foundation directory*, M. Luller and N. Luman, eds., published annually.
*The foundation directory, Part 2*, Luller, M. and N. Luman, eds., published annually.
*The foundation directory supplement*, M. Luller and N. Luman, eds., published
    annually.
*Guide to U.S. foundations, their trustees, officers, and donors*, published annually.
*The foundation 1000*, published annually
*National directory of corporate giving*, published annually
*Corporate foundation profiles*, published biennially
*National directory of grantmaking public charities*, 1st edition
*Guide to greater Washington DC grantmakers*, 2nd edition
*New York State foundations: A comprehensive directory*, published biennially
*Directory of Missouri grantmakers*, 1st edition
*Foundation grants to individuals*, published biennially

## Grant Directories

*The foundation grants index* (most recent edition)
*The foundation grants index quarterly* (most recent edition)
*Who gets grants: Foundation grants to nonprofit organizations*

## Guidebooks, Manuals, and Reports

*The foundation center's grants classification system indexing manual and thesaurus*,
    (newest edition)
*The foundation center's user-friendly guide: A grantseeker's guide to resources*, (most
    recent edition)
*The foundation center's guide to proposal writing*, (most recent edition).
*Program-related investments: A guide to funders and trends*

## Additional Resources

*Most of the following may be obtained from* The Foundation Center:

Berstein, P. (1997). *Best practices of effective nonprofit organizations: A practitioner's
    manual.*

Cohen, L., & Young, D. (1989). *Careers for dreamers and doers: A guide to management careers in the nonprofit sector.*

Firstenberg, P. (1996). *The 21st century nonprofit.*

Freeman, D., & the Council on Foundations (1991). *Handbook on private foundations.*

New, A. (1991). *Raise more money for your nonprofit organization: A guide to evaluating and improving fund raising.*

Olenick, A., & Olenick, P. (1991). *A nonprofit organization operating manual: Planning for survival and growth.*

Salamon, L. (1992). *America's nonprofit sector: A primer*

Seltzer, M. (1987). *Securing your organization's future: A complete guide to fundraising strategies.*

Skloot, E. (Ed.) (1988). *The nonprofit entrepreneur: Creating ventures to earn income.*

Young, D., & Steinberg, R. (1995). *Economics for nonprofit managers.*

CHAPTER 13

# Marketing and Promotion

## Learning Objectives

1. To learn the components of a marketing plan
2. To determine the characteristics of a promotional mix
3. To identify the pros and cons associated with the different elements of a promotional strategy
4. To conceptualize the program you are designing and developing
5. To develop the marketing plan and promotional mix for your program

## Key Terms

1. Marketing
2. Sales Promotion
3. Promotional Mix
4. Advertising
5. Publicity
6. Public Relations
7. Direct Selling/Personal Selling
8. Marketing Logic
9. Market Analysis
10. Networking
11. Free Ink/Free Air
12. Press Release

In the simplest terms, **marketing** is the process of letting your potential consumers know that you have services that may be of interest to them. We may not think that we're selling a "product" but, in reality, our "product" is the attainment of goals and the satisfaction of "need." In fact, product is "anything that can be offered to a market for attention, acquisition, use, or consumption and that might satisfy a need or want." (Kotler and Armstrong, 1991; p. 7) Marketing also includes an intent to "sell" the services to the potential market/consumer (even if the services are free). This marketing aspect of selling is often referred to by the more aggressive term **sales promotion**, and those areas that are selected to promote your services are referred to as the **promotional mix**. In her discussions of marketing yourself as an occupational therapy practitioner, Gilkeson (1997) describes this promotional mix to include the three areas of advertising, publicity, and personal selling. Gerson (1991) utilizes a more conventional list preferred by business to include advertising, public relations, direct selling, and sales promotion. Richmond (2003) would remind us that although marketing is often used synonymously with selling or advertising, it is much more than that. Marketing can be defined in terms of exchanging products and values with others; however, unless those products (programs) are visible and accessible to the consumer, the exchange can't take place (Richmond, 2003; p. 179).

Writing for the potential small business entrepreneur, on the other hand, Ryan, Ray, and Hiduke (1999, p. 99) include all of these areas in their promotional mix. In their words, mix "refers to all the elements that are blended to maximize communication with the target customer or population." An important aspect of promotion for these authors is the advancement of the "image" of your practice, or displaying for the potential consumer the "quality" of your services.

**Advertising**, of course, includes all of those marketing methods we have come to take for granted in our lives, such as visual media (television), print media (magazines and newspapers), radio, and now the Internet. We hardly notice media ads, billboards, or bus signs, yet we are influenced by their messages. **Publicity** may be positive or negative and is usually not targeted by the marketer; rather, it is received by the marketer. The receipt of positive publicity, for example, could be in the form of responses to a public presentation we have done or to a community service event we have organized and/or in which we have participated. Of course, there is also the negative potential of such publicity as the announcement of a malpractice suit or other legal sanctions having to do with unethical or unsafe practices. **Public relations** describes the direct intent of interfacing with your public in such a way that the image of you and your service delivery remains positive.

**Personal selling** has been emphasized in earlier chapters, and it may begin when we interface with potential partners or collaborators; or perhaps earlier. Let's examine personal selling in consideration of our marketing mix from the perspective of personally going out to make others aware of our program. Drucker (1973) has long been a compelling voice in the wilderness of business management. He suggests that if the marketing process has been well organized and carried out effectively, personal selling might not be necessary. For our purposes, however, personal selling is a critical—perhaps the most critical—part of health promotion, intervention, and the extensive scope of most of the program development described in this text. A few minutes taken to meet the pediatricians, teachers, and parents in your community, coupled with the delivery of a well-appointed brochure describing your pediatric occupational therapy services is well worth the time.

Although your new program or practice may represent one of those circumstances where you will open your doors and they will come, this is not likely. If others in the community have a vested interest in your program (such as our examples of the cooperative gardening project for the mentally ill who are homeless or the sanctuary program for runaway adolescents), then they will likely assist you in attracting clients and in getting them to you. Anytime you have the enthusiasm, interest, and support of an agency or organization, you will have less marketing to do in order to get your clients through your doors; certainly your collaborators and your partners will be strong allies in this effort.

As we mentioned earlier in the text, your first marketing task was to *sell yourself* to the people who required a planner. If they were not yet aware that they needed a planner, then you sold them on the idea. We assume that you have already done this, but the process of selling yourself never quite ends. Even if you have the support of an agency to start the program, you will have to continue "selling" the idea and, more importantly, making people aware of how effective your programming is. As described by Gilkeson (1997), this is **marketing logic**, or the representation of an attitude that supports the principles of selling yourself and the belief in your ideas. It is the belief that you are the "program" and that the program is an extension of you. It represents your beliefs, your ideas, and your ethics.

If you are developing a new program under the sponsorship of your employer, then the marketing task will not be yours alone. It is likely that you have already proven your worth or you would not have been invited to develop a new program. In addition, assuming the development is responsive to an expressed need, part of the marketing/promotion has probably already been accomplished. In a case such as this, the primary marketing task—as it is for all programs—will be one of proving effectiveness weighed against cost.

Sometimes a program is initiated because someone else has recognized the need but does not have the expertise, or perhaps the interest, to provide it. That person might come to you, or you might hear of it and go to them. The marketing task then is to sell yourself as the best one to do the job.

Let's consider the following scenario.

You are attending an open house of a new cardiac care unit and happen to overhear one of the attendees ask if there would be a cardiac "wellness" program to complement the surgical practice. You are an astute marketer/planner and later ask one of the cardiac surgeons if you could meet with him or her regarding your ideas for supplementary services organized around occupation; after all, you are an occupational therapy practitioner (or "therapist" if that is a more marketable term in this environment). Needless to say, after some planning, promotion, and negotiation with the corporation, you will develop a maintenance and wellness program that may include providers of information and skills in the areas of balanced lifestyle, work, nutrition, relaxation (maybe yoga), graduated exercise, and perhaps sexuality and you have further marketed this program to other cardiac caregivers and surgeons. This is an example of a "success" story.

Of course, you are not finished; you must keep careful formative and summative outcome data to market your program's effectiveness in "lengthening life" and in "enhancing quality of life." The goal of a program such as this could be not only the promotion of longer lives but also the assurance of longer *meaningful* lives. This is a burgeoning area of interest and research in occupational therapy, so part of your task is to keep abreast of all the work that is being accomplished to support the establishment of meaning in one's life and to provide potentially valued options for how one chooses to live, perhaps to include the *redesign* of one's life (Mandel, Jackson, Zemke, Nelson, and Clark, 1999).

The most challenging marketing task may be for the private practice. Many therapists who initiate private practices do so a bit cautiously while still being employed by other organizations. As we said earlier, a private practice is a business, and there are risks to be considered. If you were an entrepreneur as a child or adolescent and started a successful business (a lemonade stand, babysitting service, or anything else), you know something about marketing and promotion. You may have been selling a product or a service or maybe both.

For example, neighborhood children might collaborate to climb trees, retrieve mistletoe, package it, and sell it door to door during the holiday season. The mistletoe was likely hanging on the trees of most of the people who purchased it. The marketing mix would include an attractively wrapped product and a service (retrieval of the "product" from the trees), and most people would probably buy it. There is little doubt that known neighborhood children are a strong component of the promotional mix, regardless of what they are selling. Consider how many subscriptions, packages of candy, and holiday cards you have purchased from a child at your door. This example may seem a bit remote from our interests as occupation-centered practitioners, but it clearly shows how an effective promotional mix is developed, and it is not unlike what you will do.

You will be selling a product and a service—thoughtful, skilled intervention that is well packaged in a comfortable and welcoming environment. In addition, you can and will prove that this particular intervention makes a difference. Your clients/patients/members may be able to do for themselves some of what you do, but certainly not as effectively or as efficiently. Consider why people go to clubs to exercise when they could exercise at home. Could some of their reasoning also apply to your clientele? You are the professional skilled in understanding and utilizing meaningful occupation, so your marketing brochures and your business card should reflect this. If you find that people misinterpret what you do as an occupational therapist or as an occupational therapy assistant, include a meaningful explanation of your services on a brochure or an explanatory phrase on your business card. You may want these materials to be focused toward the population you wish to serve. For example, a pediatrics program might be described as providing "supportive play through small-group interactions."

In an earlier chapter we discussed the many levels of assessing need. The term **market analysis** is related in that information is gleaned to "define the market and determine if the organization's perception of the wants and needs of the market are valid" (Shoemaker and Wheeler, 1996; p. 10). Richmond (2004) reminds us that we must be responsive to the "bottom line;" you must have clients to stay in business. She goes on to describe the target markets that you must be aware of as you conduct your analysis: the clients/potential clients, referral sources, and the payers (Richmond, 2004; pp. 83–86). You might think of the market analysis as a "check" on the validity of your research and your collective needs assessment results. According to Richmond (2004) the market analysis is organized within two main assessment methods: assessment of the organization, and assessment of the environment (Richmond, 2003; p. 182). The goals of the analysis incorporate the identification of trends, opportunities, and potential threats, as well as competition and position of the organization (offering programming) in the market.

## The Promotional Mix

What are the choices available to us as we prepare to let others know about our program, and how do we select the options that will be most advantageous? Consider the following possibilities adapted from Ryan, Ray, and Hiduke (1999):

| Promotional Element | Pros | Cons |
| --- | --- | --- |
| 1. Paid media advertising (radio, television, Internet, newspapers, and magazines) | Quick, effective | Expensive |
| 2. Direct mail (to your potential consumer) | Affordable, efficient | Can be wasted if you have a fragmented market; difficult to write |

*(continued)*

| Promotional Element | Pros | Cons |
|---|---|---|
| 3. Professional literature (become a source of information in your specialty and an expert in your field, and write about it) | Little or no cost; respected by colleagues and consumers | Will take work and experience |
| 4. Free ink and free air (reviews, features, interview shows, press releases, newspaper columns to talk about what you do) | No cost and effective | Takes time to "market" to media |
| 5. Promotional products (products with the name of your program, such as key chains, pencils, mugs, shirts, etc.) | Targeted and effective; can be very creative | Can be costly |
| 6. Working visibility (develop and maintain a positive presence in the community; stand out from the competitors because you are better) | Common sense | You have to be good! |
| 7. Personal selling and networking (business cards distributed at events, meetings); displays | Personal and effective | Takes time and can be costly |

Consider these alternatives as you develop your promotional strategies. For most nonprofit community programs, the planner will rely on those with low cost. Communicating with others in the community about your program is known as **networking**, or getting to know others in the community who can and will help you remain a viable community resource. Sometimes this is accomplished through very informal means such as going to the same coffee shop as those you wish to know, and living in the community is certainly a plus. Networking also might be more formal and can include attending professional meetings or town meetings, or if you have a private practice, you may wish to join the Chamber of Commerce. Getting free media coverage, or **free ink/free air**, by providing a news item or story is excellent advertising. Writing a human-interest story about one of your clients or a client's family and then sending the story along with a photo to the media in the form of a **press release** will not only let the potential consumer know about your services but also will let those who may be able to offer financial assistance know as well. Always keep in mind working visibility and the process of becoming a professional authority in your specialty; certainly these are substantial facilitators to a successful private practice. Consider offering to do presentations, workshops, or seminars to Parent-Teacher Associations, Lions or Kiwanis Clubs, and community religious groups. These are excellent ways to market your program and to give the potential consumer a way to see how you work and to know whether or not they wish to engage your services. You may also target some referrals in this way as well. Public service activities such as community health fairs are yet another way to interface with potential consumers and those who may wish to refer consumers to your program.

# Promotional Products and Advertising

Regardless of the nature or size of your program, you will likely wish to develop a logo with accompanying business cards and letterhead/envelopes and perhaps a brochure. You may also want to place your logo on a t-shirt for campers, on the side of a transportation van, or on "Halloween" candy wrappers that your clients give to local businesses in a marketing "reverse trick or treat."

Business cards (always carried with you) and brochures (distributed where your potential consumer or family/friends of the consumer will see them) always should be professional. In many ways, these may be considered as print advertising, and they are a representation of your practice. If they are less than serious, your practice will be assumed to be less than serious. In addition, your informational materials (flyers/brochures) should not be overly dramatic, and never make claims you cannot support.

Some therapists put advertisements in the telephone yellow pages and in newspapers (particularly neighborhood or community newspapers). Again, these must be professional. Brochures, pamphlets, or flyers made available directly to the consumer, to consumers' family members, and to other professionals from whom you may get referrals is sometimes enough to initiate a practice, particularly when start-up funding is limited. Physicians will often permit other practitioners to place brochures in their reception area (after marketing to them and with their approval, of course). A marketing/networking visit to teachers, psychologists, clergymen, and other therapists and a brochure or business card left behind may also generate referrals. Of course you would not try to advertise in the offices of competitors, but consider whether your services can supplement or complement those of other occupational therapy practitioners (for example, day camps to complement pediatric practices).

Once you have established programming, consider sending holiday greetings with your logo on the cover. A holiday greeting may be coupled with an end-of-the-tax-year "invitation" for dollars to support programming (such as tuition for camp attendance). If you and your clients/members go into the wider community either as part of your services or to do exhibits and community fairs, a logo on a shirt can go a long way to make your services known. If you choose to do this, you may wish to remind your clients/members that they are your best advertisements—a very persuasive enabler for a goal of personal efficacy.

See Figure 13–1 and Figure 13–2 for examples of marketing flyers, brochures, and logos.

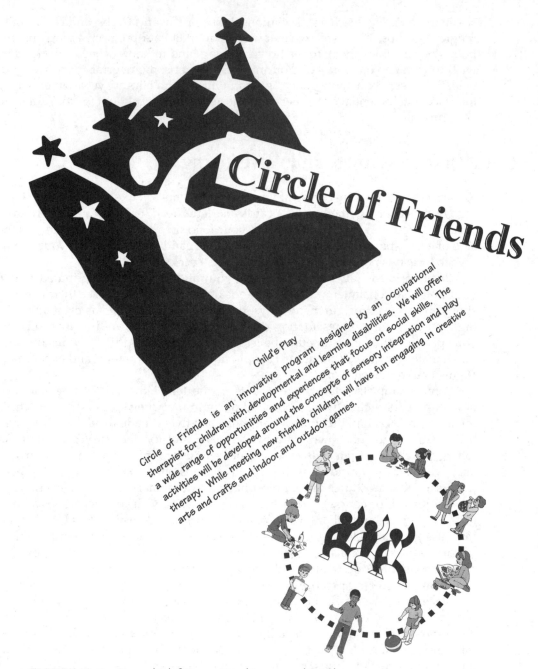

Child's Play

Circle of Friends is an innovative program designed by an occupational therapist for children with developmental and learning disabilities. We will offer a wide range of opportunities and experiences that focus on social skills. The activities will be developed around the concepts of sensory integration and play therapy. While meeting new friends, children will have fun engaging in creative arts and crafts and indoor and outdoor games.

**FIGURE 13–1**    Examples of Promotional Logos and Brochures

REGISTRATION

PLEASE FILL OUT AND RETURN TO:_____

Phone: _____ Camp Voice Mail: _____ Fax: _____

Name of Child: _____ Name of Child: _____
Birthday: _____ Birthday: _____

Phone: _____

Session Preferred: _____

✂ — — — — — — — — — — — — — — — — — — — — — — — — — — —

PLAY AWAY YOUR DAY!! A SUMMER DAY CAMP FOR CHILDREN

PLAY AWAY YOUR DAY! is a day camp offered from 10:00 A.M. to 3:00 P.M. for children with special needs between the ages of four and seven (and their siblings of the same age range).

Each week will offer a theme around which the activities, games, arts, and crafts are designed and organized. A field trip complementing the theme will offer children and their parents the chance to share a fun experience in the community.

Through arts, crafts, games, and activities, the campers will be encouraged to actively play and learn together.

Each camp group will be staffed by an occupational therapist, an occupational therapy assistant, and volunteers to ensure that each child's needs are acknowledged and respected.

Dates:  Session 1   May 31–June 11
Session II   June 14–June 25
Session III   June 28–July 9
Session IV   July 12–July 23
Session V   July 26–August 20

Location: Sunset Park in Alta Vista Ranch

**FIGURE 13–2**   Examples of Promotional Flyers

PLAY AWAY YOUR DAY!!

...... a summer day camp for children with special needs and their siblings.

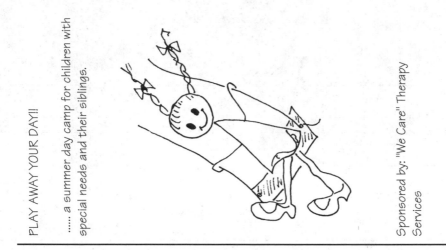

Sponsored by: "We Care" Therapy Services

TO:

PLAY AWAY YOUR DAY!!

Fill out and return the attached registration form along with your $25.00 deposit. Priority will be given to children who are currently receiving services in our clinic or are clients of a regional center.

Camp fees:

$600.00 per 2-week session

Funding options:

* Private pay (may be considered day care for tax purposes)

* Regional center (consult with your caseworker)

* Some scholarships (based on financial need)

**FIGURE 13–2**   Examples of Promotional Flyers—continued

## Exercise 1

### Conceptualizing Your Program

1. Think about the program you are designing and developing. How would you like to represent it to potential consumers or other professionals? Referring again to your goal(s) and your objectives, write down a few words or phrases that sum up your program in user-friendly terms. Consider *what* you will do for the client/patient/member, *how* you will do it (your programming), and *who* will do it (the expertise of your staff):

_____

_____

_____

_____

_____

2. Consider now what your marketing mix will be. Will you use direct mail and/or personal distribution for brochures? Will you and your employees carry business cards? Will you create some kind of specialty advertising/promotional products? Will you use paid media advertising? Will you rely on free ink/free air? In what ways will you ensure visibility in the community? Note your ideas below:

_____

_____

_____

_____

_____

Now that you have selected your marketing mix, you may find it helpful to collect advertisements from the telephone book or newspapers or a few brochures or promotional items from organizations or professional offices that you visit in your weekly round of activities. Most professionals are finding it necessary to advertise these days. How do they conceptualize the services that they offer? Which ones do you like and why? Which ones do you not like and why?

## Exercise 2

**Developing Marketing Materials for Your Program**

Based on the previous exercise, think about a logo that will symbolize your programming. Consider how it will be expressed on your letterhead, envelopes, and business card. Before you begin, collect some examples, and with your group or colleagues note why some appeal to you and why some do not. Is there too much information? Not enough? Do you consider the font, color, and paper quality to be professional? What might you do differently?

On a sheet of paper, or on your computer:

1. Sketch some ideas for your logo.

2. Consider your letterhead, envelopes and your business card. How will you use your logo? Will you use any terms or phrases to define your services? Sketch how you would like the letterhead, envelopes, and business card to look.

3. Draft some ideas for a brochure highlighting your program (consider color, photos, font style, as well as the information you will include). Keep it simple, but include everything your potential consumer will need to know.

When you have formulated your ideas, go to your computer and complete the brochure.

## *Summary*

We have explored the elements of marketing a program to the community and to the potential client/consumer. Our first interests are in the "selling" of ourselves as program planners, developers, and practitioners. From this stance of personal selling, we have gone on to identify ways we might promote our program. Several elements of the promotional mix have been identified, which include paid media advertising, direct mail, promotional products, and free ink/free air. We have also described low-cost ways we might promote our program, including doing the job well and letting others see what we do (or working visibility). Promoting ourselves as authorities on a particular element of practice following the development of our expertise and some accumulated experience through the professional literature is also recommended as a further way to legitimatize our programs and our practices. We have also developed a marketing/promotional plan that includes a logo, business card, and a brochure to describe our program. With the completion of the marketing plan, we are now ready to firmly establish the time line for the initiation of our program.

# References

Drucker, P. F. (1973). *Management, tasks, responsibilities, practices.* New York: Harper and Row.

Gerson, R. F. (1991). *Writing and implementing a marketing plan.* Los Altos, CA: Crisp Publications.

Gilkeson, G. (1997). *Occupational therapy leadership: Marketing yourself, your profession, and your organization.* Philadelphia: F. A. Davis.

Kotler, P., & Armstrong, G. (1991). *Principles of marketing* (5th ed.). Englewood Cliffs, NJ: Prentice-Hall.

Mandel, D., Jackson, J., Zemke, R., Nelson, L., & Clark, F. (1999). *Lifestyle redesign: Implementing the well elderly program.* Bethesda, MD: American Occupational Therapy Association.

Richmond, T. (2004). Marketing Plan. In T. Richmond, & D. Powers, (Eds.), *Business Fundamentals For the Rehabilitation Professional* (pp. 81–97). Thorofare, NJ: Slack Publishers.

Richmond, T. (2003). Marketing. In G. McCormack, E. Jaffe, & M. Goodman-Lavey, (Eds.), *The occupational therapy manager,* (4th ed., pp. 177–192). Bethesda, MD: AOTA Press.

Ryan, J. D., Ray, R., & Hiduke, G. (1999). *Small business: An entrepreneur's plan.* Fort Worth, TX: The Dryden Press.

Shoemaker, T., & Wheeler C. (1996). Marketing, In F. McCarrey, & M. Fisk, (Eds.), *The occupational therapy manager,* Bethesda, MD: American Occupational Therapy Association.

## Internet Resources

Information on Web advertising and building a Web site: www.e-land.com
Information on Direct Mail Advertising: www.dmworld.com
SCORE, a nonprofit association of retired and active business owners and executives providing education for entrepreneurs and to encourage small companies, is located in Washington, D.C. and is sponsored by the U.S. Small Business Administration. Volunteers offer counseling in the areas of writing a business plan, managing cash flow, and obtaining capital. Workshops are offered around the country. Contact SCORE at www.score.org or at 1-800-634-0245 (for SCORE chapter information).

CHAPTER 14

# Program Evaluation: How Will Outcomes Be Measured?

## Learning Objectives

1. To understand the purpose of program evaluation in achieving and maintaining quality services
2. To identify various methods that may be used to measure program effectiveness
3. To understand the link between the goal(s) and objectives of the program and the evaluation of outcomes
4. To evaluate outcome measures in earlier researched evidence-based practices with similar goals and populations
5. To consider the formative and summative measurement of individual progress to facilitate the measurement of program outcomes
6. To explore the rationale for selecting both quantitative and qualitative measures to evaluate program outcomes and to ensure quality
7. To distinguish between the various levels of evaluation
8. To appreciate the value of participatory action in development and evaluation of community programs
9. To develop an evaluation plan for the program you are designing and developing

## Key Terms

1. Program Evaluation
2. Stakeholders/Participants/Clients
3. Program Effectiveness
4. Outcome Evaluation
5. Formative and Summative Measures of Outcome
6. Baseline Assessment Measures
7. Quantitative Measures of Outcome
8. Qualitative Measures of Outcome
9. Pretests and Posttests
10. Program Logic Models for Evaluation
11. Project Level Evaluation
12. Cluster Evaluation
13. Participatory Action/Participatory Action Research

What is program evaluation and why should it be done? C. MacDonell (1996, p. 398) describes **program evaluation** first of all as a "system" that is put into place "to provide information that an organization can use to improve performance to an agreed-on level that meets desired outcomes." Therefore, we know that program evaluation is intended to improve programming performance and that it does so in the process of meeting our desired outcomes (our goals and the accompanying objectives). Brownson, C. (2001) reminds us that an evaluation plan is a strategy; and, that it is developed as part of the overall program plan. Such a plan is only effective if it is done with the input of key **stakeholders** (partners, supporters) and, of course, present and potential **participants** or **clients** (Scaffa, 2001; p. 113).

For occupational therapy practitioners and other health care providers, the impetus for scrutinizing the effectiveness of our services began some thirty years ago with the then newly developing social programs, but it has only been in the last ten years that evaluation has become imperative for programs to remain viable. Certainly, through our unfolding history, we have placed the provision of quality patient care at the top of our priorities, and in providing that care we have focused our attentions on the process of therapy. In many ways, this attention to process at the exclusion of outcome has created inefficiency in our treatment styles and a tendency to trust in the effectiveness of our services rather than devise ways to effectively measure those outcomes.

The field of physical rehabilitation was perhaps most effective in the 1970s and 1980s in the refinement of outcome measures, but effective measurement of outcomes did not quite happen for psychosocial practices; we now see the results with shrinking service provision for the mentally ill. Since much of our work in the community considers the needs of those persons with severe and persistent mental illness, it is imperative that we work to refine outcome measures and determine the most efficient programming to obtain results. If our future is to include occupation-centered community-based programs in the areas of prevention and health maintenance, we will have an even greater challenge as we design and implement outcome measures. It is not only our obligation to be aware of the evidence that exists to support positive results of practice models, but to contribute to this work as well through publication of our designs, methods, and outcomes.

# Methods of Evaluation

Let's investigate further the different ways to evaluate **program effectiveness**. Forer describes **outcome evaluation** as the method of evaluation that "concentrates on the *results* of services, programs, treatments, or intervention strategies" (1996, Introduction). Our primary goal in all of our programming efforts is, of course, the evaluation of the effectiveness of our program—the full component of services. Weiss (1972) emphasizes that program evaluation is a broader concept than outcome evaluation and suggests that the components of program evaluation be expanded beyond outcome evaluation to include the following: needs assessment, process evaluation, program efficiency, program effectiveness, impact of the program, and outcome evaluation.

If you have worked with the guidelines of The Commission on Accreditation of Rehabilitation Facilities/Rehabilitation Accreditation Commission (CARF) or the Joint Commission on Accreditation of Healthcare Organizations (JCAHO), you know that these organizations place a great deal of emphasis on outcomes. CARF documents define program evaluation as "a systematic procedure for determining the effectiveness and efficiency with which results are achieved by persons served during the service delivery phase and following program completion . . . as well as the individual's satisfaction with them" (1995).

The programs' performance is always measured against the goals and objectives established by the planner or planning group. Therefore, the careful and accurate expression of the goal and the objectives coupled with a well articulated and comprehensive plan to achieve them will not only provide accurate guidelines for measurement of outcomes but also will ensure that those outcomes compare favorably with the intent of the planner and with other similar programs.

It is timely to revisit the evidence you've gleaned to support the goal(s), objectives, structure, and content of your programming. In the evidence-based practices, you reviewed what outcome measures were used to determine effectiveness. Are these appropriate for your circumstances? Using similar measures of effectiveness and reaching similar results will strengthen your programming and options for continued or new funding. Karsh and Fox (2003, pp. 166–167) and Knowles (2002, pp. 70–82), in discussions of program evaluation for successful grant applications, consider two levels of evaluation. The first level is evaluation of program implementation—carefully reviewing and evaluating what you've done—the process. The second level is that of program impact. What differences has the program made? Is there a strong indication that you've reduced the "need?"

# Will You Evaluate Individual Clients?

Certainly one cannot design a program with accompanying goal and objectives without considering the needs of the client/participant. Those needs collectively provide the basis for the program. All programs deliver services to a client/participant group and, for most programs, monitoring individual process and progress provides us with incremental measures that ultimately contribute to our evaluation of the program's effectiveness. These measures contribute to the **formative** evaluation process that is occurring at intervals throughout the program, both for the progress of the participants and the "process" of programming. These measures allow us to know how the group is responding to the objectives and goal of the program, and to the programming itself. Formative evaluations can identify where changes may be required in the process of delivering services. These formative measures are then coupled with **summative** measures that occur at the end of a programming cycle. You may wish to develop your own evaluation instrument(s) based on the goal and the objectives of your program. In some cases, you also may choose to purchase evaluation instruments for individual participants that are designed to accompany the theoretical orientation or frame(s) of reference you have selected to guide your programming.

You may need to research what is available for your population and your theoretical orientation and what will meet the needs structured by your objectives and your goal. Some assessments can be copied from texts or articles, while others are restricted. Hinojosa and Kramer (1998) have provided an excellent resource for client evaluation in their text, *Occupational Therapy Evaluation: Obtaining and Interpreting Data*. Another excellent resource is Asher's (1996) *Occupational Therapy Assessment Tools: An Annotated Index, 2nd edition*. You may wish to review both of these texts should you consider individual evaluation of clients/patients as part of your formative and/or summative program evaluation process. You may also want to review the extensive list of studies utilizing various outcome measures in Moyers' (1999) "The Guide to Occupational Therapy Practice" as well as your occupational therapy textbooks for lists of assessments appropriate to particular populations.

Your decision regarding individual assessments will be based on what the results of these will tell you about the effectiveness of your *program*. Your *program evaluation* is linked to the progress your individual clients make, so some consistent **baseline measure** of their performance must be made. In some instances, that measure will be made by other agencies/practitioners, and you will need to access the information.

For example, if we are providing day camp services for children who are presently being seen by other therapists, then we might assume that these children have already been evaluated. There is no need for us to further evaluate each child (at least not in the same way). Certainly we would collaborate with the therapist who is continuing to see the child or perhaps sees the child through a school year; we would have initiated this process with the needs assessment. The camp will provide intervention to "enhance" the treatment the child is receiving from the referring therapist and to assist in meeting the therapist's goals for the child. In addition, the camp experience might "supplement" the child's individual therapy with opportunities to learn socialization through structured group play.

In this example you might wish to go further and consider establishing baseline measures and continuing formative and summative measures around the goal of socialization/group play. Certainly your marketing efforts for such a camp would be enhanced if you could demonstrate indicators of success in addition to what you expect the child's primary therapist might identify.

In some kinds of programs, a structured interview may also be used to establish a baseline assessment. You would likely establish the interview format yourself, which certainly would be based on your goal and on your chosen theoretical orientation.

## Other Measures to Consider

In many of the programs described in this text, there is not individual measurement of progress as we may be accustomed to in our traditional models of evaluation and intervention, but we are always aware of the progress of individuals and that their goals and objectives are reflective of and companion to those of the program. For example, a program goal may target the development of moral judgment in adolescents as they transition to young adulthood. The goal may specifically target the development of skills to negate law-breaking in the community. Accompanying objectives may focus on skills to find work and a residence or perhaps the provision of opportunity to explore and engage in alternative meaningful occupations. All of these objectives are measurable, and all are related to outcomes. Not all of the adolescents participating in such a program may be successful in the attainment of each objective, and all may not accomplish the goal. It is important to remember, however, that a *program* may still be successful even if all of the participants are not. In some cases we will establish a measure of objective attainment at 80 percent of the participants; in some cases perhaps 100 percent can be realistic. We know that pretests and posttests can measure acquired information, and perhaps skill acquisition. Frequently, though, we attach further measurement to information and skill acquisition through monitoring such things as employability, graduation from school, and perhaps reports (or not) of delinquency or law breaking. Intermediate measures to get at changes enroute to other outcomes such as the measurement of efficacy, locus of control, perceived well being, and life satisfaction are helpful to see if our theoretical model supports anticipated outcomes.

Mandel, Jackson, Zemke, Nelson, and Clark (1999) utilized several measures of primary outcomes in the USC Well Elderly Research Study. Utilizing a pretest/posttest format with follow-up six months following completion of the programming, several instruments and measures were selected. Overall, the intent of programming was to improve health and slow aging-related declines in the elderly. Selected measures were the Functional Status Questionnaire (Jette and Cleary, 1987); Life Satisfaction Index-Z (Wood, Wylie, and Sheafor, 1969); Center for Epidemiologic Studies (CES) Depression Scale (Radloff, 1977); Medical Outcomes Study (MOS) Short Forms General Health Survey (Stewardt, Hays, and Ware, 1988); and RAND 36-Item Health Status Survey, Short Form-36 (RAND SF-36; Hays et al., 1993; Ware and Sherbourne, 1992). Collectively, these measures provided a comprehensive picture of the general health and well-being of the participants in the clinical trial before programming and following programming. The RAND SF-36 is particularly useful in measuring responses to much of our adult programming with populations seeking to maintain wellness and health. It is a self-report measure of health-related quality of life (HRQL) that was designed to measure health status efficiently from the consumer's perspective. (Mandel, Jackson, Zemke, Nelson, and Clark, 1999; pp. 57–58; McHorney, Ware, and Raczek, 1993). The RAND SF-36 groups question items into eight domains: general health, mental health, physical functioning, social functioning, role limitations attributable to physical health problems, role limitations attributable to emotional problems, bodily pain, and vitality.

The best way to evaluate the objectives and ultimately the goal of your program is to ask yourself the following questions: How will I know if *that* actually happens? When and how will I measure *it* when it does? All programs must be able to evaluate effectiveness in order to justify their continued existence. Such evaluation will not only justify their continuation, but also will provide the information that is needed to continue to improve the match between the goal, the objectives, and the programming. This is the function of formative evaluation. The day-to-day program enables you to meet the program objectives and ultimately the goal. If objectives are not being met, then alterations, adjustments, and fine-tuning may be made in day-to-day programming. If the goal is not satisfied, then likely these adjustments are required in the objectives as well.

There are several dimensions or tiers of measurement needed to fully evaluate a program. We begin program evaluation by determining the dimensions within which we will establish measure of program success.

# Measuring Outcomes in a Head Start Program for Children

To provide an example of outcome measurement in an occupation-centered community-based program, we will highlight a program established to support the mission and goals of Head Start. As you may know, Head Start is a federally mandated program designed to aid preschool children in the attainment of skills that have been determined to be necessary for successful achievement when they enter school.

Children who qualify for Head Start programs are those considered to be "at risk" with regard to lower economic status, some level of involvement with social services-child protective services, or physical and/or emotional disabilities.

As with all program design, the Head Start program was initiated with the community and population profiles followed by the needs assessments. The mission and philosophy of the Head Start program was discussed with the director and teaching staff of the selected site. In this first phase of needs assessment, which also included teachers in the district schools these children would attend, several unmet needs were identified that were appropriate for occupation-centered programming. The teachers expressed a strong desire to assist parents in assuming the role of prime educator of their child; through this process they would help to identify potential problems the child might be experiencing. They specifically identified the need for fine-motor/prewriting skill development and the additional need for early screening to determine which children might require more specific intervention before they enter school as opposed to those who might benefit from a little extra help in school or at home. In the focus group utilized for Phase II and performance skills deficits assessment, parents were concerned that they did not know what behaviors they should look for in their child that might present problems in school. If they did suspect problems, they did not know what to do about them. All parents concurred that they would like to help their child be ready for school if they knew what to do.

The goal of the program was essentially the same as that of the larger organization: To enhance the children's successful entry into school through parent-teacher-child teamwork.

The objectives to enable the accomplishment of the above program goal were:

1. The parents and teachers will be provided with information and activities to assist them in identifying deficits in the child's development that may indicate potential problems in school.
2. The parents and teachers will be provided with games and activities to engage in with children to encourage the development of fine-motor/prewriting skills.
3. Early developmental screening by occupational therapy practitioners will be conducted to assist in determining which children may require more extensive assessment and intervention.

The program provided a number of training sessions to parents and to teachers. Materials were developed to meet the needs of both groups in their efforts to help their children prepare for school. In addition, home and Head Start program visits and observations by occupational therapy practitioners and occupational therapy students assisted both parents and teachers in learning to identify potential problems. These visits were coupled with developmental screening of each child in the Head Start program. This program provided what might be considered both indirect and direct services. In community programming—perhaps in all occupation-centered programming—it is important to provide services that will empower the recipient and the family to share in meeting the responsibilities required to satisfy the program goal.

# Initiating Program Evaluation

Now that we have our goal and our objectives and we have conducted the program for a period of time, we must ask ourselves the following questions: Is the program effective? Does it do what we think it does? Did we satisfy our objectives? Did we meet our goal? Were we successful? There are several steps to be accomplished before we can answer these questions and determine whether or not we are successful in meeting our goal. First we must measure the objectives we have established to permit us to meet our goal. If our objectives are accurate in their expression of our goal and if they are measurable, we will have no problems in accomplishing this first phase of evaluation.

To return to our example, there were three objectives for the Head Start occupation-centered program. All three objectives are measurable:

1. Parents and teachers **will be provided with information and activities** to assist them in identifying deficits in the child's development that may indicate potential problems in school.
2. The parents and teachers **will be provided with games and activities** to participate in with children to encourage the development of fine-motor/prewriting skills.
3. **Early developmental screening by occupational therapy practitioners will be conducted** to assist in determining which children may require more extensive assessment and intervention.

Regardless of the parameters of time established (such as one month, six months, one year, and so on), we should be able to measure these objectives. Did we provide the parents and teachers with information and activities to assist them in identifying deficits in the child's development that may indicate potential problems in school? Did we provide parents and teachers with games and activities to participate in with children to encourage the development of fine-motor/prewriting skills? And did we provide early developmental screening by occupational therapy practitioners to assist in determining which children may require more extensive assessment and intervention?

Even though we always begin by measuring the objectives established for our program, this alone is not enough. Even if we can clearly answer yes to all of the above objectives, we really know nothing about the effectiveness or success of our program. We simply know that our program has provided the services that we promised. A positive evaluation of an objective that is designed to measure the dissemination of information and materials is only as meaningful as the *quality of the materials* and the *mode of dissemination*. Our professional knowledge, skills, and experience contribute to our clinical reasoning in helping us to provide the programming (the information and materials) that will be effective.

Recall our example of the Denver sanctuary program. The goal of encouraging self-efficacy was enabled through an objective of providing developmentally appropriate information and skills with which to make informed choices about practiced sexual behaviors. As was mentioned previously, this is very different than simply offering condoms. The success of this program is contingent on all of the embedded "clues" known to occupation-centered practitioners. By linking efficacy to cognitive and moral development and to the expression of sexuality as occupation, our clinical reasoning guides us to arrive at a program that does far more than provide information and skills; rather, we can provide information and skills that result in the program's success.

## Exercise 1

### The First Step in Program Evaluation: Measuring Objectives

1. Considering the previous examples, discuss with your classmates or colleagues ideas for how you will measure the program you are designing. Revisit your goal and your objectives. In the space provided, write the goal or goals for your program, your objectives to support your goal, and the time you have established for measurement.

Your goal:

_____

_____

_____

Your objectives:

_____

_____

_____

_____

_____

Reexamine the evidence gleaned in your early research that was used to support your programming model. What measures of outcome were used? Were individual assessments/measures utilized in gathering outcome data? Consider whether or not you will use individual assessments and, if so, what you will use. Will you be able to obtain baseline assessment data for your population from other sources?

For each of your objectives noted above, determine the quantitative measures that you will utilize.

---
 

---
 

---
 

---
 

---
 

---

Clearly the first step in evaluating any program is to meet the objectives we have established as our first line of measurement. These first measures are **quantitative**; that is, we determine who received the services and how often. Without first knowing that everyone has received the services specified in our objectives, we cannot go further to determine the **qualitative** measures necessary to evaluate whether or not our services met our expectations and therefore were effective.

By carefully logging contact hours with parents and teachers and by videotaping the informational meetings, it was clear that the foundation (the quantitative measure) of the first two objectives for the Head Start program had been satisfied (27 parents and 4 teachers had received the information).

Over the course of six weeks, all of the children (23) had been screened to determine if any of them might require more extensive assessment and intervention. Following review of the screening results, 6 children were referred for further occupational therapy assessment.

Following review of the three objectives that were established, it was determined that the third objective required no further evaluation. There were no qualitative measures required to further assess this objective as it was written. In fact, it is arguable whether or not this objective relates to the goal for the program, which was "to enhance the children's successful entry into school through parent-teacher-child teamwork." Though nothing in this objective directly relates to parent-teacher-child teams, there is certainly an assumption that early screening and any resultant intervention will enhance the child's successful transition to school. In any further work with this program, and to ensure funding for this objective, it would be necessary to evaluate this assumption through extensive literature review and by following each child's progress in school either by single case or compared to children who did not receive assessment and intervention.

The question of how we measure the outcomes to determine whether or not the program is effective, however, still remains. There are several methods—both quantitative and qualitative—we can use to accomplish this task.

## Pretests and Posttests

When we use the term *outcome*, we are referring to the results that were obtained at the completion of our program and, perhaps, at intervals after programming has ceased for the participant. However, as we've indicated previously, one cannot measure the result of a program, or a treatment for that matter, without first obtaining some kind of base measurement. If we were to use this method in our Head Start example, at the first meeting of parents, teachers, and occupational therapy practitioners, a brief **pretest** or questionnaire would be developed and administered to determine how much the teachers (one group) and parents (one group) knew about the developing child generally, how much they knew about the identification of potential deficits, and how much they knew about the development of fine-motor skills related to prewriting specifically.

For our example, the pretest would ask specific questions regarding the developmental markers for fine-motor coordination in children between the ages of 3 and 4 (the ages of the children in the program). A video might be used in conjunction with the questionnaire to provide examples of motor skills.

The same questionnaire/test (a **posttest**) would be given following the in-service or series of in-services. The comparison of responses to the pretests and posttests provides a further marker for how successful the intervention (the in-service) was in meeting the objective of providing information, games, and activities. Our posttest will also provide us with information as to how effective we were in developing materials that were appropriate to the needs of each group—parents and teachers. From this information, we could return to the materials and the way they were provided to make necessary changes to enhance their receptivity.

Since the first objective of our example suggests that the information we provide will assist the parent and teacher to identify any deficits in the child's development that may indicate potential problems in school, we will want to evaluate whether this happened or not in order to further ensure the effectiveness of our program. We might do so by asking the parents and the teachers to note any deficits they observe on a chart or check-sheet. This information might then be correlated with the results of the occupational therapy practitioner's screening. Positive correlations would add further strength to the results provided by this objective. If these correlations were not found, then we might wish to return to our programming to determine how we might be more effective. Stronger and more definitive research designs might also be employed to measure the effectiveness of this program (see the reference list at the end of this chapter for examples of such measures).

Meeting the second objective goes beyond the quantitative measure of providing games and activities and assumes participation by parent-teacher-child to encourage the development of fine-motor prewriting skills. To provide a valid measurement of this objective, each child's fine-motor prewriting skills would need to be measured before the program (pretest) and again following the program (posttest). Although these tests would not provide enough information to definitively say that our program supported improvement in these skills, such test results could strongly suggest such a finding, particularly if we had measures of normative parent-child or teacher-child participation in our suggested games and activities.

## Revisiting Goals

It is wise to continue to revisit our goal to be sure that our evaluation of objectives has not caused us to become blind to our purpose. Although the objectives for our example are sound and do relate clearly to the goal, it is likely that we will want to have one or two more. None of the objectives truly address the idea of *teams* mentioned in our goal, and as indicated in earlier chapters, teams can be empowering. Teamwork assumes a sharing of responsibility and equal distribution of rewards. Without a specific objective, we do not know whether we have established programming that will encourage the formation of teams or the philosophies and ideas that support teamwork. Without such an objective, the child appears to be the targeted "problem" in this program rather than a shareholder in the outcome. Although not formally tied to an objective, videotaping all aspects of the program offered a potential opportunity to qualitatively evaluate the formation of teams from the early stages of program design through actual programming, and the elements of teamwork did emerge. You might like to write an objective that would target the development of parent-child-teacher teams to help us more fully support our goal. Our goal also uses the subjective term "successful" to describe the desired transition from Head Start to school. Our objectives translate the results of our needs assessment into the skills we believe to be necessary for this transition to successfully occur. The results of the needs assessment also identified the need for children to be socialized to the school environment before actually entering, although we did not develop an objective to meet this need. Can you suggest one?

## Exercise 2

### Going Beyond Quantitative Measures . . . to Measure Quality

1. Again review your objectives and your goal(s). Are there further measures you will need to make in order to determine the effectiveness of your program? How will you measure the quality of your program? First consider other quantitative measures, then more qualitative ones. Note what additional measures you will require below.

_____

_____

_____

_____

_____

2. Do you have a mode of measurement for every aspect of your objectives? Will the results of these measures determine whether or not you have met the goal(s) for your program? Will they help you determine if changes in programming may be necessary? Make notations below for any alterations you may need to make now.

_____

_____

_____

_____

_____

Continuing program evaluation at whatever interval you've determined— three months, six months, yearly (or all of these)—will also be the time you reevaluate your goals. Even a year is likely too soon to alter the original goals and certainly too soon to throw them out and start over, but it is not too soon to make changes in objectives and/or programming. This will also be the time to evaluate staffing, costs, and the program environment. How do these factors impact the quantity and the quality of your intervention? Most federal granting agencies expect at least yearly outcome reports and provide the program a two- or three-year running period before reapplying for continuation. This offers a reasonable time to measure outcomes and make minor alterations in programming. Consider, too, repeating your phases of needs assessment as a way of evaluating the connection between need, your goal(s), and your program design. You may wish to conduct a focus group as a qualitative measure of program effectiveness whether or not you used this technique in assessing need. Such a group can provide a strong measure of how you are doing. A focus group of parents and one of teachers would be extremely useful as a formative or a summative measure for our Head Start example.

## Outcomes Over Time

It is often of interest and/or critical to determine if your program has lasting effectiveness after the program has been terminated for the participant. We have alluded to this in our Head Start example with the recommendation that the children be followed through their school experience to effectively determine whether or not we have enhanced their progress and success. Evaluation over time is more difficult to achieve and will require more manpower and financial resources than formative and summative short-term evaluations. A long-term follow-up evaluation will require a system to track participants and a set of measures related to your original goals. If follow-up effectiveness seems critical to what you want to achieve, then your original goal(s) should state the follow-up outcomes as well as the immediate measures of success.

If you intend to manage numerous outcome measures, particularly over time, then you will need an effective data management system to do so. Forer (1996) also offers a substantial reference section that provides a list of publications describing programming in a variety of disability areas as well as outcome evaluation techniques appropriate to differing kinds of programming. Review the discussion of sample programs in Part V for examples of program evaluation plans and instruments.

## Present and Future Trends in Evaluation

There is little doubt that our present emphasis on establishing programs that ensure successful programatic outcomes will continue, and with more expectation of rigour than ever before. Outcomes and funding will not likely ever be separated. The Kellogg Foundation (2001) is reflective of present interest in evaluation. The Foundation identified their core mission "to help people help themselves through the practical application of knowledge and resources to improve their quality of life and that of future generations" (Intro). In line with its core mission, as early as 1998 the Foundation made evaluation a priority.

Their recent guide to evaluation is designed to assist programmers in the use of the **program logic model** to facilitate evaluation. The program logic model is defined as "a picture of how your organization does its work . . . the theory and assumptions underlying the program" ". . . such a model links both short and long-term outcomes with program activities/processes and the theoretical assumptions/principles of the program" (Introduction). The approach to programming described in this text (need, goal, objectives, theory) establishes a sound foundation to layer the language of a logic approach to evaluation.

In its simplest form, the logic model begins with a picture of your program (the multiple profiles, the structure, the programming). This picture includes your theoretical base and the rationale for your approach, and what you put into the program (action—inputs), will result in an anticipated outcome (outputs). This is a sequence of "if-then" relationships and may be considered the core of planning and evaluation. Outputs, then, are a result of what we do (activities) and who we do it for (participation). Outcomes, according to the logic model, are what results for individual participants, for organizations, and ultimately for communities.

Evaluation is recommended at three levels. The **project level** is where we have focused in this text; measuring the effectiveness of our specific programming as efficiently as we can. The second level is **cluster evaluation**; aggregating outcomes of projects with similar goals across the country to monitor change. The third is to use the levels of outcome measurement to influence policymaking (1998, p. 14).

The planner may choose differing approaches to utilization of the logic model. The theory approach models emphasize the theory of change that has influenced the design and plan for the program. The outcomes approach models focus on the early aspects of program planning and attempt to connect the resources and/or activities with the desired results in a program. These models likely measure change (outcomes prompted by a given set of activities) over time: short term (1–3 years), long-term (4–6 years), and impact (7–10 years) (Kellogg, 2001; pp. 9–10). The activities approach models pay the most attention to the details and specifics of the implementation process. These models describe what a program intends to do and, as such, are most useful for the purpose of program monitoring and management. The reader is encouraged to visit the Kellogg (2001) Foundation Web site and others listed at the close of the chapter for current information on evaluation, particularly as it is linked to potential funding of programs.

# Service Development and Program Evaluation

## Participatory Action Research

**Participatory action research**, in fact, informs several sections of this text. It is placed here because it can be extremely useful as a method/process to support program evaluation; however, as an extension of empowerment theory, it informs much of our goal development in community-based practices. Participatory action research is particularly well suited to community intervention as it involves consumer participation, power, and leadership. It can inform the development, implementation, and evaluation of services (Reason and Bradbury, 2001; Taylor, Braveman, and Hammell, 2004; Suarez-Balcazar, Martinez, and Casa-Byots, 2005).

Just what is this mode of inquiry and practice we're describing as participatory action? In their edited text, Reason and Bradbury (2001) emphasize the intent with the suggestion that knowledge is always gained through action (2005, p. 4). Not that this is a unique idea; however, the participation of all stake-holders and the empowerment that is intrinsic in this participation is unique. Action research, as a method, may be described as a participatory democratic process concerned with "developing practical knowing in the pursuit of worthwhile human purposes" (Reason and Bradbury, 2001, Introduction). Such a method seeks to bring together action and reflection, theory and practice, in participation with others. It can be described as a practical method because it seeks solutions to practical problems (what people grapple with every day of their lives); and, in fact, practical problem solving is the venue of community practitioners.

"Community" implies "people" mutually involved in identifying problems and seeking solutions. First identifying and then solving problems requires collective "action;" sharing strategies, information, and skills. Thus participatory action is the crux, whether it contributes to the development of a community-based program, and/or the evaluation as well as contributing to the research base for scaffolding further understanding and inquiry.

## Participatory Action Research: Some Examples

Participatory action research has been a central methodology to both rural and urban development in the third world for more than two decades. Huizer (1997) describes projects to enhance people's participation in development on their own behalf in Thailand, Sri Lanka, Zambia, and Sierra Leone. Sharing in common, empowerment of the poor, all of these examples were described as grass roots efforts for peasant organization and adult education (Huizer, 1997; p. 2). It is with these same interests that the programming descriptions shared by Kronenberg, Algado, and Pollard (2005) offer us examples of a kind of community practice driven exclusively by the expressed needs of the people involved. The practitioner is there to provide what is needed to help people (empower them) to solve their own problems—guidance, encouragement, information, skills training, and effective ways to disassemble the bureaucracies. Is this not what all community practices should be?

Occupational therapy practitioners are also using participatory action methods in community programming, evaluation and research. Taylor, Braveman and Hammel (2004) describe their recent work utilizing this approach with two case examples: one with persons who have chronic fatigue syndrome and the other with persons who have autoimmune deficiency syndrome (AIDS). As in other successful participatory action approaches, services and outcomes were consumer driven and relevant. Participants in both projects were empowered to "recognize, use, and build upon their existing resources to accomplish their goals" (Taylor, Braveman, and Hammel, 2004, p. 81). Addressing the needs of an underserved Hispanic population in the Midwest represents the participatory action research of Suarez-Balcazar, Martinez, and Casas-Byots (2005). Community residents participated in five public forums or focus groups intended to elicit needs, establish action agendas, and brainstorm solutions to address health and community needs that included the lack of affordable bilingual dentists and youth involvement in gangs, drugs, and alcohol (Suarez-Balcazar, Martinez, and Casas-Byots, 2005; p. 146).

Both of these examples emphasize the collaborative relationship between participant and practitioner. Both groups broadened their skills and knowledge through participation/action.

## A Call to Contribute to the "Evidence"

Chapter 8 offered a description of how one may go about retrieving evidence that programs such as the one you're considering are effective. Implicit in this description is the obligation that we all share, as community programmers, to contribute to this body of evidence through publication of our own comprehensive evaluation measures. You may do this independently in presentations and/or articles or in collaboration with others who are doing similar work. As you explore the existing practice evidence, note the practitioners and researchers who are doing the work; talk to them about supporting their efforts through your own data gathering. Always remember that effective and comprehensive program evaluation is key to ongoing program success.

## *Summary*

This chapter has provided the rationale for program evaluation. The reader is reminded always to link the goal or goals of the program and the objectives to the evaluation of outcome. Not only is program evaluation necessary to determine the effectiveness of a program, but it also can provide a measure of the quality of the programming. Both measures of effectiveness and quality are necessary to enhance the successful future of a program and often are necessary to guarantee its continuation. These measures will also provide information with regard to the effectiveness of your staffing and the impact of your intervention environment and may also help you reevaluate costs. You have also been introduced to various tools and approaches for measuring outcomes, as well as present and future trends in evaluation measures.

# *References*

Asher, E. (1996). *Occupational therapy assessment tools: An annotated index* (2nd ed.). Bethesda, MD: American Occupational Therapy Association.

Brownson, C. (2001). Program development for community health: Planning. Implementation, and evaluation strategies. In M. Scaffa, (Ed.), *Occupational Therapy in Community-Based Practice Settings.* Philadelphia: F. A. Davis (pp. 95–118).

Commission on Accreditation of Rehabilitation Facilities (CARF). (1995, January). *Survey standards for medical rehabilitation.* Tucson, AZ: Author.

Forer, S. (1996). *Outcome management and program evaluation made easy: A toolkit for occupational therapy practitioners.* Bethesda, MD: American Occupational Therapy Association.

Hays, R. D., Sherbourne, C. D., & Mazel, R. M. (1993). The RAND 36-Item Health Survey 1.0. *Health Economy,* 2, (217–227).

Hinojosa, J., & Kramer, P. (Eds.). (1998). *Occupational therapy evaluation: Obtaining and interpreting data.* Bethesda, MD: American Occupational Therapy Association.

Huizer, G. (1997). Participatory action research and people's participation: Introduction and case studies. Third World Centre, Catholic University of Nijmegen, The Netherlands.

Jette, A. M., & Cleary, P. D. (1987). Functional disability assessment. *Physical Therapy,* 67, (1854–1859).

Karsh, E., & Fox, A. (2003). *The Only Grant-Writing Book You'll Ever Need.* New York: Carroll and Graf Publishers.

Kellogg, W. K., Foundation. (2001). *Logic Model Development Guide.* Battle Creek, MI: W. K. Kellogg Foundation.

———. (1998). *The Evaluation Handbook.* Battle Creek, MI: W. K. Kellogg Foundation.

Knowles, C. (2002). *The First-Time Grantwriter's Guide to Success.* Thousand Oaks, CA: Corwin Press.

Kronenberg, F., Algado, S., & Pollard, N. (2005). *Occupational therapy without borders: Learning from the spirit of survivors.* London: Elsevier.

MacDonell, C. (1996). Program evaluation. In AOTA (Eds.). *The occupational therapy manager* (pp. 398–410). Bethesda, MD: American Occupational Therapy Association.

Mandel, D., Jackson, J., Zemke, R., Nelson, L., & Clark, F. (1999). *Lifestyle redesign: Implementing the well elderly program.* Bethesda, MD: The American Occupational Therapy Association.

McHorney, C. A., Ware, J. E., and Raczek, A. E. (1993). The MOS 36-Item Short Form Health Survey (SF-36): II. Psychometric and clinical tests of validity in measuring physical and mental health constructs. *Medical Care,* 31, (247–263).

Moyers, P. (1999). The guide to occupational therapy practice. Appendix F: Outcomes. *American Journal Of Occupational Therapy,* 53 (3), 298–322.

Radloff, L. (1977). The CES-D Scale: A self-report depression scale for research in the general population. *Applied Psychological Measures,* 1, (385–401).

Reason, P., & Bradbury, H. (2001). Handbook of action research: *Participative inquiry and practice.* London: Sage.

Suarez-Balcazar, Y., Martinez, L., & Casas-Byots, C. (2005). "A Participatory action research approach for identifying health service needs of hispanic immigrants: Implications for occupational therapy. In P. Crist, & G. Kielhofner, (Eds.), The scholarship of practice: Academic practice collaborations for promoting occupational therapy. Occupational Therapy in Health Care, Vol. 19, No. 1/2. Binghamton, NY: Haworth Press.

Stewart, A. L., Hays, R. D., & Ware, J. E. (1988). The MOS Short-Form General Health Survey. *Medical Care,* 26, (724–735).

Taylor, R., Braveman, B., & Hammel, J. (2004). Developing and evaluating community based services through participatory action research: Two case examples. *American Journal of Occupational Therapy,* 58(1), 73–82.

Ware, J. E., & Sherbourne, C. D. (1992). The MOS 36-Item Short-Form Health Survey (SF-36): I. *Medical Care,* 30, (473–481).

Weiss. C. (1972). Evaluation research: *Methods for assessing program effectiveness.* Englewood Cliffs, NJ: Prentice Hall.

Wood, V., Wylie, M. L., & Sheafor, B. (1969). An analysis of a short self-reported measure of life satisfaction. *Journal of Gerontology,* 24, (465–469).

## Internet Resources

W. K. Kellogg Foundation web site: http://www.wkkf.org

Joint Commission on Accreditation of Healthcare Organizations (JCAHO) web site: http://www.jcaho.org

Logic Models Information and Examples: University of Nevada, Reno Western CAPT web site:
     http://www.unr.edu/colleges/educ/captta/prev/evaluate.html

Rehabilitation Accreditation Commission (CARF) web site: http://www.carf.org

United Way of America's Outcome Models web site:
     http://www.unitedway.org/outcomes/contents.htm

## Additional Resources

Bickman, L. (Ed.). (1987). Using program theory in evaluation. *New Directions for Program Evaluation Series (no. 33).* San Francisco, CA: Jossey-Bass.

Rossi, P. H., Freeman, H. E., & Lipsey, M. W. (1999). *Evaluation: A systematic approach.* Thousand Oaks, CA: Sage.

Schmitz, C. C. & Parsons, B. A. (1999). *Everything you wanted to know about logic models but were afraid to ask.* Battle Creek, MI: W. K. Kellogg Foundation.

Wholey, J. S., Hatry, H. P., & Newcomer, K. E. (Eds.). (1994). *Handbook of Practical Program Evaluation.* San Francisco, CA: Jossey-Bass Publishers.

CHAPTER 15

# Programming to Support Meaningful Occupation and Balance for the Disenfranchised and Homeless: The Development of a Proposal

## Learning Objectives

1. To appreciate the condition of homelessness
2. To understand the impact of homelessness on the program participants' choices and on their participation in occupation
3. To appreciate the impact of severe and persistent mental illness on the occupations of homeless persons
4. To identify how a shelter may be utilized as a site for occupation-centered programs
5. To follow the development of a programming proposal from identification of need to outcomes

## Key Terms

1. Disenfranchised
2. Homelessness
3. Homelessness and Severe/Persistent Mental Illness
4. The Sunshine Mission

# Introduction and Background

According to *Webster's Dictionary* (1975), the definition of **disenfranchised** is "to deprive of the right to vote or some other right of citizenship." Therefore, the use of the word in connection to the homeless population is not entirely accurate, although it does carry with it an assumption as to the *rights of a citizen*. If the citizen has obligations to the community (such as governance, taxation, and so on), does not the community have obligations to the citizen? Having access to shelter is the foundation for any attention to meaningful occupation and must be attended to for the achievement of purpose.

Approximately 7 million people (men, women, and children) experienced **homelessness** in the latter half of the 1990s (National Coalition for the Homeless, 1997; CalWorks: Homeless Families, 2005); and, at any one time, approximately 20 to 25 percent of the single, adult homeless population are considered to be experiencing some form of **severe and persistent mental illness** (Koegel, 1996). The general deinstitutionalization of the mentally ill during the 1950s and 1960s may have initiated some of the developing increase in homelessness; however, the vast increases in homelessness did not occur until the 1980s (Federal Task Force on Homelessness and Severe Mental Illness, 1992). Why did this occur? Koegel (1996), Kaufman (1997), and the report of the Federal Task Force on Homelessness and Severe Mental Illness (1992) attribute the cause, among other things, to the general decrease in incomes and to the loss of housing options for the marginalized populations. The mentally ill experience these causes as well as those associated with debilitating illness and frequently the inability to access or receive therapy services. They are also likely to remain homeless for longer periods of time and have less contact with family and friends than others who are homeless. Their opportunities for employment are fewer, and they tend to be in poorer physical health than their homeless peers (Federal Task Force on Homelessness and Severe Mental Illness, 1992). Although it has been a widely accepted belief that the homeless mentally ill refuse rehabilitative services, Oakley and Dennis (1996) reported that homeless individuals with serious mental illness are willing to use services that are easily accessible and that meet their perceived needs. Of course, there are others who are homeless and have debilitating illness such as drug and alcohol abuse and Human Immunodeficiency Virus (HIV). These persons require similar access to services as do the mentally ill. When rehabilitation includes active case management, therapy, housing options, and long-term follow-up and support services coupled with *meaningful daily activity in the community* (including work), homelessness can come to an end (Oakley and Dennis, 1996).

According to the Federal Task Force on Homelessness and Severe Mental Illness (1992), only 5 to 7 percent of homeless persons with mental illness need to be institutionalized; most can live successfully in the community but not without supportive services that include housing options. Unfortunately, there are currently not enough of either in any of the large urban areas of the United States. We are not without options, however; such programs as the Projects for Assistance in

Transition from Homelessness, or PATH (Wells, 1996), and the many community-based programs across the country of which occupational therapists are an active part can make a difference.

There are also homeless who are living with Acquired Immunodeficiency Syndrome (AIDS) and other illnesses caused by HIV. These persons, an estimated 36 percent of whom have been homeless since learning that they had HIV or AIDS, experience many of the same problems of avoidance and stigma as do those who are mentally ill (O'Connell, Lozier, and Gingles, 1997; Robbins and Nelson, 1996). In many ways there may be less public support for this population than for the seriously mentally ill, particularly when it comes to employment and supportive housing. A related problem is experienced by homeless adolescents who often engage in sex in exchange for food, clothing, and shelter, for they are at great risk for contracting HIV-related illnesses. Robertson (1996) reported on the results of a series of studies performed in four cities across the United States in which a median HIV-positive rate of 2.3 percent for homeless persons under age 25 was found.

We have identified some of the problems of the homeless who are ill, but who are the homeless who are not ill? Do they share common characteristics whether they are found in urban areas or in rural ones? Do the homeless populations in the East, Midwest, South, or West have common characteristics? Even though we are able to make estimates of the numbers of homeless persons based on the numbers of people in shelters and on the street, those estimates are undoubtedly below the actual numbers. Many people who lack a stable, permanent residence and, for example, are living from friend to friend or in a car have fewer shelter options and remain uncounted. In fact, in a recent study of homelessness in 50 U.S. cities, the estimated number of homeless people greatly exceeded the number of emergency shelter and transitional housing spaces (National Law Center on Homelessness and Poverty, 1996). As reported by Waxman and Trupin (1997), there is a nationwide shortage of emergency shelters. In addition, Aron and Fitchen (1996) reported that, although there are significant numbers of homeless in rural areas of the United States, there are virtually no shelters. Where there are few shelters, it is also likely that there are fewer support programs.

Most of the adults who are homeless, particularly the families, have experienced loss of employment. This loss, coupled with little formal education or vocational training, often prompts moves across the country in search of opportunities, which often results in becoming homeless in a strange city. Women with children may also become a part of this scenario when they are abandoned or divorced and have no resources or employment skills. Loss of employment is certainly not the only contributor to homelessness, but it is a significant one.

Programming for the homeless or near homeless can take many forms, ranging from those that are conducted within shelters that provide the basics of comfort and safety to day shelter programs that provide temporary housing and a balance of occupations for at least the waking hours. Dear (1996) noted that the homeless are sometimes referred to as the service dependent. By intention or neglect, those services that are accessed by the homeless, including health care, social welfare, emergency shelter, and job training, are most often localized to those areas of the city known as skid row or a similar term. This area, which becomes the *community* of the homeless, is where they live, eat, talk to friends, and oftentimes work. According to Dear, it is a well-defined time-space prism, and it is a coping mechanism for the homeless (Dear, 1996; p. 109). Perhaps this *community* is a sanctuary just as your home may be after a long work week. Most likely any occupation-centered programming, as an extension of this service network, will also be part of this *community*. Any effort to move programming outside of the location where homeless people are congregated is often met with resistance from those living in the outside neighborhood or community. Whether this resistance is merited or not, if programming is to occur outside and a new community is to be created, we would expect that there are related goals to make this the most desirable circumstance. If this is the case, we must consider accessibility and motivation, and a transitional program might be the best way to initiate services.

Programs can be provided for children and adolescents within various educational formats (formal or shelter schools), but attention must be focused on the needs and concerns of these children who have lived without homes and the safety of a stable shelter. Neville-Jan and associates describe one such program that included foster care children who had experienced homelessness (Neville-Jan, 1997; pp. 144–157). Although this program included a broad range of children with varying needs, during the course of the programming it was noted that the children who had experienced what might be described as the culture of homelessness were more likely to engage in protective negative social behaviors such as hoarding of supplies, lying, and petty theft—attributes that were likely extremely adaptive on the street. Certainly these characteristics challenge the practitioner beyond what might be expected when programming focuses on the development of social skills and behaviors that enhance and support learning.

Chapters 18 and 19 will describe several programs that were designed for and conducted with homeless and near homeless persons. The following example is a description of student-designed programming for a homeless women's shelter. This example will provide you with a step-by-step discussion, from the first examination of the site and the population to the final steps of evaluation. This example describes the process recommended for your own programming plan and proposal development, although the order and depth may vary. This description will be followed by less inclusive examples of several other programs targeting persons in varying situations of homelessness and illness; as well as programs for those who are believed to be at risk for illness, injury, and delinquency. All of these should provide you with ideas you can use for programming with similar populations in your area.

# Programming for a Homeless Women's Shelter

## The Site

Founded in 1941 by radio evangelist Sister Essie Binkey West, the **Sunshine Mission** began to offer shelter to homeless women in downtown Los Angeles. In later years the city condemned the downtown facility and another was purchased just north of the University of Southern California campus. Functioning first as a school, then as a hotel, and then a USO facility, this building, Casa de Rosas, enjoyed a colorful history. In 1951, Sister West moved her entire Old Time Faith programs, including her radio broadcasts, publications, and services to the homeless and needy, to this site, and she remained there until her death in 1976. The Old Time Faith operated with donations from Sister West's followers, and some of them continue to support the Sunshine Mission with donations today.

In 1989 the organization ended its religious affiliation and reorganized itself into Casa de Rosas, Inc.; a tax-exempt California corporation. The volunteer board of directors and management team initiated numerous programs to restore the agency both physically and financially. Support presently includes a range of government contracts, corporate charitable grants, fund-raising events, and regular individual donations. The physical structure was recently renovated by the city and the state as a historical residential project. The building now is an example of the community's architectural history and an example of modern, safe housing for its homeless and low-income citizens.

Today the Sunshine Mission provides housing, food, and life necessities to adult single women for periods of thirty to sixty days. The Mission can comfortably house 20 women per night, and each woman is expected to work with the shelter manager to develop and implement a plan to assist her in returning to independent living.

Adjoining the Sunshine Mission is the Casa de Rosas Hotel (1996), which provides single-occupancy accommodations for the near homeless. Residents include senior citizens, the disabled, people in recovery, and working people of low income. The hotel can house 45 tenants who pay low monthly rents.

The above information incorporates the mission statement of Casa de Rosas, Inc. (1996), portions of the Agency Effectiveness Report, and Phase I needs assessment interview material provided by the manager.

## The Community Profile

The Sunshine Mission is one of several connected buildings surrounding a central plaza and is secured from outside entry. It is located in South Central Los Angeles, approximately seven miles from downtown. The area is bordered by the 110 Freeway, the 10 Freeway, Vermont Street to the North, and the USC University Park campus to the South. The area is diverse with a mixed population of African

American and Hispanic low-income families. There are several gangs occupying territory in the adjacent neighborhoods, and although the Mission is secured, it is considered to be in a high-crime area. According to 2004 and 2005 Los Angeles Police Department (LAPD) statistics, nearly 50 percent of all crimes committed in Los Angeles County are perpetrated in the South Central area where the Mission is located (http://www.lapdonline.com).

## The Target Population

From our earlier discussion, it would appear that there are multiple factors that contribute to and sustain the problem of homelessness. Many of these are no different in Southern California than in the larger United States. According to a 1993 Report of the Glendale, California Task Force on Homelessness, some of these factors include illiteracy, lack of competitive job skills, substance abuse, emotional trauma from histories of child abuse, extensive employment layoffs, deinstitutionalization of the mentally ill, working poverty, and lack of affordable housing. Much of the reported information deals with the male homeless population, but it is not difficult to draw the assumption that women fare far less successfully when measured against the above list of factors. A recent report of CalWorks Homeless Families (2005) demonstrated that African American and Hispanic females headed most homeless families in Los Angeles County, and that females were more likely to seek shelter services than males.

Recent statistics provided by the Mission show that 60 percent of the women in residence were African American, 20 percent were Caucasian, and 20 percent were from various other cultural groups. The typical age range was from 26 to 45 years of age. Fifteen percent of the women reported a background of domestic violence, and 12 percent had a history of alcohol and/or drug abuse. The average educational level was completion of elementary school, and some had differing amounts of vocational training. Most of the women had held previous jobs (http://www.sunshinemission.org).

## The Needs Assessment

The shelter manager was contacted by student representatives to gain a perspective on what programs were currently being offered and what needs the residents might continue to have that could be considered in designing a useful and meaningful occupation-centered program. The manager was also questioned regarding past, present, and future trends concerning homeless women at the Mission.

The students then did further research to develop the service profile and determined that in 1995 the homeless population in Los Angeles was estimated to be approximately 83,900. The Shelter Partnership of Los Angeles (1995) estimated this population to be even larger. Statistics for the same area in 2004 demonstrated a slight increase. This information, coupled with a review of national as well as local community statistics over time, seemed to support a trend that the numbers of homeless would only increase and that their needs would become greater. In addition, women were becoming more proactive in seeking services and were advocates for other women. All of this information pointed to an increased demand for information and services tailored to the needs of women, and was useful when resources were required.

A search for evidence to support the direction of successful programming for women, or women with families, who were homeless resulted in a review of programs currently in place to include: Solutions at Work, Cambridge, MA; homeless shelter programs in Maryland to include Baltimore, Capital Heights, Frederick, Hagerstown, and Westminster; and personal contact with programs in Los Angeles County (see websites at the close of this chapter). A search of the occupational therapy literature resulted in descriptions of programming with similar populations reported by Tryssenaar, J.; Jones E. and Lee, D., "Occupational Performance Needs of a Shelter Population" identified first from the web site for the Canadian Journal of Occupational Therapy Abstracts, Vol. 66, No. 4, Oct. 1999.

According to the manager, during the Phase I assessment of need, the Mission and the residents would be most interested in programs to prepare the residents for the job-search process. A review of shelter programs and the report of CalWorks (2005) supported the need for programs with a work (or) return to work emphasis. Following this comprehensive review of the needs of shelter populations in general and women's shelters in particular, brain storming to generate ideas for programming that might be useful adjuncts to the present programs, and considering the manager's perspectives, a Phase II needs assessment was developed for distribution to the current residents.

Following a trial distribution, it was soon discovered that the Phase II assessment instrument was too broad and open-ended; residents requested services that the students were not prepared to provide or were beyond the scope of the program being considered. Thus, a second version of the Phase II needs assessment survey instrument was designed and distributed to residents in the dining hall. See Figure 15–1 for the Phase II needs assessment. The students distributed the assessment personally, answered questions, and collected the assessments before leaving the site. Distributing the needs assessment at a time when the majority of residents were available, answering questions, and collecting the completed assessments before leaving the site were all ways to ensure a maximum number of responses.

This second assessment instrument was aimed at identifying what realistically could be provided in a mission environment with very little financial support, but still meeting the needs identified in Phase I. This instrument incorporated the ideas of the students and the concerns of the manager. The students wanted to ensure that the programs could be utilized and were also cognizant of the need to design programs that could be conducted by volunteers from the community and perhaps by occupational therapy students without loss of the goal structure.

Results of this second questionnaire indicated that the largest percentage of residents identified employment skills and money management as being of greatest concern to them. Coping skills, followed by life skills, completed the ranking of the results.

FIGURE 15–1  Needs Assessment Survey

## Sunshine Mission Survey

We are interested in providing programming that will assist you in preparing for your return to the community. To do this we would like to know what activities you would find most useful. Please fill out this survey to help us identify your needs and interests.

### Check all that apply:

I am most interested in activities that will help me:

(Rate 1 through 6, with 1 being the area you are most interested in and 6 the area you are least interested in)

_____ learn how to get a new or better job

_____ meet people I can do things with

_____ learn about free or low-cost services in Los Angeles

_____ take better care of myself

_____ relax and enjoy life more

_____ develop new interests and/or skills

Things I would be interested in trying:

_____ arts and crafts

        anything in particular _____

_____ home skills

        _____ apartment hunting: how and what to expect

        _____ cooking/baking

        _____ nutrition/healthy meal planning

        _____ shopping/how to find coupons and discounts

        _____ small plot (or) community gardening

        _____ budget decorating

        _____ sewing

        _____ other (please describe): _____

_____ learning about the community

        _____ seeing Los Angeles on a budget

        _____ the Los Angeles library services

        _____ riding public transportation

        _____ activities of 'singles' organizations

        _____ assisting others in need of help

---

**Sunshine Mission Survey** (continued)

_____ Los Angeles community social services
_____ religious outings
_____ other (please describe): _____
_____ pre-employment skills
_____ how to "job search"
_____ developing a resume
_____ how to fill out a job application
_____ how to interview well
_____ other (please describe): _____
_____ self-care
_____ exercise classes
_____ how to relax and manage stress
_____ safety education/women's self-defense
_____ grooming and hygiene
_____ other (please describe): _____

Thanks for your time; you'll be seeing programs posted by the end of the month. See you there!

_____

_____

---

## Selection of a Theoretical Orientation to Support Goals and Programming

A collection of theories derived from occupational behavior perspectives is likely to be of most use in helping to understand and structure the selection of a rationale to guide programming for the women at the *Sunshine Mission*. Two are of particular importance: The Model of Human Occupation; and Occupational Adaptation. The Model of Human Occupation (MOHO) is useful in that it helps to structure our thinking as we approach our participants in those processes of occupational adaptation described as volition (personal causation, values, and interests) and the volitional processes incorporated under the broader category of habituation (habits and roles). (Kielhofner, 2002; Kielhofner, Forsyth, and Barrett, 2003). MOHO addresses motivation for occupation, the routine patterning of occupations, the nature of skilled performance, and the influence of environment on occupation

(Kielhofner, Forsyth, and Barrett, 2003; p. 212). All of these features are of significance for the women at the Mission as they engage in a normalizing round of daily activities in preparation for finding employment and living independently. Programming to encourage personal causation, engagement in activities of interest, awareness of the multi-contexts for performance, and the development of skills seems on target to meet the "needs" and to ensure positive outcomes.

The model of Occupational Adaptation is from the work of Schultz and Schkade (2003) and complements our interpretation of the Model of Human Occupation. Occupational Adaptation considers the person—(the interaction)—and the occupational environment. Their emphasis on the desire for mastery, the press for mastery, and the demand for mastery as translated through these interactions is appropriate for our understanding as we design programming that will present an occupational challenge and a resulting occupational response. It will be our task to provide mediating opportunity and assistance for adaptive response formation (through the design of programming) that will help our participants reach their goals and achieve successful long-range outcomes.

## Drafting Goals and Objectives

Following careful review of the results of the needs assessment, the mission statement, characteristics of the facility, and the characteristics of the population, two goals for the program were drafted and were followed by measurable objectives, as shown by the following examples. Goals and objectives are intended to support programming that will result in employment and in independent living.

### Program Focus: Attention to Healthy and Balanced Independent Living

*Goals:*

1. *To be healthy and balanced* by increasing awareness of healthy living strategies to include nutrition, personal care, exercise, relaxation, stress management, job and apartment search, self-defense, and safety.
2. *To control one's destiny* by increasing the individual's sense of personal causation, self-esteem, and self-efficacy, resulting in sustained employment and independent living.

*Objectives:*

1. (a) Fifty percent of the residents at the Sunshine Mission will attend four out of the six sessions (nutrition, personal care, exercise, stress management, job and apartment search, self-defense, and safety).
   (b) Of the women attending each session, 80 percent will demonstrate knowledge of information and techniques provided in that session.

2. (a)  Of those women attending all of the sessions, 80% will demonstrate increased self-efficacy, self-esteem, and personal causation by the time they leave the Mission programming.
   (b)  Of those women attending all sessions, 80% will find employment.
   (c)  Of those women finding employment, 80% will sustain such employment for six months.

## The Program

Single-session workshops that lasted approximately 1½ to 2 hours were developed in each of the above-identified areas (nutrition, personal care, exercise, stress management, job and apartment search, self-defense, and safety). These areas were selected from the four broader areas of the needs assessment: employment skills, money management, life skills, and coping skills. Nutrition was added by the planners when it became evident that concerns regarding appearance, healthy activities, and self-esteem could be somewhat alleviated with attention to nutrition.

### Nutrition

The session on nutrition was initiated with a verbal survey of how and what the residents preferred to eat and what, if any, problems they were experiencing that they thought might have a relationship to their nutritional likes and dislikes. Most of the residents preferred "fast food" when they were not receiving Mission meals, and many were either under or over their preferred weight.

From earlier discussion with the manager and some of the residents, the students were prepared with materials gleaned from the fast-food restaurants regarding their own statistics for calorie, fat, and salt content. This information was coupled with some suggestions for balancing fast-food meals and some hints for ways to reduce cholesterol and calories. Meeting the residents' basic needs was important to the success of this session and provided a good foundation from which other nutritional sessions such as healthy meal planning and cooking could develop.

### Personal Care, Exercise and Stress Management

Personal care in the forms of personal hygiene and makeup were important as a segue to job searches. Enthusiastic volunteers were solicited from neighborhood shops to provide demonstrations of manicure and pedicure techniques and application of makeup. A local beauty school provided no-cost hair cuts and styling techniques.

A group walking program was established both for exercise and stress management, and an aerobics dance class was initiated. Both quickly came under the direction of residents. Relaxation techniques and guided imagery sessions rounded out the program.

### Job and Apartment Search

Job-search skills consisted of exercises in learning how to read the classified section of the newspaper, how and where to access other job announcements, how to develop a skills-based resume that would not negatively highlight periods of unemployment, and how to write a cover letter. Videotaped role-playing provided practice in interviewing. A similar format was used in finding and evaluating apartments for location (near public transportation, shopping) and cost.

### Self-Defense and Safety

A community martial arts studio volunteered the time and expertise of a female instructor to provide instruction in physical self-defense techniques. Small-group discussions followed the self-defense instruction to assist in the emotional buffering necessary for some women who had histories of physical abuse.

Representatives of the Los Angeles Police Department and the University Crime Prevention and Rape Awareness Group provided information verbally and in the form of handouts to assist the residents in being safe on the street and in the neighborhood, including safety precautions to follow if they were living on the street.

Since the residents frequently rotate, a set of programs can be repeated. This is positive in that the students have time to develop and enhance existing materials; but it can be something of a disadvantage when relying on volunteers from local shops and agencies.

## Staffing

As noted previously, staffing for the sessions/workshops was provided by neighborhood volunteers in the form of representatives from local shops and agencies. Residents were trained to become facilitators whenever possible—not only to assist in providing "womanpower" but, more importantly, to provide as many residents as possible with leadership opportunities.

Another important source of assistance for the ongoing success of the program was the linkage to the Student Occupational Therapy Association and the O.T. Student Residence, as well as the University Housing Residential Advisors and Coordinators. All of these organizations "adopted" the Mission as an ongoing service project. Occupational therapy graduate students may also obtain service-learning credit for participation in and expansion of the programs and activities. The on-site manager supports student involvement and acts as a liaison between the occupational therapy student programs and the needs of the residents. All activities are supervised by a Department faculty member, as well as the resident advisors who live in all University student residences.

## Space

When the students first went on-site to conduct the tentative needs assessment, they explored the space (including storage) and materials/supplies that would be available to them. Two rooms provided the space and work tables necessary for the planned programming—the existing dining room and a conference room. In addition, the outside courtyard and kitchen could be used for some activities.

All space was used for multiple purposes and had to be scheduled at the convenience of the Mission. For the convenience of all concerned, it was determined that the preferred time for activities was after the evening meal (although it was a competitive time with television). Weekend times offered additional possibilities.

Tables could be moved aside for activities that required floor space. There was one file cabinet where some space could be provided, but secured storage was limited and could not be relied upon. The rooms contained electrical outlets that could accommodate a radio, VCR, and/or CD/DVD player, and the adjoining kitchen was well supplied with utensils. A small storage area contained rulers, pencils, and paper, and a typewriter and personal computer were available for the residents' use (donations). Secured parking for volunteers was limited.

## Supplies and Equipment

Efforts were made to design activities requiring minimal equipment and supplies and little, if any, requirement for storage. Equipment (see above) was available through the Mission facilities. All activities utilized the existing tables and chairs in the dining area and/or conference room, the kitchen, and the floor space in the dining area.

## Cost

Even though most of the activities relied on donated supplies, a cost breakdown of supplies and equipment was done in order to anticipate replacement costs (if required) and to assist those who wished to donate by establishing a cost/value for items.

## Funding

Since residents of the Mission were provided services and information free of charge to assist them as they prepared for independent living, this was clearly a service program. The program required the Mission to absorb minimal cost, if any, for supplies, and these costs were incorporated into the existing budget.

The occupational therapy students explored the processes of fund-raising, including those activities already in existence through the Mission. Successful efforts were made to build collaborative bridges with local shops and agencies for ongoing relationships to provide volunteer staff and donated supplies. A sense of *community* and *community responsibility* was created between the University, the local residents, and the local businesses and agencies; all partners in encouraging success for the residents.

In addition to the above efforts, the creation and maintenance of *community* was of equal importance to the occupational science and occupational therapy academic programs that assumed some fiscal responsibility for the student-related Mission activities as part of their Occupational Therapy-Los Angeles (OT-LA) community service and community service-learning programs and projects.

## Marketing

There is some marketing to be done, even with community service programs. The first marketing, of course, was to the Mission manager who, in turn, brought the ideas to the board of directors. This first effort was accomplished in the initial on-site meeting. The students were prepared with appropriate and relevant questions and could offer a brief scenario of their interests in working with the residents. This was also an excellent opportunity for the students to market some of the basic tenets of occupation, meaningful engagement in activity, and occupational therapy. In addition, they were able to link their interest in occupation with the work of the Mission.

Secondly, the residents needed to be informed of the program's activities. This was done initially through the needs assessment and the verbal/visual introduction to the students who would be involved. When plans for programming were finalized, the students prepared colorful flyers advertising the full program and giving information about the activities as well as how residents could benefit. These were supplemented by weekly flyers highlighting the "program of the week." Programming was offered whether there was one participant or twenty participants. There was also marketing to the potential students and residents who might wish to become involved in programming. Flyers were posted in dormitories and program planners/coordinators attended floor meetings at the beginning of the semester to explain the program.

The next phase of marketing required some substantial networking as well as leg work. The purpose of the Mission's activities and the goals and objectives of the students' programming was taken to the shops and agencies that the students had targeted as providing services that would benefit the residents of the Mission. The idea of volunteering time and, in some cases, supplies had to be "sold" to the shop owners and employees. The students found this to be the most disconcerting aspect of marketing the program, but in many ways it turned out to be the easiest.

It should not be lost that this third phase of marketing strongly involved the encouragement of responsibility—and perhaps obligation—to the *community*. This was made even stronger through the residence of the programmers within the neighborhood where the Mission existed. Certainly students are transients, but the responsibility that is created by an investment in the shared premise of *community* can become a legacy handed from one student group to another through the investment of the institution (the University) and the department.

## Outcomes

Taking time to work and rework program goals and objectives is worthwhile when it comes to determining how effective the program has been and continues to be. Of course, to really know long-term effectiveness, it is necessary to follow the residents' progress in obtaining employment and acquiring suitable housing. This follow-up is attempted by the Mission but for numerous reasons it is difficult to accomplish. Record of first employment following completion of the program can be attained, and six month follow-up can be accomplished; however, if the participant leaves employment, or is fired (and doesn't return to the Mission) it is not likely she would be identified for follow-up. As the occupational therapy student's programming continues to attract residents, and if that programming is effective, then we would expect to see this reflected in any data the Mission is able to obtain.

The goals and objectives of the student's programming can be measured for short-term effectiveness in the following ways:

*Goal:*

1. *To be healthy* by increasing awareness of healthy living strategies to include nutrition, personal care, exercise, stress management, job and apartment search, self-defense, and safety

*Objective:*

1. (a) Fifty percent of the residents at the Sunshine Mission will attend four out of six sessions.

*Measurement*
This objective is measured simply by an organized system of attendance marking and is compared to the number of women who are in residency during the programming. The relationship of the objective to the goal carries the assumption that being present during the session does, in fact, increase awareness. Since awareness is a fairly superficial goal, the objective is likely being measured adequately. Measurement of this objective could be strengthened with the use of an observer/participation checklist similar to the one shown in Figure 15–2 which can be used to note the level of each participant's engagement in the session.

*Objective:*

1. (b) Of the women attending each session, 80 percent will demonstrate knowledge of information and techniques provided in that session.

## FIGURE 15–2 Observer Check-Sheet for Participation Level

### Client Attendance and Performance Rating Form

| Name | Session 1 | Session 2 | Session 3 | Session 4 | Session 5 |
|------|-----------|-----------|-----------|-----------|-----------|
|      |           |           |           |           |           |
|      |           |           |           |           |           |
|      |           |           |           |           |           |
|      |           |           |           |           |           |
|      |           |           |           |           |           |
|      |           |           |           |           |           |
|      |           |           |           |           |           |
|      |           |           |           |           |           |
|      |           |           |           |           |           |
|      |           |           |           |           |           |

**Key:**

| Rating | Performance |
|--------|-------------|
| 0 | Did not attend |
| 1 | Attended session but did not participate in activity |
| 2 | Quietly participated but not interactive with others |
| 3 | Engaged, active participation, interaction with others |

*Measurement*

This objective is best measured in two ways. A brief questionnaire can be distributed following each session to focus on the information that the facilitator wishes to convey, or a brief structured interview can be utilized for participants in a small group. It is important that the facilitators think carefully about the content and reflect the main ideas in their questionnaire/interview. Always ask the following question: What is really important to assist the participants in meeting the goal?

If there are demonstrated techniques, as there were with the sessions on personal care, exercise, job search, and self-defense, then an observer checklist is again appropriate. The facilitator must determine the level of competency that is desired to assess achievement of the objective and measure at that level. An actual resume was required as part of the session(s) on job search—either this was accomplished or it was not. If a particular level of quality is expected when something is actually produced, then this must be reflected in the checklist.

Pretests and posttests could be utilized to get a truer measure of information the participants bring to a session as opposed to new information they acquire in a session. For the purposes of this program, it was thought that a pretest was most useful to determine at what level to introduce information. (See Figure 15–3 for an example of pre-post tests.)

*Goal:*

2. *To control one's destiny* by increasing the individual's sense of personal causation, self-esteem, and self-efficacy.

*Objective:*

2. (a) Of those women attending all of the sessions, 80 percent will demonstrate increased self-efficacy, self-esteem, and personal causation.

*Measurement and Supporting Rationale*

An important aspect of this objective is the requisite that all of the sessions be attended. The selection of content, or enabling activities, was made with the belief that mastery would, in fact, increase the participant's self-esteem, self-efficacy, and sense of control over her environment or personal causation. Further, it was assumed that the participants were deficit in these characteristics (validated through pre-test measures) and that this could be the area that would make a difference in their future successes in seeking employment and living independently.

In this case, pretest and posttest measurements were selected. The Generalized Expectancy for Success Scale, or GESS (Fibel and Hale, 1978; Asher, 1996), and the Self-Efficacy Scale, or SES (Asher, 1996; Sherer, Maddox, Mercandante, Prentice-Dunn, Jacobs, and Rogers, 1982), were given to all participants at the first session in the series, and individual scores were calculated. The measures again were given to all participants (those who had attended all of the sessions) at the last session of the series. It is doubtful that improvement in these measures would be sustained over time with such a short programming window; however, if all

---

**FIGURE 15–3 Safety Self-Assessment Check-Sheet**

## SAFETY SELF-ASSESSMENT

Please read the following statements carefully. Rate each statement using the following scale:

**1 = strongly agree**
**2 = agree**
**3 = doesn't apply/don't care**
**4 = disagree**
**5 = strongly disagree**

1) I feel that I can protect myself.                                          _____

2) I feel that I DON'T give up easily when faced with problems.               _____

3) I feel safe when walking to the store.                                     _____

4) I feel comfortable saying "No."                                           _____

5) I understand the difference between verbal abuse and physical abuse.       _____

6) I feel comfortable when a stranger approaches me.                          _____

7) I feel that I know how to deal with confrontation.                         _____

8) I feel that I can rely on myself.                                          _____

9) I feel confident that I would survive an attack.                           _____

10) I know when to use my words and when to use my fists to protect myself.   _____

11) I feel that I have control over my life.                                  _____

12) When I want something, I work hard to get it.                             _____

---

Mission programming was considered as contributing to efficacy, then a post-test previous to leaving the Mission might be more valid.

Differences in individual scores were calculated for participants. Although the numbers attending all sessions were small, there was improvement in each set of scores. Of course, there may have been many factors affecting the increased scores. Some formative questions we could consider are: Why did some residents attend one session and not another? How did the women who attended all sessions differ from those who did not? How did their initial scores compare? Did the content of some sessions affect the scores more than others (for example, self-defense or personal care)? These are all legitimate questions that would strengthen the measures, both formative and summative.

## Time Frame

The programs were prepared over the course of an academic semester (15 weeks), with student groups meeting one time each week for 2-hour periods. The initial program, healthy living, was conducted in 2-hour sessions, one time per week, over a 6-week period.

Minimal supplies were required, and there was no substantial lag time for acquisition. The most difficult aspect of the time line was the substantial marketing effort to those organizations that would provide volunteer time and the scheduling of sessions for their convenience and for the convenience of the residents. Since their initiation, the programs have continued to be conducted with new ideas and new participants.

## *Summary*

The disenfranchised and homeless include children, adolescents, and adults and the numbers are growing daily. Homelessness is sometimes by choice, but most often it is a product of the individual's loss of control over his or her life. Matters of economics and loss of income are integrated with loss of meaningful occupations and hope. One program has been described to provide an example of services for the homeless and/or those in shelter environments. This was an in-depth description of a program provided for homeless women living in a shelter. The goals for this program included the pursuit of "health" and the development of knowledge and skills to "control ones' destiny." To support the goals and to meet the objective, programming focused on self-care, community awareness, holiday arts and crafts, home skills, and pre-employment skills.

Several program designs were combined in this program example; however, the author wishes to specifically thank the following students for their substantial contributions to this program design: Lisa Aguila, Andrea Fong, Sylvia Garciga, Yvonne Lubczynski, and Leigh Peterson.

## *References*

Aron, L. Y., & Fitchen, J. (1996). Rural homelessness: A synopsis. *Homelessness in America*. (The "series" of pamphlets/reports.) Washington, DC: Oryx Press/ National Coalition for the Homeless.

Asher, E. (1996) *Occupational therapy assessment tools: An annotated index* (2nd ed.). Bethesda, MD: AOTA .

CalWorks: *Homeless Families* (2005, May). Report to the County of Los Angeles Board of Supervisors, County of Los Angeles, Department of Public Social Services.

Dear, M. (1996). Time, space, and the geography of everyday life of people who are homeless. In R. Zemke, & F. Clark, (Eds.), *Occupational science: The evolving discipline* (pp. 107–114). Philadelphia: F. A. Davis.

Federal Task Force on Homelessness and Severe Mental Illness. (1992). *Outcasts on main street: A report of the federal task force on homelessness and severe mental illness.* Delmar, NY: National Resource Center on Homelessness and Mental Illness.

Fibel, B., & Hale, W. D. (1978). The generalized expectancy for success scale— A new measure. *Journal of Consulting and Clinical Psychology, 46,* 924–931.

Kaufman, T. (1997). *Out of reach: Rental housing at what cost?* Washington, DC: National Low Income Housing Coalition.

Kielhofner, G. (2002). *Model of Human Occupation* (3rd ed.). Philadelphia, PA: Lippincott.

Kielhofner, G., Forsyth, K., & Barrett, L. (2003). The model of human occupation. In E. Crepeau, E. Cohn, & B. Schell, (Eds.), *Willard and Spackman's occupational therapy* (10th ed., pp. 212–219). Philadelphia: Lippincott.

Koegel, P. (1996). The causes of homelessness. In *Homelessness in America.* Washington, DC: Oryx Press, National Coalition for the Homeless.

Los Angeles Police Department (LAPD). (1996, 2004, 2005). *Los Angeles county crime report.* Los Angeles, CA: Author.

National Coalition for the Homeless. (1997). *Homelessness in America: Unabated and increasing.* Washington, DC: National Coalition for the Homeless.

National Law Center on Homelessness and Poverty. (1996). *Mean sweeps: A report on anti-homelessness laws, litigation and alternatives in 50 United States cities.* Washington, DC: National Law Center on Homelessness and Poverty.

Neville-Jan, A., Fazio, L. S., Kennedy, B., & Snyder, C. (1997). Elementary to middle school transition: Using multicultural play activities to develop life skills. In L. D. Parham, & L. S. Fazio, (Eds.), *Play in occupational therapy for children* (pp. 144–157). St. Louis, MO: Mosby.

Oakley, D., & Dennis, D. (1996). Responding to the needs of homeless people with alcohol, drug, and/or mental disorders. In *Homelessness in America.* Washington, DC: Oryx Press, National Coalition for the Homeless.

O'Connell, J., Lozier, J., & Gingles, K. (1997). *Increased demand and decreased capacity: Challenges to the McKinney Act's health care for the homeless program.* Nashville, TN: National Health Care for the Homeless Council.

Report of the Glendale, California Task Force on Homelessness. (1993). Glendale, CA: City of Glendale, California.

Robbins, G., & Nelson, F. (1996). *Looking for a place to be: A report on AIDS housing in America.* Seattle, WA: AIDS Housing of Washington.

Robertson, M. (1996). *Homeless youth on their own*. Berkeley, CA: Alcohol Research Group.

Schultz, S., & Schkade, J. (2003). Occupational adaptation. In E. Crepeau, E. Cohn, & B. Schell, (Eds.), *Willard and Spackman's occupational therapy* (10th ed., pp. 220–223). Philadelphia: Lippincott.

Shelter Partnership of Los Angeles. (1995). *Annual Report*. Los Angeles, CA: Author.

Sherer, M., Maddox, J. E., Mercandante, B., Prentice-Dunn, S., Jacobs, B., & Rogers, R. W. (1982). The self-efficacy scale: Construction and validation. *Psychological Reports, 51*, 663–671.

Sunshine Mission/Casa de Rosas, Inc. (1996). *Mission statement: Agency effectiveness report*. Los Angeles, CA: Author.

*The International Webster New Encyclopedia Dictionary of the English Language*. (1975). Chicago: The English Language Institute of America.

Wells, S. M. (1996). *Projects for assistance in transition from homelessness: A summary of fiscal year 1994 state implementation reports*. Washington, DC: National Coalition for the Homeless.

## Internet Sites

CJOT Abstracts, Vol. 66, No. 4, October 1999: http://www.caot.ca
HIV/AIDS and Homelessness: http://nch.ari.net/hivaids.html
HIV/AIDS Statistics:
    http://www.ama-assn.org/special/hiv/support/aidstat.htm
Homeless Shelters: Maryland
    http://www.gtii.com/members/lannin/shelters/maryland.htm
Los Angeles Police Department (2002): http://www.lapdonline.com
Mental Illness and Homelessness: http://nch.ari.net/mental.html
National Resource Center on Homelessness and Mental Illness:
    email: nrc@prainc.com.
Solutions at Work:
    http://www.huduser.org/periodicals/fieldworks/1202/fworks4.html

# Intervention and Support Programming in Day Camps, Sleep-Away Camps, and "Adventures"

## Learning Objectives

1. To appreciate the importance of environments for intervention that support and encourage a "normalizing" experience for the participant
2. To explore potential program development within the structure of day camps and sleep-away camps
3. To identify programs that offer "adventure" as an opportunity for participants to explore meaningful challenge in their leisure occupations

## Key Terms

1. Normalizing Environments
2. Day Camp
3. Sleep-Away Camp
4. Adventures

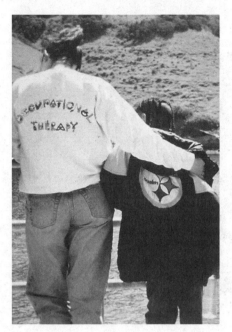

A hug on the deck of a boat, while returning home after a long day of fun, may be the best part of this "adventure."

# Introduction

This chapter will offer some examples of what might be described as programming that showcases environment-centered occupations that provide significant meaning for all ages. Although certainly not restricted to one season, this type of programming does carry with it the flavor of summer, with its games, crafts, fun, being outdoors, being with friends, and perhaps even nursing a sunburned nose, a few bug bites, and a bruised knee. Adults hold these moments of play/leisure in pockets of pleasurable memory, and children relish the time spent at play.

The selected environments for programming provide a comfort zone for children and adults with or without significant disability. They are user-friendly environments that offer all participants equal access and the opportunity for autonomy rather than dependency; in other words, they are **normalizing environments**. Day camps are probably the simplest to develop and program. Sleep-away camps, on the other hand, are more challenging and more costly but provide significant opportunities for building positive experiences, self-esteem, and efficacy for both the young and for those who are older.

What is meant by adventures, the third category of programming included in this chapter? Coming from the word *advent*, which means to begin or to commence, *adventure* is the undertaking of doing so (Random House, 1984). When participating in an adventure-oriented intervention program, it is not unusual for clients to exclaim "I'm alive again!" or "This is living!" The *adventures* of Christopher Robin at Pooh Corner, Alice in Wonderland, Robin Hood and his Merry Band, Luke

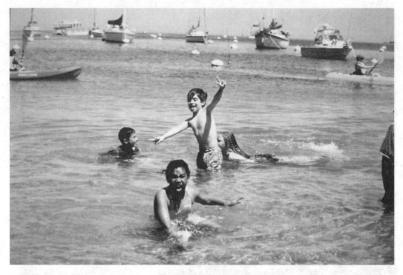

Whether in the ocean or a wading pool, water play is a significant activity for campers of all ages and abilities.

Skywalker in *Star Wars*, Zorro, or Batman conjure up exciting images of new places, new events, mysteries, and maybe a little danger. These are the attributes that put the keen edge on "meaningful occupations" for many.

Yerxa (1999) describes the need for people to become "effective managers of their own environments" and notes that through this process there is undoubtedly an accompanying need to "search for novelty," perhaps the core of intrinsic motivation. Yerxa (1999) refers to *homo occupacio* to describe man's link with occupation: "occupation helps construct who I am." What better way to initiate this construction than through the novelty imbedded in an adventure? Whether these adventures come in the form of horseback riding, spending the night on a hiking trail high in the mountains, diving in the ocean, driving with the top down, spying an unseen species of bird, or another activity of equal challenge, they are all *adventures*.

Throughout this text, we have discussed that the prerequisite to programming for any population is to "know" that population on all levels. A thorough investigation of the developmental expectations, along with the parameters of any disability or differing ability, is of absolute necessity to provide programming that will be formative or preventative. Since day camps, sleep-away camps, and adventures are typically adjunct to other programming the clients are receiving, communication with other providers is important to maintain and support the goals for intervention that are already in place.

## The Day Camp

**Day camps** can be developed for clients of any age. They can be developed for the child alone, the child and a sibling, or the child and a parent; or they can be developed for the adult alone or the adult and a caregiver, depending on the goals of the program. Although not discussed at length here, day programs for adults, particularly those with cognitive dysfunction, are actually day camps. If you think of them in that way and incorporate many of the activities of a typical children's day camp (scaled to adult needs and interests) in the adult treatment environment, goals can be attained while supporting the pleasurable attributes and nostalgia of "camp." Most adult programs for clients with Alzheimer's disease, in fact, do this by combining a routine of indoor and outdoor activity, rest, snacks, and celebration of life events (holidays, birthdays, and so on). Since the day programming offers some respite for the caregiver, much of the programming is for the client; however, selected shared adventures such as trips away from the treatment environment and the immediate community can provide an opportunity for the client and caregiver to enjoy positive experiences together. These shared experiences can assist in alleviating some of the daily stressors and often the accompanying guilt that may overpower the caregiver.

Supportive programming for children can occur anywhere; many after-school and Saturday day camp models are in the practice settings common to pediatrics. If at all possible, however, this kind of programming, particularly a day camp that occurs for a period of time (for example, daily for two-weeks), should be held at a campsite. This dissociation from the treatment environment provides an arena for children to experience new challenges and opportunities to meet these challenges in different ways. Of course, some day camp programming can be for children who have no apparent cognitive, emotional, or physical disabilities. These day camps for children who may be considered to be at risk for losing out on what we might describe as "life's rewards" are excellent ways to provide supportive and preventative programming. The "club" models described in Chapter 17 highlight programming examples of this kind.

## An Example of Programming for a Children's Day Camp

### The Needs Assessment

The program we will examine in this section came to fruition when the City Recreation and Parks Department experienced numerous requests from parents and teachers to add children with emotional, cognitive, and physical disabilities to their summer camp programming. These requests were not new, and efforts had been made previously to mainstream these children into the existing structures but with limited success.

The 1997 mission of the City of Los Angeles Department of Recreation and Parks included the following sentence: "To unify Los Angeles by providing diverse recreational opportunities, beautiful facilities, and innovative leadership for the universal enjoyment of our residents and visitors by providing a broad range of recreational opportunities at various facilities to the general population, especially youth, and to *all special need segments of the population.*" Thus, providing such a camp was well within the scope and interests of this department.

The department employed a recreation therapist (R.T.) and several adolescent assistants from the surrounding community to operate the summer day camp programs. The adolescents were thought to be at risk and had been selected to participate in an "opportunity for success" employment program operated under the auspices of the police department. The recreation therapist recognized that the potential campers identified with special needs were of sufficient number and variability to require several small groups with different programming for any meaningful outcomes to occur.

Since occupational therapy, an added partner and collaborator, became involved late in the process and the time frame was fairly short, an occupational therapist, along with other therapists who were or had been seeing the children for varying kinds of therapeutic programming, volunteered time to further develop the needs assessment. The children ranged in age from 5 to 8 years old. Some were no longer receiving therapy, and some continued to receive therapy on a weekly basis. All available information regarding individual therapeutic goals for the children was gleaned from a variety of services, and individual objectives were developed for each of the fifteen children who were expected to attend. The children were then grouped according to their objectives rather than by age or disability status.

A goal was developed for the camp and was shared by all of the children. "Camp for Friends" was designed to help each child increase his or her interpersonal and general social skills. The collective responses to the assessment of need provided assurance that the goal and objectives for the program were on target for all of the participants.

Thus, this example actually was initiated with the first expressed *need*. It would appear that the initial planning steps outlined in Part II of this text were bypassed; however, it is important to note that an enterprising and experienced programmer carries all of the process in his or her head. The therapist involved in this example recognized the trends toward inclusion of differently abled children but also recognized that inclusion requires cognizance of appropriate and meaningful goals. In addition, this therapist knew how to expand the needs assessment so that programming ensures that the goal or goals were met and resources were not wasted.

The programmer should also know that, with skillful task analysis and appropriate adaptations and modifications, a full round of camp activities can be enjoyed by every child in the program. This programmer will also be able to successfully market the uniqueness of occupation-centered intervention coupled with program evaluation methods so that a future for occupational therapy practitioners is assured in this particular community-based practice environment. When the programmer works cooperatively with the recreation therapist and other staff, a full round of therapeutic and supportive activities can be developed by this team and the concept of community can be strengthened and maintained.

## Programming

Daily programming for the campers in our example was not unlike what other summer day camps were utilizing. Programming was held Monday through Thursday

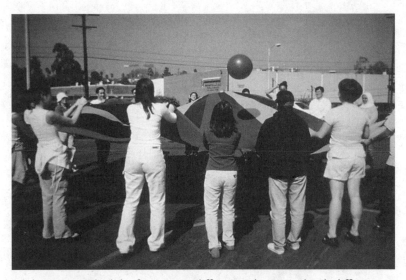

Adolescents and adults from many different cultures and with differing abilities learn to cooperate in a day camp parachute game.

from 10:00 A.M. to 4:00 P.M. and lasted for one month. Transportation to and from camp was provided by Parks and Recreation Department vehicles, which also accommodated the two children in wheelchairs.

Daily programming consisted of arts and crafts, field trips, swimming, games, and pet care combined with snacks/lunch and a short rest period. Arts and crafts were similar to those enjoyed by all summer campers (including t-shirts sponge painted with the camp logo, lanyards for ID badges, leathercraft, and an assortment of other ideas all task-analyzed and adapted to ensure full participation and successful outcome).

Cooking was also a favored activity, and it was tailored to the out-of-doors camp environment (such as chocolate, graham cracker, and marshmallow S'mores, hot dogs on sticks, toasted marshmallows, and so on). Field trips included an amusement park, the local children's museum, the beach, and the zoo. The children collected an assortment of objects from the beach for a collage to be constructed later, and the wet sand provided an interesting tactile challenge for bare feet and bodies. Swimming also offered opportunities to practice dressing in and out of swimsuits, grooming wet hair, and toweling dry.

A task-analysis pre-visit by the therapist and/or students to all of the field trip sites paved the way for successful access and the "just-right" challenge with regard to managing the terrain and crowds and avoidance of potential exhaustion with resulting temper tantrums. Bathrooms and lunch areas were also mapped so that children would not experience any potentially embarrassing accidents or be unintentionally the brunt of discrimination.

Most games were played out-of-doors with the favored ones involving the parachute and variations of the parachute with foam balls that were large enough

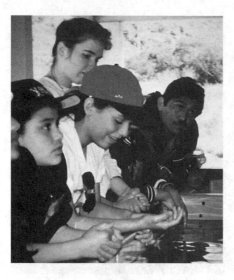

A field trip to an aquarium touch-tank transforms this camp activity into an *adventure*!

for all to grasp and throw. Pet care was actually serendipitous with the discovery of a frog, which was later joined by a duck that happened to enjoy the swimming pool and rabbits that were adopted. One of the premises supporting pet care by children is that of offering the opportunity for experiencing responsibility—relentless as it is when it comes to feeding and taking care of an animal. But more important to our community was the normalizing process of caring for a pet that most children can access and many take for granted. The campers had more often been the recipient of caretaking rather than the provider of care.

You will find a number of resources at the close of this chapter to help you with camp programming. One of these resources, *Backyards and Butterflies: Ways to Include Children with Disabilities in Outdoor Activities*, includes descriptions of several adaptations to assist with pet care (Greenstein, Miner, Kudela, and Bloom, 1993).

### Space, Staffing, and Cost

Space for this camp was in a city park with an adjoining secured building. The building provided some office space, a large gymnasium, a kitchen, and rooms for small-group activities. A playground with newly designed equipment, a swimming pool, and child-sized picnic tables and benches were adjacent to the building. All of the facilities were fenced away from other public park activities.

Since there were other camp activities scheduled at the same time as these camps, it was necessary to coordinate not only these groups through daily programming but also to coordinate with other groups as well for the use of the swimming pool, vehicles for field trips, and the use of the gymnasium. Several times each month there were opportunities for shared activities, and many of the children had siblings in the other camps.

Since the budget had already been established before the camps were conceptualized and developed, the first summer of the program the occupational therapy personnel were largely volunteer or minimum wage employees. There were also four paid adolescent assistants assigned through a separate agency. Following the first summer, an occupational therapist, an occupational therapy assistant, additional adolescent assistants, and two Level II occupational therapy and/or occupational therapy assistant students were expected to be added to the programming. It was also anticipated there would be additional campers following further marketing efforts.

Costs for the activities were subsumed under the regular camp costs. The cost of supplies for one month of programming was approximately $120 per child. These were budgeted items for craft and activity supplies and did not include transportation, field trip admissions, or lunch; nor did they include the cost of salaries or use of space. These items were part of the larger Parks and Recreation Department budget obtained from individual fees, city funds, and donations. Some of the per-child tuition was funded through therapy services, and those who were not able to pay received tuition assistance through gifts from businesses and individuals.

Keep in mind that many day camp sites make use of donated or minimal cost lease sites with summer availability, including school buildings and grounds or community buildings. While having access to a swimming pool or beach is ideal, if these are not available, then wading pools can be substituted to satisfy some of the water-related programming. We must remember that some or all staff must be responsible for the appropriate credentials to ensure safety and liability (such as water safety and instruction).

Because normalizing environments can be dangerous ones, programming efforts must provide a median, or safe, zone between risk and safety. A sufficient number of personnel is critical, and one staff member per child is not excessive. Never permit yourself to be maneuvered into enrolling too many children for your available staff; if you have a greater need than you can safely manage, then run more and shorter-duration camps (for example, one-week or two-week rotations).

## Marketing

Because the need and requests for services initiated the programming in this example, marketing was an afterthought. However, a brochure describing the occupational therapy services was sent to all recipients of Parks and Recreation Department mailings, and these services were also highlighted in that organization's newsletter. Keeping occupation, occupation-centered intervention, and, in this case, *therapy* strongly linked to the camp was a critical part of continued involvement in this setting.

Summer day camps or Saturday camp programming are excellent private practices or extensions of existing therapy practices. These may be specialty camps utilizing specific frames of reference such as sensory-integration or behavioral models for a number of differently abled children, or they might be specific to a diagnosis such as asthma, muscular dystrophy, eating disorders, spinal injury, or severe emotional disorders (SED).

As in this day camp example, camps may be mixed, without particular attention to diagnosis. In all of these cases, marketing and the other processes of program development will be followed by conceiving (as a first step) and then developing a program. Marketing will be to parents, to other professionals, and perhaps to the owner of a building and to potential donors of a tuition scholarship.

In general, most of the supply costs can be covered by tuition and donations. Tuition can be paid out-of-pocket by consumers or can be partially covered by therapy payment services and/or tuition donations. For such a freestanding camp, corporate giving can be an important contributor depending on the mission of the program and the clientele.

## Evaluation

Initial evaluation is, of course, directly tied to the goal or goals and to the objectives of the program. If campers bring with them individual therapy goals established by another practitioner or by Individualized Education Plan (IEP) goals, then these must be integrated into the goals of the programming. If they are not integrated directly, then the program goals must complement individual goals. For these children, progress will be measured by the programmer or, in some cases, by the occupational therapy practitioner who is seeing the client external to the camp. Camp experiences are excellent venues to maintain the goals and objectives of school-based therapies, for these goals otherwise may be abandoned over the course of a summer without continued programming. For goals supporting social skills development (appropriate for most participants regardless of diagnosis or functional abilities), an observer checklist provides a marker for daily observations of those behaviors determined to be appropriate to social skills goals and objectives.

For instance, for some children, making eye contact with a therapist or another child is indicative of an objective at least partially achieved; for others, giving up a toy or receiving one would merit a mark. The person recording the observer checklist can be someone who is not directly involved in programming, such as a volunteer. You could also consider the employment of a minimally cognitively impaired adult, which would be an excellent way to utilize the skills of therapy "alumni" who may be transitioning to a work environment. With some assistance and practice, they can make a significant contribution to this task that cannot be done by someone who is directly involved in activities with the children. There are other measures of social skills, but for the limited exposure of a summer camp, we are assuming that individual evaluations will occur at the primary therapy site and that our programming will enhance goal performance or at least assist in maintaining stability.

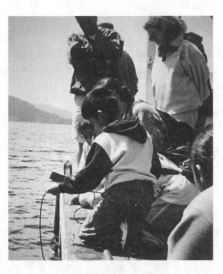

For some an adventure means fishing for Marlin; for others it's the possibility of hooking a sunfish off the dock. *Adventures* are in the "eye of the beholder"!

# Sleep-Away Camps

Anyone who has ever participated in a **sleep-away camp** knows what a life-changing experience being away from daily support systems can be for a child. There is probably no experience more frightening or more freeing for a child—abled or differently abled. Unfortunately, the differently abled child is most often restricted from such experiences. First of all, few opportunities exist, and for those that do, marketing such a camp to protective and concerned parents is quite a task. The cost of the additional and professional personnel is expensive, and ensuring accessibility and comfort in existing away-camp structures is difficult.

Although not carried to fruition (more because of time constraints than anything else), a pilot plan for a sleep-away camp was developed as a programming proposal by graduate students. This camp was designed to accommodate 8- to 10-year-old children with mild to moderate cognitive and physical disabilities but of such significance that they would not likely be permitted to join most sleep-away camp groups. Programming was developed for the pilot group of ten children to be at the camp for a period of one week. The reader may wish to explore the *Hole in the Wall Gang* system of sleep-away camps for children who are terminally ill. This organization, sponsored initially by Paul Newman and Joanna Woodward is an excellent example of what can be accomplished with such a model; and with effective and persuasive fund-raising efforts (www.HITWGCAMPS.org).

### Goals

The broad goals for this occupation-centered program included 1) team building; 2) positive interaction with others; 3) exploration of new interests; 4) development of new skills; 5) accepting and meeting responsibilities; and 6) having *fun*.

### Programming

Programming should provide a set of activities that is as normalizing as possible. A typical daily routine might include the following:

Wake-up call at group tents (three children and a counselor)
Get ready for the day (morning routines and dressing)
Breakfast in the dining tent
Animal care/pet therapy
Morning exercise according to individual abilities and needs
Activities to include hiking (also wheelchair hiking trails), water sports, paddle boating, and burro trail riding
Lunch in the dining tent
Kitchen cleanup and help routines
Rest, sleep, and/or story telling
Preparation for Family Day skits/mini plays
Camp craft, gardening, pet care, and games
Dinner in dining tent
Campfire stories and activities
Preparation for bed and "good night"

### Staffing

Staffing for a program such as this is best when overlaid on an existing camp structure with staff such as employed cooks, kitchen help, horse/burro wranglers, and lifeguards. In fact, many organizations such as the Young Men's Christian Association (YMCA) and the 4-H Clubs have such camp facilities. There are also similar camp facilities located in national parks and forests and in some state and city parks and recreation facilities.

Overlaying occupation-centered programming on such existing structures is far easier than trying to do the whole thing yourself. If you would like to develop a pilot camp such as this, first do a thorough two-phase needs assessment to other care providers in the community and to potential parents/caregivers, then locate a suitable existing camp facility and market your proposed program there.

The facility's administrators may be able to offer you funding or at least support funding for their services if you can obtain tuition for your attendees and perhaps some matching funding for the programming you are suggesting and for the additional specialized personnel you will require.

You will likely need one-to-one counselors (preferably high school or college students) under the supervision of an occupational therapist or an occupational therapist and an occupational therapy assistant. In addition, prerequisites include any specialized staff to ensure safety and personnel with the therapeutic skills to be sure that each child is meeting the goals and objectives of the camp experience. The credentials and experience of your professional staff will be of extreme importance in your marketing efforts to parents.

### Supplies and Cost

Assuming you are able to get the support services to offer the sleep-away experience, supplies and materials will not be unlike those described for day camp programming. Many parents would pay tuition out-of-pocket for such a camp experience for their child; for those who could not, corporate sponsorship could probably be obtained through your marketing and fund raising efforts.

For an ongoing camp such as the one described here, the primary cost would be in the professional personnel and perhaps for some initial physical alterations in camp structures that may be required to ensure accessibility (for example, ramps, bathrooms, and wheelchair-accessible trails). Volunteer groups, parents, and patient advocacy groups are generally more than willing to assist with meeting these requirements, and Wilderness Adventure organizations and conservation groups can assist with cutting wheelchair-accessible trails and trails adapted for others (such as emphasis on scents and sounds for the vision-impaired camper).

A camp such as this offers an excellent Level II fieldwork opportunity for student involvement at all levels of development and marketing as well as in actual programming.

# Adventures

Of course, camps are adventures in the making, but we will also explore ideas for **adventures** programming geared toward young adults and "not so young" adults. Most likely the *adventure* is identified and defined by the participants themselves. As was mentioned earlier, the client and the client's family are the best advocates for services. In these circumstances, the occupational therapy practitioner is the "coach" who provides information, access, and strategies for success. It is the practitioner who orchestrates the "just right challenge," or that set of circumstances where challenge and skills are exquisitely matched (Csikszentmihalyi, 1982).

## Disabled Divers

Disabled Divers is a program that combines the services and expertise of the Office of University Disability Services and Programs, the Handicapped Scuba Association (HSA), associated fund-raising organizations and programs for University handicapped athletes, and the Student Occupational Therapy Association (SOTA). Strongly motivated by the athletes with disabilities themselves, the purpose of this program is to encourage and develop students with disabilities who have an interest in water sports to become certified scuba divers. Although strongly supported by spinal-injury participants in her California coastal occupational therapy practice, Dowd (1993) has also reported scuba diving interest from not only paraplegics and quadriplegics but amputees and the vision impaired as well. Water, at least for those who can swim, is truly a normalizing and equalizing environment. A certified scuba instructor herself, Dowd represents a common link among occupational therapy practitioners to mobilize the meaningful occupations they have selected in their own lives to motivate and encourage their clients.

In many universities, colleges, and YMCAs, there is strong participant support for the differently-abled to access sports such as wheelchair basketball, rugby, skiing, and snowboarding. Recent interest on a national and international level in the Paralympic Games has offered further support for the model of adventures through sports and, in many cases, competitive sports.

The Disabled Divers program has provided an incentive to many men and women with disabilities whose opportunities for engagement in their choice of meaningful occupations have been obliterated or at least threatened. Remember that occasionally you may have to exceed your own occupational boundaries in considering the world of your clients. Do not limit their engagement in adventure and their pursuit of meaningful occupations by not being aware of the opportunities that exist for them. For example, although you may not want to go near the water, if your client does, then you should find the best avenues possible to assist him or her in reaching that goal. Of course, safety must be a primary consideration, and for programs such as the one just described, every precaution is taken to protect the participant. Certified and quality instruction is critical, and your task and that of your client is often to educate the instructor with regard to the disability so that he or she can be prepared for the additional precautions that may be required.

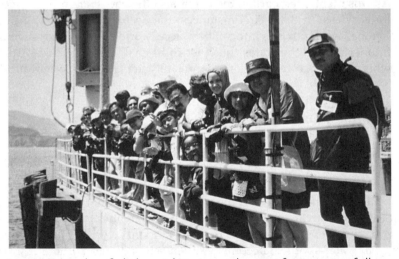

Anticipating a day of whale-watching is an adventure for campers of all ages and abilities.

## Healing Through Surfing and Ocean Activities

The newest of our programs that have come to fruition through the hard initial work realized in a student project is sponsored by the *Jimmy Miller Memorial Foundation*. The mission statement for the newly developed foundation is:

> the Jimmy Miller Memorial Foundation is a non-profit 501(c)(3) Foundation dedicated to honoring the life of our inspiration, Jim Miller, by supporting the healing of mental and physical illness through surfing and ocean related activities. Through recreational, educational and mentoring programs, the Jimmy Miller Foundation will bring together surfers, educators, therapists, lifeguards and friends to help people affected by mental and physical illness feel the joy and healing power of the ocean and surfing. The Foundation also supports other charities that support the protection, preservation, appreciation and safe enjoyment of the oceans, beaches and marine environment. Our mission is to carry on the legacy of Jim's pure love of surfing by showing the ocean's power to heal (www. jimmymillerfoundation.org).

The final proposal for the program was designed by an occupational therapist; initiated while she was a student in the author's "development of occupation-centered programs" class in the Department of Occupational Science and Occupational Therapy at USC. Knowing she was an ocean lifeguard, a surfer, and an occupational therapist, the Foundation approached her for suggestions, and accepted her proposal for programming. Although changed somewhat from the initial idea, the "story" of the early development of this program is described in some detail in a chapter by Fazio (2008; in press). Another program that seats "adventure" in the ocean environment is "Therapy in Ocean" owned and operated by Bethany Brown, OTR. In this program, provision of occupational therapy services include children and adults with a variety of special needs in a safe and therapeutic ocean environment (BethanyLBrown@msn.com; URL: http:// sheldonbrown.org/ocean/). Mentioned earlier in Chapter 6, Israel "Izzy" Paskovitz's non-profit surfing program "Surfers Healing" offers free camps during the summer months for autistic children from Malibu to San Diego, California (www.surfershealing.org).

In your investigation of potential *adventures* with your patient or client, also consider such venues as wilderness outings, kayaking, sailing, or boating. Look to align yourself with organizations that offer such programming to the general public in your community. Also consider the activities of organizations such as the Sierra Club or Elderhostel for those still seeking adventure but perhaps less gregariously. Although Elderhostel and Sierra Club activities are not specifically designed for populations with disability, careful choice of programming can help your clients achieve goals directed toward the accomplishment of a camera safari, wild flower viewings, and numerous other activities with these organizations. Adventure, after all, is in the eye of the beholder!

# Summary

The opportunity for a child, adolescent, or adult to participate in what has been described as normalizing experiences is considered to be significant in providing meaningful engagement in occupation. These experiences may consist of the conventional model for day camp that might include weekly, after-school, or weekend programming. The day camp example provided demonstrates the relationship between the assessment of need, the programming, space, staffing, cost, marketing, and evaluation. Although sleep-away camps are more challenging for the planner, they are recommended as a way to provide opportunities for the achievement of autonomy and skill building for the camper.

"Adventures" are novel, challenging experiences and are defined as such by the participant. For some, adventures might involve diving in the ocean as our "Disabled Divers" program describes, or surfing, or perhaps kayaking or a camera safari. For others it may be viewing wildflowers from a wheelchair-adapted hiking trail.

The opportunity to play, have fun, find challenge and freedom in the out-of-doors defines the occupations highlighted in this chapter. In this regard they are those experiences that promote "normal" engagement in life—experiences that are of importance for the abled and the differently abled child, adolescent, and adult.

# References

City of Los Angeles. (1997). *Mission Statement*. Department of Recreation and Parks.

Csikszentmihalyi, M. (1982). Toward a psychology of optimal experience. In L. Wheeler, (Ed.), *Review of personality and social psychology*, Vol. 2. Beverly Hills, CA: Sage.

Dowd, D. (1993, Sept.–Oct.). Aquatic heaven. *California Active: The Guide to Health, Sports, and Fitness*, 1, 32–33.

Fazio, L. (2008, *in press*). Developing and evaluating occupation-centered community programs. In M. Scaffa, M. Reitz, & M. Pizzi, (Eds.), *Occupational therapy in the promotion of health and wellness*. Philadelphia: F. A. Davis.

*The Random House Thesaurus* (College Edition). (1984). New York: Random House.

Yerxa, E. (1999, April 9). Confessions of an occupational therapist who became a detective. Lecture. University of Southern California.

You will find the following references helpful in designing and implementing camp programming:

Ashton, M., & Varga, L. (1995). *101 games for groups*. Tucson, AZ: Communication Skill Builders.

Breines, E. C. (1995). *Occupational therapy: Activities from clay to computers*. Philadelphia: F. A. Davis.

Brown, O. (1983). *The metropolitan museum of art activity book*. New York: The Metropolitan Museum of Art and Harry N. Abrams.

Campbell, J. (1993). *Creative art in groupwork*. Bicester, Oxon, United Kingdom: Winslow Press.

Carlson, L. (1993). *EcoArt: Earth-friendly art and craft experiences for 3- to 9-year olds*. Charlotte, VT: Williamson.

Cohen, J. G., & Wannamaker, M. (1996). *Expressive arts for the very disabled and handicapped for all ages*. Springfield, IL: Charles Thomas.

Crist, J. (1996). *ADHD—A teenager's guide*. King of Prussia, PA: The Center for Applied Psychology.

Dikengil, A. T., & Kaye, M. E. (1992). *Building functional social skills: Group activities for adults*. Tucson, AZ: Therapy Skill Builders.

Drake, M. (1992). *Crafts in therapy and rehabilitation*. Thorofare, NJ: Slack.

Ettinger, J. (1995, July 27). Scuba diving surfaces. *O.T. Week*, 22–23.

Furrer, P. J. (1982). *Art therapy activities and lesson plans for individuals and groups*. Springfield, IL: Charles Thomas.

Goldstein, S., & Goldstein, M. (1991). *It's just attention disorder. User's manual, study guide, and video*. Salt Lake City, UT: Neurology, Learning and Behavior Center Publishers.

Gomez, A. (1992). *Crafts of many cultures*. New York: Scholastic.

Gray, L. (1990). *Something special: Seasonal and festive art and craft for children*. Twickenham, England: Belair Publishers. (Distributed by Incentive Publications, Nashville, TN.)

Greenstein, D., Miner, N., Kudela, E., & Bloom, S. (1993). *Backyards and butterflies: Ways to include children with disabilities in outdoor activities*. Ithaca, New York: State Rural Health and Safety Council.

Harwell, J. (1989). *Complete learning disabilities handbook: Ready-to-use techniques for teaching learning-handicapped students*. West Nyack, New York: The Center for Applied Research in Education.

Henkes, R., & Smith, D. (1991). *Art projects around the calendar*. Portland, ME: J. Weston Walch.

Jones, C. B. (1994). *Attention deficit disorder: Strategies for school-age children*. Tucson, AZ: Communication Skill Builders.

Kamiya, A. (1985). *Elementary teacher's handbook of indoor and outdoor games*. West Nyack, New York: Parker.

Kay, J. G. (1977). *Crafts for the very disabled and handicapped for all ages*. Springfield, IL: Charles Thomas.

Knoth, M. (1995). *Activity planning at your fingertips*. Lafayette, IN: Valley Press.

Korb-Khalsa, K., Azok, S., & Leutenberg, E. (1991). *Life management skills I (II, III, and IV)*. Beachwood, OH: Wellness Reproductions.

Korb-Khalsa, K., Azok, S., & Leutenberg, E. (1995). *Self-esteem and life skills (S.E.A.L.S.+PLUS)*. Beachwood, OH: Wellness Reproductions.

Korb-Khalsa, K., Azok, S., & Leutenberg, E. (1996). *Self-esteem and life skills, Too! (S.E.A.L.S. II)*. Beachwood, OH: Wellness Reproductions.

Lamport, K., Coffey, M., & Hersch, G. (1993). *Task analysis handbook*. Thorofare, NJ: Slack.

Morris, L. R., & Schulz, L. (1989). *Creative play activities for children with disabilities: A resource book for teachers and parents*. Champaign, IL: Human Kinetics Books.

Nelson-Jones, R. (1993). *Lifeskills helping: Helping others through a systematic people-centered approach*. Pacific Grove, CA: Brooks/Cole.

Nelson-Jones, R. (1993). *Student manual for lifeskills helping*. Pacific Grove, CA: Brooks/Cole.

Orlick, T. (1982). *The cooperative sports and games book: Challenge without competition*. New York: Pantheon Books.

Parker, H. C. (1988). *The ADD hyperactivity workbook for parents, teachers, and kids*. Plantation, FL: Impact Publications.

Rider, B. B., & Gramblin, J. (1987). *The activity card file*. Kansas City, KS: Rider and Rider.

Rider, B. B., & Scharfenberg, C. (1999). *The book of activity cards for DD adults: Designed for groups*. Kansas City, KS: Rider and Rider.

Rodriguez, A. (1984). *The special artist's handbook: Art activities and adaptive aids for handicapped students*. Palo Alto, CA: Dale Seymour.

Rohnke, K. (1984). *Silver bullets: A guide to initiative problems, adventure games and trust activities*. Dubuque, IA: Kendall/Hunt.

Rowland, A. (1995). *How I learned to make friends: A workbook of activities to help children make friends*. King of Prussia, PA: The Center for Applied Psychology.

Sattler, H. R. (1987). *Recipes for art and craft materials*. New York: Beech Tree Productions, William Morrow and Company.

Sayne, J. T. (1996). Ability awareness day: Summer day camp disability-education program. *Parks and Recreation, 31*, 24.

Sher, B. (1995). *Popular games for positive play: Activities for self-awareness*. Tucson, AZ: Therapy Skill Builders.

Smead, R. (1995). *Skills and techniques for group work with children and adolescents*. Champaign, IL: Research Press.

Sobel, J. (1983). *Everybody wins: 393 non-competitive games for young children*. New York: Walker.

Tedrick, T., & Green, E. (1995). *Activity experiences and programming within long-term care*. State College, PA: Venture.

Terzian, A. M. (1993). *The kids' multicultural art book: Art and craft experiences from around the world*. Charlotte, VT: Williamson.

Tobin, L. (1991). *62 Ways to create change in the lives of troubled children*. Duluth, MN: Whole Person Associates.

Wankelman, W. F., & Wigg, P. (1993). *A handbook of arts and crafts*. Dubuque, IA: William C. Brown.

Watson, D. (1997). *Task analysis: An occupational performance approach*. Bethesda, MD: American Occupational Therapy Association.

Witoski, M. L. (1992). *It's not just a parachute: Integrative activities for children of all abilities*. Tucson, AZ: Therapy Skill Builders.

Wnek, B. (1992). *Holiday games and activities*. Champaign, IL: Human Kinetics Books.

## Internet Sites

Ocean Therapy/Carly Rogers, M. A., OTR/L, Redondo Beach, CA: www.jimmymillerfoundation.org

Therapy in Ocean/Bethany Brown: http://sheldonbrown.org/ocean

Surfers Healing/Israel "Izzy" Paskovitz: www.surfershealing.org

Elderhostel, United States and Internationally: www.elderhostel.org

The Association of Hole in the Wall Gang Camps, Inc.: www.HITWGCAMPS.org

Sierra Club: www.sierraclub.org

# Prevention and Wellness Programming Within Existing or Newly Formed Clubs: Collaboration and Partnering

## Learning Objectives

1. To understand the significance of the "club" as a structure within which to place occupation-centered programs
2. To appreciate how the structure of a "club" is defined by the developmental age and resulting needs of the child or adolescent
3. To appreciate the opportunities for collaboration and partnering with existing community organizations
4. To identify examples of existing clubs and associations whose mission and goals are compatible with occupation-centered programs
5. To consider the importance of gender in developing the goals and structure of club-based programs
6. To explore program examples housed in existing club structures and associations
7. To examine the design and development of freestanding club structures to meet the occupation-centered program needs of children, adolescents, and adults

## Key Terms

1. Clubs
2. Middle-Childhood
3. Adolescence
4. Gender-Specific Clubs
5. 4-H Club
6. Jane Goodall "Roots and Shoots" Clubs
7. Boys and Girl's Clubs of America
8. YMCA/YWCA
9. Freestanding Clubs

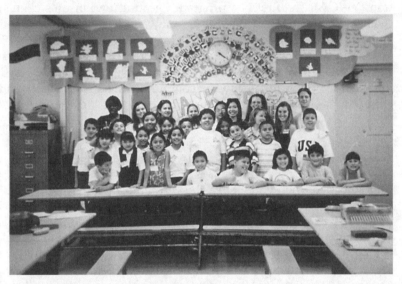

The "Roots and Shoots"/4-H club members and student planners share a moment of pride!

# Introduction

This chapter will focus on the concept of *club* as a community within a community and will describe new and existing structures appropriate for the placement of occupation-centered programs. Included will be program examples that offer a combination of preventative and restorative goals appropriate to the children and adults involved, and one—the "Jazz" club—demonstrates the specific intention of strengthening and reaffirming *community* for the members.

A foundation for understanding why the context of club is appropriate for occupation-centered programming will be established, and examples will be provided to describe the characteristics and goals of several organizational structures based on the concept of *club*. To highlight the importance of collaboration and partnering with other community organizations and structures, examples of programs for children, adolescents, and adults will be offered that have been incorporated into existing clubs with missions and goals that are compatible with our own occupation-based views of effective programming. Two examples will be provided where a new, freestanding club was established to support the proposed programming.

The first example for children and adolescents is occupation-centered programming that utilizes the Roots and Shoots project sponsored by Jane Goodall, which is then placed within an urban 4-H Club. Secondly, a program that exists within the structure of a Boys and Girls Club will be described, which is followed by two brief examples of programming under the umbrella structures of the Young Men's Christian Association (YMCA) and the Young Women's Christian Association (YWCA). The first is a program for adult Parkinson's clients/members and their spouses, and the second is a "Mommy and Me" program for adolescent mothers. The last two examples are of clubs created for the purposes of enhancing the goals and objectives of the developing occupation-centered programming. One is the middle-school "Ice Cream Cart" club, and the second is the "Jazz" club intended to "create"or "establish"community in a group of older adults disenfranchised by the changing city and urban culture that surrounds them.

# Why Clubs?

Think back to when you were a child. You most likely sought membership in both formal and informal **clubs**. Why are clubs so appealing to children? Perhaps some of the answers to this question can be found by exploring what is known of the social, behavioral, and cognitive development of children and adolescents that for each group would permit the club to be such a powerful motivator and, in that regard, a powerful agent for positive change. Florey (1998; 2003) and Florey and Greene (1997) discuss the occupation of play in middle childhood (ages 6 to 12) and the transition in social groups toward increasing structure and elaboration of membership requirements. Citing Boy Scouts and Girl Scouts as examples, Florey recommends that occupational therapy programming for children—particularly for children in middle childhood—include an emphasis on clubs to meet the inclusion needs of this age group.

## Middle Childhood

In particular, the earlier years of **middle childhood** (ages 6 to 7) in most cultures appear to be the time that both adults (parents and caregivers) and peer groups alike place fairly stringent demands on children for new and more sophisticated social behaviors. This is particularly so in societies where formal schooling is a central occupation for this age group. Even more than the often-stringent parental expectations for more *grown-up* behaviors, the peer group moves into position as perhaps the major context for continued development—particularly in the social and behavioral domain—during these years. Although adult control may appear to be absent in these peer groups, covert parental/adult sanctions are realized through the rules attached to games and, perhaps more specifically for our examples, through memberships in clubs or organizations. These club/organizational selections are often more formal in nature and are supported by the parent or adult caregiver. The peer-selected and peer-organized clubs are of a more informal nature but nevertheless have a tremendous impact on the child's social development.

Why do the child and adult parent both gravitate toward the idea of club? The work of Piaget (1960) would suggest that cognitive changes—particularly those that serve to mediate social and behavioral learning—are occurring in middle childhood. These changes permit children to appreciate actions and views of others that may be in disagreement with their own, and through this awareness they may learn to mediate their actions to get along with adults and peers. The demands of this developmental "window" can best be realized through play, most likely through such forms of organized play as soccer, hockey, and baseball and the clubs organized around these sports. Membership and participation in such clubs have a set of prescribed rules/expected behaviors accompanying membership, and the rules for sports clubs might support cooperation, fairness, participation, spirit, and team building.

## Adolescence

Many developmental theorists, including Piaget (1960), Inhelder and Piaget (1958), Erikson (1968), Havighurst (1972), Kohlberg (1984), Keating (1980), Siegler (1981), Gilligan (1982), and Sigelman and Shaffer (1995), have proposed numerous ways to define and understand development from childhood to older adulthood and, of course, including **adolescence**. Their varying theoretical perspectives describe development from an organismic view (biological, psychoanalytic, or cognitive-developmental) or an environmental view (sociological-anthropological or social learning-behavioral). Although agreeing on the general parameters, the developmental theorists differ in the emphasis they place on the influences that biology, cognition, social factors, environment, and culture have on the phases of development and on the psychological characteristics attached to it. As you review these theorists and others, you will likely find that you will be more influenced by some views than by others, and your programming goals and objectives will reflect this.

If middle childhood seems to hold the most opportunity and challenge for social behavior/rule development and seems to offer the strongest support for clubs, then the period of later childhood or adolescence, which begins at around age 12 and continues to age 20 or so and is accompanied by expectations for adult responsibility, is likely one of even greater potential social change. Numerous theorists, including those mentioned previously, have applied their knowledge to the period following middle childhood. This is the period that we have come to know as adolescence, which is derived from the Latin verb *adolescere* and means "to grow to maturity." Most agree that it is a developmental passage of fairly dramatic changes in all of the domains (physical, cognitive, psychological, and social). Expanding cognitive availabilities often invite the adolescent to think about worlds he or she does not yet have the physical and social development to master. The adolescent is not quite an adult but also is no longer a child. The potential frustration and impatience prompted by this discrepancy coupled with the "adult" desire for independence and the "child's" need to self-validate through belonging offer support of carefully structured club programming for the adolescent as well as for the child.

According to Keating (1980), adolescents are developing ways of thinking that are different than those of middle childhood, and these ways of thinking must be considered and encouraged as we write programming. Adolescents are capable of 1) thinking about possibilities; 2) thinking ahead; 3) thinking about hypotheses; 4) thinking about thought (that is, thinking about one's own thought processes or meta-cognitive thinking and second-order thinking such as developing rules about rules); and 5) thinking beyond conventional limits (Keating, 1980, p. 609; Piaget, 1960).

These characteristics are in contrast to the middle childhood years, when much thought in response to choices and circumstances may be spontaneous and more self-centered. This is not to say that all adolescents have achieved the same level of thought or social/behavioral responsiveness, nor does this suggest that all younger children have not. Rather, it is always necessary to know the child regardless of chronological age expectations, for there may be broad ranges of variation between developmental and chronological expressions of age.

Another developmental factor that may influence programming for adolescents is their generalized ability to consider questions regarding the social order, values, and ethics (Kohlberg, 1984). For example, a club membership may have an entirely different meaning for an adolescent than it might for a younger child. The opportunity to meet with peers in a club format for projects and discussions dealing with issues of moral responsibility and global concerns might not only engage the adolescent in positive peer interactions, but also might assist in the achievement of the underpinnings necessary for choosing all present and future occupations holding meaning and personal fulfillment. For example, the Roots and Shoots club may be equally appealing for younger children and for adolescents, but programming within the goals of the club would take on quite different features to hold the interest of the two age groups. Csikszentmihalyi and Larson (1984) have researched the lives of adolescents in order to provide a picture from the "inside-out," or the adolescent's internal dimensions of experience. They explore many areas that can assist us in organizing programming for this age group, but much of the adolescent experiences appear to be ones of conflict between instinctual choices (perhaps more similar to middle childhood) and emerging values. This transition reinforces the use of activity experiences to assist in clarifying thinking with regard to daily and long-term occupational choices and to value systems that may be in the process of development.

Whether one supports the view of adolescence as a generally unpleasant and stormy period of transition or not, it is surely recognized as a period of considerable stress and responsibility as the child prepares for new roles requiring independence. This is a time when intervention in the form of education, information, skill building, and supportive coaching/mentoring is needed to encourage self-efficacy and a smooth transition toward positive choices. You may wish to review the developmental theories of childhood and adolescence in depth as you prepare to work with these groups and as you select your conceptual framework or "window" through which to view your community group. When we consider the ideas for community programming with adolescent populations—whether these populations are thought to be at risk (note that some theorists believe this is such a difficult period that *all* adolescents may be *at risk*) or whether we are working with adolescents who have recognized psychopathology—we must utilize what is known developmentally about these children to build the goals for our programs.

If you are designing programming for children with known psychosocial dysfunction or children with delayed cognitive and social development, then you must be familiar with the literature on seriously emotionally disturbed (SED), autistic spectrum disorders, attention deficit disorder, and cognitive disabilities. Although it will not tell us much about the individual child's problems, the *Diagnostic and Statistical Manual for Mental Disorders, V* (American Psychiatric Association, 2003) is widely used to describe the clinical manifestations of these disorders. Florey (1998, 2003) and Florey and Greene (1997) however, caution us that there is confusion in identifying children with emotional problems. The reasons for this dilemma may include such factors as fear of stigma, financial constraints, and general lack of identification, which often results in children being inappropriately labeled collectively as "learning disabled."

The school system, which is where the child's primary occupation is enacted, is likely the "community" where much of your child-adolescent programming will take place (if not directly in the school, then in environments adjacent to the school). Alternative schools and detention centers are also excellent sites for programming; these are sites where children and adolescents may be placed following engagement in risk factors (such as substance abuse, delinquent behavior, and youth pregnancies) that may accompany SED or learning disability.

## Gender-Specific Clubs

When considering the structure of a club or "community within a community," one must consider how much the structure/organization should mirror the so-called "real world" or expected environment of the child and how much it should be adapted to provide opportunities for learning and preparation for a reality not yet attained. Young (1992) and Batsleer (1996) support the idea of community programming as a way to support young girls' and women's concerns separate from those of young men, and they offer an agenda to challenge what they describe as sexism in community work—at least from a social service perspective. Although their particular examples are from England, there is likely cross-cultural validity in their findings. Hooks (1984) proposes the use of the forum of community programming to assist in advocating for women and their emancipation and to assist in obtaining justice. In her view, community programming can support feminism in its effort to end oppression. In fact, community work with young women who have been abused, are pregnant in childhood, are young single mothers, or have been accustomed to becoming sexually and emotionally support to or codependent with young male gang members may have such an awareness and intention as an obvious or, more likely, covert agenda.

Women and men as "communities" may share some but not all social experiences. Mixing same sex but different ages and cultures may offer new interpretations of experience and new identities. Taking risks and acknowledging differences and similarities may result in creativity in problem solving and resultant strength (Batsleer, 1996). Batsleer goes on to support offering young women relevant information in an environment where they feel comfortable and secure. The comfortable and secure environment may be the strongest support for **gender-specific clubs**. Beetham (1991) and Arendt (1986) refer to these community groups as "empowering," which is triggered by acting in concert. Arendt (1986) notes that "power is never the property of an individual; it belongs to a group and remains in existence only so long as the group keeps together" (Arendt, 1986; p. 64). Arendt goes on to say that same-sex groups (women in her examples) can exercise power by rules of exclusion. This exclusion of not only the opposite sex but also members of the same sex by arbitrarily changing "passwords" for entry or other such exclusionary rules is, in fact, part of the appeal of informal clubs in middle childhood.

Safe houses and other examples of community programming for abused women and their children are examples of what Arendt (1986, p. 64) might describe as "empowering practice." These are intended to be safe places to teach and support strategies for resisting or avoiding violence but perhaps more importantly to establish links to the legal and social systems and to other women.

With any community, group empowerment seems to be a desirable agenda even if it is not the primary or even visible one. Programming that includes informed choices, self-reflection through the telling of life stories, and survival techniques offers empowering opportunities. The "Mommy and Me" Story Quilt Club program is an example. One should also note that empowerment is certainly not only for the young, for older adults are often disenfranchised when it comes to issues of power and efficacy as well. An important feature of the study on aging performed by Clark, Azen, Zemke, Jackson, Carlson, Mandel et al. (1997) was that wellness was supported in part by knowing how to access the occupations in which one wanted to engage. In this way, the occupational therapists offered information and opportunity with regard to access not only to such things as public transportation but, more importantly, to power and efficacy.

If these arguments seem too political for you, consider the work of several developmental theorists concerning gender and minority-group development. A number of researchers have studied identity formation as a critical stage of adolescent development, and several of these studies have focused specifically on gender differences (Abraham, Feldman, and Nash, 1978; Markstrom-Adams, 1992; Markus and Kitayama, 1991). Others have focused on minority differences where there appears to be much stronger evidence than for gender-based differences. Spencer and Markstrom-Adams (1990), for example, have researched identity formation among minority-group children in the United States. For these children the progression through childhood and adolescence is further complicated by negative social stereotyping by their majority peers and often by lower incomes that push them to a social status lower than their majority peers. If you consider these factors alongside Marcia's stages of identity formation, then the children in this group may be at risk for altering their development through what he describes as foreclosure, or adopting an externally-based identity and prematurely committing to roles rather than to goals and values (Marcia, 1966; p. 556).

Earlier theorists, including Freud (1935/1953) and Erikson (1968), believed there were significant sex differences in the process of forming an identity. More recent research offers mixed support for this earlier contention. In their work on identity development, role-taking skills, occupational knowledge, and career development in adolescence, Grotevant, Cooper, and Kramer (1986) and Grotevant and Durrett (1980) reported that adolescent girls scored higher levels of identity achievement than boys with regard to friendship. Their work was supported by Archer (1982, 1992), who found that girls score higher in areas of choice with regard to combining career and family. Based on this somewhat limited research, support for gender-based clubs is not as compelling as support might be for minority-based programming. If one considers other measurements of development in addition to identity formation, however, then perhaps a stronger case can be made. Certainly gender-based and minority-based programming will likely have a different mission, goals, and objectives than those where the population is more diverse. Neville-Jan, Fazio, Kennedy, and Snyder (1997) offer a description of a middle school program that focuses on transition. The programming interweaves the developmentally related needs of these children along with minority-based concerns that extend into the family and the community.

# The Clubs

Although this is certainly not an exclusive listing, there are many opportunities for programming across the country offered in conjunction with the following five organizations or clubs: the 4-H Club; the Jane Goodall Roots and Shoots Program; the Boys and Girls Clubs of America; the Young Men's Christian Association (YMCA); and the Young Women's Christian Association (YWCA). These organizations have been selected specifically because of the compatibility of their missions with our interests as occupation-centered practitioners. The following descriptions will provide you with some general background information on these four groups. As you read about the organizations, think about compatible occupation-centered programming that you might develop.

## The 4-H Club

I pledge my HEAD to clearer thinking, my HEART to greater loyalty, my HANDS to larger service and my HEALTH to better living.

Perhaps you recognize this as the motto, or pledge, of the **4-H club**. The beginnings of the twentieth century also witnessed the beginnings of what might be described as the demise of the rural American lifestyle, which was represented through a sense of "rugged individualism" coupled with a concern and kindness translated as "neighborliness." The young people of rural America were rapidly leaving for the cities and perceived brighter futures in industry. Beginning as early as the late 1800s, several factors brought about the beginnings of the 4-H club. These included a growing concern for the quality of rural education and the relevance of the public schools to country life and a concern for advancing agricultural technology that was being developed by land-grant universities but was not gaining rapid favor in most agricultural communities (www.4h-usa.org).

4-H appears not to be the idea of any one person; rather, it was developed as a widespread grass-roots movement to encourage rural youth to "stay on the farm" but to do so while embracing new ideas for productivity as well as sound values and behaviors. By 1904 clubs were formed to teach life skills and learning-by-doing projects. Community service projects were developed to capture the joint efforts of adults and youth, first by appealing to boys through activities such as rewarding the best corn crop and then to girls by fostering sewing, canning of vegetables, and baking projects. Interest spread throughout the Midwest and Texas, and in 1906 Thomas M. Campbell, an assistant of George Washington Carver, organized clubs with similar goals for Black farmers and their children in the south. These so-called "corn" and "sewing" clubs came under the sponsorship of the Cooperative Extension System established by the Smith-Lever Act in 1914, and 4-H clubs soon were started in nearly every state. The clubs for boys and girls tended to be organized separately. While boys were being encouraged to adopt new agricultural techniques and methods to increase production, the girls' groups were evolving to examine the roles of women in the rural home and community. Self-confidence and a commitment to community became shared goals.

Clubs were not only in rural areas but in cities as well. Many of the city-based clubs were organized to encourage activities between rural and city youth, and by 1948 the exchanges were matched by those between American and European club members through the International Farm Youth Exchange.

Today the 4-H club movement continues to be strong and is more centered on the personal growth of the child. 4-H boys and girls clubs are most often combined under similar interests. Projects continue to be utilized in the development of life-long skills, and efforts are rewarded. It is intended that participants become contributing, productive, self-directed members of society. Making decisions, learning to communicate, learning the characteristics of leadership, and learning how to cope with change are goals of today's clubs.

The 4-H club remains a largely federally organized group with county and states retaining control over its programs. International programs are presently active in more than 80 countries. A wide and diverse range of interests was represented in the listing of the National Training and Events Activities of Clubs in 1997–1998; these included such topics as Partnerships for Preventing Violence; Habitat Evaluation; Engineering, Science, and Leadership; Dairy Conference; Safety Council Congress and Exposition; and the Poultry and Egg Conference (www.4H-usa.org/history.htm; world.htm).

Today's clubs, which have expanded to become some of the most successful youth clubs in existence, range from the community club model to urban interest groups, community resource development, special interest groups, school enrichment, camping, and interagency learning experiences. The most recent 4-H initiative, in 2002, was the 4-H Afterschool (www.4hafterschool.org), a volunteer driven program designed to help kids find something fun, constructive, and safe to do in the hours after school. It is not difficult to recognize the similarities between the purposes and goals of 4-H and those of occupational therapy. An occupation-based program focused on health promotion, social skills enhancement, and emotional risk reduction can be comfortably placed within the existing structures of 4-H club programming while retaining the vitality of both. Opportunities for creative programming based on the principles of occupation are boundless.

## Roots and Shoots

**Roots and Shoots** was established in the summer of 1960 by the internationally recognized ethologist Jane Goodall. Dr. Goodall is best known for her research on chimpanzee behavior in Tanzania, but she is becoming equally recognized for her substantial interests in conservation, education, and animal welfare. Roots and Shoots is an international environmental education and humanitarian program for young people. The program encourages and empowers children and young adults to coordinate constructive activities that promote care and concern for the environment, for animals, and for the human community. Roots and Shoots was the name selected to recognize that "children are the fertile ground in which seeds are planted" (The Jane Goodall Institute for Wildlife Research, Education, and Conservation, 1995).

Once seeds germinate, of course, their roots spread in all directions and establish a firm foundation. Important work can be accomplished when each child is recognized as important to the future of all children. Clubs currently exist in 38 states and more than 30 countries around the world. The fundamental concepts and philosophy of Roots and Shoots include "care and concern for the environment; care and concern for animals; and community enrichment through constructive service projects" (The Jane Goodall Institute for Wildlife Research, Education, and Conservation, 1995).

The example we will explore a bit later in this chapter is one of a club within a club, that is, Roots and Shoots within the structure of a 4-H club. Although the interests of the occupational therapy providers/occupation-based practitioners were in the enrichment of and concern for the individual child, all of the concepts and philosophies of both the 4-H club and the Roots and Shoots organization were utilized as tools in the development of programming.

## Boys and Girls Clubs of America

The Boys and Girls Club movement is a nationwide affiliation of local autonomous nonprofit organizations. The mission of the Boys and Girls Clubs of America is "working to help youth from all backgrounds, with special concern for those from disadvantaged circumstances, develop the qualities needed to become responsible citizens and leaders" (www.ncnatural.com/UCYOUTH/youthweb.htm).

It is important to note that the Boys and Girls Club has a physical location, usually a neighborhood-based building where local community youth may congregate to participate in organized programs and activities. This is an important concept, for the intention is to keep children off the street and preferably not at home when adult supervision is absent. The clubs are open every day after school and on weekends. Every club has paid, full-time, trained youth-development professionals who are selected to be mentors and positive role models. Volunteers are relied on for key supplementary support. Children pay a small amount of dues per year, but supportive moneys are provided through campaigned gift donations based on the club's proven delinquency-prevention programs.

There are currently approximately 2,013 club facilities located in all fifty states, Puerto Rico, the Virgin Islands, and domestic and international military bases. In 1996 operating budgets for all clubs amounted to approximately $432,000,000 (www.bgca.org/html/numbers/html).

It is interesting to note that of the 2,800,000 boys and girls served in 1996, 71 percent lived in urban/inner-city areas, 53 percent were from single-parent families, 51 percent were from families of three or more children, 56 percent were from minority families, and 42 percent were from families with annual incomes below $22,000. Ages of members range from 7 years and younger (16 percent) up to 18 years of age (21 percent are between the ages of 14 and 18), with the largest group (34 percent) between 8 and 10 years of age. Boys make up 62 percent of the children and girls the remaining 38 percent.

Boys and Girls Clubs are another excellent site for occupation-based programming with general goals supportive of the prevention of behaviors leading to patterns of crime and delinquency.

# A Programming Example of Multiple Collaborations: A "Club" Within a "Club" Within a "Club"

This example of the Jane Goodall Roots and Shoots programming was developed at two sites—in the 4-H Club after-school enrichment program established through the partial support of the Los Angeles Housing Authority and the County

Parks and Recreation Department and at a Los Angeles Boys and Girls Club. There is likely no better example of layered and embedded collaborations and partnering. These programs were the result of the shared efforts of the Jane Goodall Institute's Roots and Shoots programming, the 4-H Clubs of America, the Los Angeles Housing Authority, the Los Angeles County Department of Parks and Recreation, the Los Angeles Zoo, the University of Southern California's Department of Occupational Science and Occupational Therapy, and the Boys and Girls Clubs of America—Los Angeles.

The two sites selected serviced similar populations, which included Hispanic boys and girls between the ages of 7 and 11 who were from low-income families. The community profiles presented similar pictures of apparent neighborhood neglect as evidenced by graffiti, numerous gang signs, and garbage. More optimistically, it was noted that two parks were in the process of being repaired and landscaped by the city.

The two occupation-centered programs were identical in their after-school structure and in their affiliation with existing clubs. The Phase I needs assessment at both sites demonstrated an interest in programming that would support the existing goals of both the 4-H club and the Boys and Girls Club. Both groups expressed interest in improving their community and suggested several ways they might do so that ranged from picking up trash to planting flowers to helping older residents run errands in the neighborhood. Because of its supportive structure for understanding and building *community* through attention to one's habitat (that is, in our case, neighorhood) and its already-developed programming ideas along these lines, the Jane Goodall Roots and Shoots structure was selected as a vehicle for the occupation-centered intervention. The success of the existing after-school 4-H Club at the Housing Authority site and the Boys and Girls Club, as well as the chronological and developmental ages of the children involved, supported the choice of a club format embedded within the existing programming.

Although not necessarily articulated, the combined message of all of the clubs was *empowerment* to *affect change* first in one's community and secondly in oneself. In addition, building a community of caring and concerned children whose example would encourage those around them to also build rather than destroy was equally important. A review of the purposes of both organizations demonstrates that the goal of "empowerment through positive change" and the objectives to demonstrate care and concern for the community through such enabling activities as conducting a community celebration of "Earth Day" are appropriate. The specific activities of exploring the habitats and migrations of butterflies and birds through research and field surveys, planting butterfly gardens on windowsills of nursing care facilities and in backyards of public housing, trash patrols, and "acts of kindness" patrols all targeted care for the community and were visible enough to encourage the participation of other children and adults in the activities.

The Jane Goodall Roots and Shoots clubs frequently form a liaison with local zoos, which offers additional programming opportunities. In this example, the Los Angeles Zoo provided an opportunity to study and assist with the design of a chimpanzee habitat for the zoo and to attend the "official" opening. What does that have to do with an inner-city Los Angeles community? It is very applicable if the programmer makes good use of the opportunity to demonstrate community as a common and global concern. In addition, if the club can be visited by Jane Goodall or by the local media news team or has the opportunity to join in world-wide conservation-environmental activities with children from other cultures and countries, then our goal of empowerment is enhanced through recognition and group consensus. These clubs also developed programming slogans around the ideas that human life—or at least the quality of life many enjoy or would like to enjoy—may be endangered. The similarities in the way that other endangered or extinct species used or abused their habitats was impetus for research and for planning.

For both programs, the low-budget activities were subsumed under existing resources in bimonthly programming. Existing space was utilized with all regular after-school club participants who were also participating in the Roots and Shoots activities. The personnel consisted of students who received service learning course credit for their contributions. At the Boys and Girls Club, older participants (teens) were paid by the club to assist with programming. At the 4-H club, paid staff was also involved with programming. In both of these cases, the consistency in programming was maintained by the paid staff when students were not available. This is a critical adjunct whenever students are involved in community-based programming so that continuity is maintained when students are not enrolled. Having volunteers or paid staff who are members of the community where programming occurs also encourages participation and investment over time. Equally important is the presence of a consistent faculty or clinical advisor/supervisor to provide

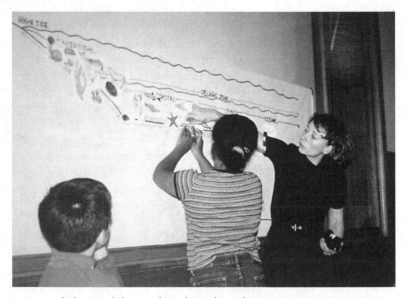

Roots and Shoots club members learn how their conservation projects in the inner-city positively impact life in the ocean.

direction as goals, objectives, and programming is turned over to others less invested. It is also an important feature when there are many "partners" sharing in the goals for programming, and in the outcomes.

In order to accurately evaluate the effectiveness of the program, it would likely need a more consistent format and perhaps some way to distinguish it from the value of the 4-H programming. A measure of the effectiveness of the combined programming, however, might be acceptable since the goals and objectives are so compatible. Evaluation of these two programs consisted of two levels: 1) information and skill building in protecting and building community (immediate); and 2) personal empowerment (long-term outcome). For the first level of evaluation, pretests and posttests of questions to determine what the children knew before and after each programming session were used to obtain immediate factual information. For example, an activity named "Take a Closer Look" (1998, p. 26) was designed to sharpen their observation skills and to serve as a reminder of individual differences. The pretest asked the children to carefully view color photos of the chimpanzees at the zoo (also identified by name), and the posttest consisted of matching the distinguishing characteristics of each and the names to the actual chimps in their habitat on a field trip to the zoo. This lesson was coupled with other activities supporting the importance of distinguishing ourselves as individuals while supporting the functions and roles of a group/community.

Teasing out the meaning associated with "empowerment" is much more complicated, and takes much longer. In these instances, the Nowicki-Strickland Locus of Control Scale for Children (1973) was used at the beginnng and end of the programming cycle, and was recommended as follow-up six months to one year later. The scale was used in an attempt to distinguish each students' sense of internal personal control over his or her life and actions. This link between perceived control and empowerment is supported by the research of Gibson (1993) and by Chamberlin (1997), who broadened the link to include community involvement and group participation. The use of the instrument appeared to produce positive outcomes, but the population was too small and the programming too inconsistent in the earlier phases to provide a sound measure. However, continued work with the instrument seems advantageous as a potentially effective measure of the program's goal. In work on self-concept formation, Harter (1982, 1985, 1990a, 1990b) developed the Perceived Competence Scale for Children, which also would be an appropriate measure of the goals for the children in these programs, as would the work of Battle (1981), Battle and Blowers (1982), Bruininks (1978), and Bryan and Pearl (1979). As an additional measure to further define the factors that contribute to community-building, empowerment, and personal control, one of the programs was videotaped to be qualitatively coded for further investigation. The programmer must always take into consideration the length of time children (or adults) are exposed to programming and the realistic time span to measure anticipated outcomes. How long before "change" will occur? How long will it last?

Another consideration to keep in mind is that whenever you select a group as recipients of your programming (in the examples here, children), you must be very aware of the meaningful occupations those recipients (children) engage in during their normal round of activities. These children were primarily engaged in a combination of schoolwork and play during their week—not an uncommon combination for any child in early and middle childhood. The task of these programs was to support the goals of schoolwork and the developmental need for play through activities that supported and enhanced "community." All of the selected programming did this, although not without some trial and error. If you would like to learn more about the use of "play" in occupational therapy, review Parham and Primeau's discussion of play (1997) and Florey and Greene's discussion of play in middle childhood (1997).

At the Boys and Girls Club site, continued programming for older participants that is external to the 4-H Club structure included the development of a Newsletter Project as well as other similar group projects to produce one shared outcome. These projects were designed to meet the goals of developing skills in the realm of leadership, communication, vocational choice, and writing and organization—all within and in support of the basic parameters of community.

As you develop your own programming, if you elect to support occupation-based goals for children to encourage the enhancement of normal development, support of school-room performance, or as a deterrent to negative-outcomes ("clubs" in the form of gangs), you may wish to more carefully examine the goals of 4-H, Boys and Girls Clubs, and, specifically, Roots and Shoots. As the Roots and Shoots programming was developed, planners discovered a number of conservation-concerned groups that provided volunteers and dollars to enhance programming. These groups included Wildlife on Wheels, Seeds of Simplicity, Heal the Bay, Tree People, The Audobon Society, and numerous parks, gardens, zoos, and museums. You will likely find similar organizations in your area.

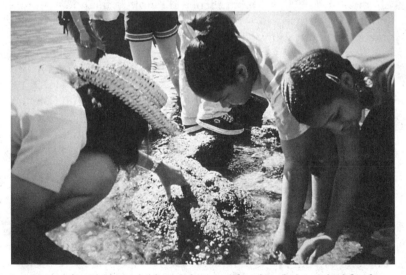

Parents work with their children in learning first-hand about the life of sea creatures as they participate in a "Heal the Bay" project.

# The Young Men's Christian Association (YMCA)

The **YMCA** was founded in London in 1844 by Sir George Williams (knighted in 1894 for his lifelong service to boys). Impetus for the establishment of the organization was the unhealthy social conditions of the times apparent in the large urban cities at the end of the Industrial Revolution. The founding young businessmen wished to help young workers avoid the social "dangers" of idleness (such as gambling and drinking) through Bible studies and prayer meetings. The organization quickly gained popularity and spread to the industrial centers of North America and throughout Europe. The first YMCA to be established in America was in Boston in 1851, and by 1854 there were 26 associations in the United States and Canada.

In 1862 the attention of the association was turned to the welfare of American Civil War prisoners. This was the first civilian volunteer organization dedicated to the welfare of war prisoners and other servicemen, and this work continued through World War I and World War II. The YMCA continued to work not only with prisoners of war but also with displaced persons, refugees, and soldiers. In 1941 the YMCA joined with five other organizations to form the United Service Organizations (USO).

The post-war YMCA continued to evolve by incorporating libraries, gymnasiums, summer camps, colleges, night schools, swimming pools, mass swimming instruction, and hotel-type rooms. It is of interest that to meet the need for a "vigorous recreation suitable for indoor winter play," an instructor at the Springfield, Massachusetts YMCA, Mr. James Naismith, invented basketball in 1891 (www.tased.edu.au/tasonline/ymca/history1.htm). At this YMCA, which is now Springfield College, volleyball was invented in 1895 by Mr. William G. Morgan, the physical education director of the YMCA in Holyoke, Massachusetts. The YMCA also assisted in the development of other groups such as the Red Cross, Boy Scouts, the Student Christian Movement, World Council of Churches, and CampFire. The years between the 1930s and the 1960s were marked by diminished interest in the activities of the YMCA and difficult financial times. In the late 1970s, however, there was renewed public interest in health and fitness, and child care was added to the organization's programs to meet the demands and needs of young mothers.

Presently the YMCA serves approximately fourteen million people a year. Local YMCAs are independent and autonomous and are dedicated to *local community needs and service* and have as their goal the provision of *values-based experiences that nurture the healthy development of children and teens, support families, and strengthen communities*. Their mission is "to put Christian principles into practice through programs that build healthy spirit, mind, and body for all" (www.ymca.net/d/1/1.html). Each YMCA is a charitable, nonprofit organization.

# The Young Women's Christian Association (YWCA)

The **YWCA** is the largest and oldest women's organization in the United States (www.ywca.org/). Its mission is to empower women and girls and to work to eliminate racism. The YWCA opened the first day nursery in the United States in 1864 and today continues to train child care providers and baby-sitters. Other child-related services are found in the forms of resource and referral agencies, child care for homeless children, services to family day care homes, and parenting education. Services for women include basic life skills training, GED courses, adult education, welfare-to-work programs, nontraditional employment, and other related services. It should be noted that women worked in the YMCA military canteens in World War I, but it was not until after World War II that they were admitted to full YMCA membership. The YWCA, however, establishes specific goals to meet the general needs of women.

Globally, the YWCA represents more than 25 million women throughout 101 countries. The YWCA provides shelter, child care, employment training, racial justice, physical fitness, youth development, leadership training, and world relations. Each year more than 650,000 people come to the YWCA for services and support to overcome violence (www.ywca.org/mission/world_relations.html).

Two examples of programming utilizing the YMCA and YWCA will be described. One program was established with the YMCA for older adults with Parkinson's disease and their spouses, and another was established for young, single, inner-city mothers under the umbrella of the YWCA. Both are quite different but well within the missions of the two organizations.

# Programs in Collaboration With the YMCA and the YWCA

Programs can be developed within the mission of an umbrella organization but also can be very different in their goals and objectives and in the population that they serve. There is no "recipe" for programs within the 4-H Club, the Boys and Girls Club, or the YMCA/YWCA. The ability to see opportunities for creative expression of an organization's mission through the exercise of occupation is entirely at the pleasure of the programmer. We will now briefly contrast two programs, each carefully articulated with the mission and goals of the YMCA/YWCA. The first, an exercise program for client/members of the YMCA with Parkinson's disease and their spouses, is described in the following section.

## A Shared Exercise Program for Client/Members With Parkinson's Disease and Their Spouses

An exercise program for client/members of the YMCA with Parkinson's Disease and their spouses, was initiated in a fairly common way—at the request of a participant in an out-patient occupational therapy program. This participant was also a member of a YMCA in an affluent neighborhood where he had long been a strong advocate for his community in many ways. He expressed to his occupational therapist a concern that he would like to return to his YMCA for an exercise group. At the time there was no such group that took into consideration the specific needs of people with Parkinson's disease. But there was another agenda as well; "meaning" for this patient was not only a wish to resume what for him had been a fairly normalizing activity ("adult play at the YMCA"), but also there was a need to continue or perhaps to encourage the expression of bonding and support by including his spouse. As a skillful and intuitive occupational therapist elicited this patient's story, he or she would recognize other meanings being expressed as well. Perhaps the patient wanted to not only engage in exercise and spend time with his spouse but also and, more importantly, wanted to return to a more proactive role in his life and his community (to be an advocate and someone who can still get things done). Perhaps he also wanted to return to a more normalizing spousal role in which he could engage in an activity with his spouse where she was not the caregiver but the partner. Oftentimes personal collaborations are as worthy of encouragement as are the larger, professional shared ventures.

With some guidance the client/member (or, simply, the community-member) developed an advocacy plan to encourage the initiation of a couples exercise/dance program for himself, his spouse, and others with similar needs. The program was developed much like what has been described in this text. When a needs assessment demonstrated that there was enough interest to start with several classes a week, the YMCA added the classes for a fee in a similar structure to other programming and took care of the promotion and marketing. The occupational therapist, who was also an aerobics instructor and an avid "line-dancer," was hired to develop the programming along with the assistance of the participants. This program demonstrates a nice bridge between the treatment setting (one of the arenas of occupational therapy) and the community (one of the arenas of the occupation-centered practitioner). It also demonstrates the true art of the practitioner—that of recognizing and enabling the strengths of the participant to once again put them in control of their own lives.

## The "Mommy and Me" Story Quilt Club

Another example appropriate to our discussion is that of a "Mommy and Me" program established in a YWCA in a far less affluent neighborhood than the one described previously. Affluence does not have much to do with these two stories, except that it does seem to go hand-in-hand with one's perceived sense of control over one's destiny, which makes for some difference in the selection of goals and objectives for a successful program. Following its own somewhat informal needs assessment, this program was initiated at the request of the YWCA. The YWCA was interested in two programs—one for young mothers (13–16 years old) and another for these mothers and the fathers. The program for the mothers was designed to also actively include the babies. The format consisted of classes, which was similar to other programming at this facility but fees were not charged directly to the participants. The mother and baby classes involved the shared and enmeshed occupations surrounding the physical care of the baby and also the "learning how to play together" emotional care of both mother (an adolescent) and baby.

Perhaps the most successful activity associated with this program (as reported by the mothers) was one that focused on meaningful occupation and self-advocacy, which was a theme in the previous example as well. The activity consisted of making an over-sized quilt block that was large enough to function as a baby coverlet. The design of the block was developed as the mother's "story" that she wished to give her baby as her legacy or gift. The story was an expression of the mother's meaningful occupations, her values, her interests, and the things about life she most wanted her baby to know and remember. An important piece of the block also carried the theme of what the mother still wished to do with her life. Although the blocks were constructed individually, the activity was carried out as a group—the "quilting club" —and this community of young storytellers shared and validated their experiences and came away with a tangible record. This class was conducted by student volunteers as a residential life community service project; and, later, became the full responsibility of the YWCA.

# Free-Standing Clubs

The last two examples we will explore are again quite different from each other in terms of population, intention, and geography and are both examples of **free-standing clubs**, although collaboration and partnering with other service providers and organizations in the community were strong factors in both. The Ice Cream Cart Club was a rural, midwestern venture, while the Jazz Club was an inner-city urban experiment.

## The Ice Cream Cart Club

The Ice Cream Cart Club was developed in response to a need, which was expressed primarily by teachers in the beginning, to better integrate children with learning disabilities and autistic spectrum disorders into the student life activities of the middle school environment. All of the students identified first by the teachers were described as "socially isolated." The program was developed as a club in consideration of the developmental needs of this group (chronologically aged 11 to 14 ), and this idea was also strongly supported in the second level of needs assessment accomplished with the children who wished to be involved. All of the children first identified by the teachers were invited to be members but none were required to be. By consensus the children elected to start a lunch-time ice cream cart business. The programming involved multiple skill development in sales, marketing/promotion, accounting, and personnel management. Although significant in helping students to focus future goals and staying in school (long-range outcomes), foundational goals were centered again around empowerment, advocacy, and self-esteem—a theme that continues to resurface in much of our programming, particularly with children and adolescents. Weekly club meetings were facilitated by a school-based occupational therapist who helped develop individual goals for each child as well as goals for the collective club. The club meetings were often indistinguishable from the goal-directed adolescent psychosocial group model (the goal being the business to be accomplished for the week). Continued programming includes the addition of several high school mentors for the group to assist in the transition from middle school as well as mentors from local businesses.

## The Dunbar Hotel Jazz Club

The second example of the development of a club model—in this case to *create* community—is that of the Jazz Club. The Dunbar Hotel is located in downtown Los Angeles and is part of the Dunbar Economic Development Corporation. In 1975 the Dunbar Hotel Black Cultural Historical Museum was established to save the Dunbar Hotel. Through these efforts, the Hotel was designated as a city and national historical landmark (The Dunbar Economic Development Corporation, 1996).

In recognition of low-income housing needs, in 1988 the hotel was financed for mixed use to include housing (73 units of low-income senior housing), commercial facilities, and cultural facilities. The intent of the occupation-based programming that was later to be developed was to create a sense of shared "community" for these residents. In order to identify the characteristics of "community" and the meaning these residents assigned to their lives and their history, it seemed appropriate to investigate the history of the hotel. Oftentimes a building or a neighborhood has forgotten history that, when resurrected, can structure the goals and objectives of a program. In this case, the history was that of jazz. In its original 1920s state, the hotel was a first-class accommodation for African American guests. It was surrounded by jazz clubs and became the hub of Los Angeles night life. As

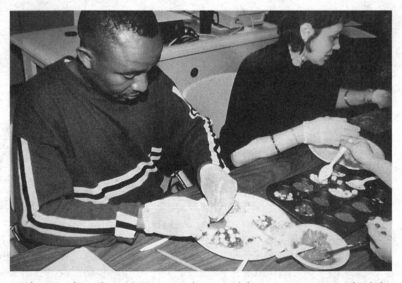

Students and residents decorate cookies to celebrate a "jazz artist's" birthday.

integration grew into the 1950s and African American entertainers and club goers were no longer restricted to downtown, the hotel and the neighborhood drifted into decay. One of the occupational therapy students, a jazz historian, took an interest in the hotel and in the present residents. Upon closer investigation and a cursory needs assessment, accomplished with the assistance of the social service coordinator, it was determined that the general health and well-being of the residents could likely be enhanced if they could be encouraged to become less isolated and share in some kind of activity programming. Although there was a space designed for shared activities, no one frequented the room and attempts at programming by volunteer groups had not been successful.

Upon further investigation, it was discovered that many of the residents had been participants in the vibrant neighborhood of the jazz era, and a number were musicians themselves. Although we cannot assume that everyone continues to assign meaning to their own histories, with the kind of shared interests evident at the Dunbar it was a fair guess that jazz , in some way, continued to have meaning for many of the residents. With the resources of the museum, a Jazz Appreciation Club was organized first to plan and celebrate birthdays of African American jazz performers and then to organize jam sessions and mini-concerts. Residents were first involved as the audience, but those who were able quickly became more active participants and/or contributors.

Again, this example includes the theme of "meaning" as the significant indicator of well-being and therapy. In this example, the meaning is assessed through linkages with history, and those linkages weave the fabric of community.

## Summary

Clubs are examples of a community within a community. They offer the child, the adolescent, and the adult structures that support and encourage their cognitive and social development. In this way, they provide the potential for powerful interventions. The cognitive and social development of middle-childhood and adolescence has been discussed to provide a foundation for understanding how the structure of clubs can be utilized to support a program that is developmentally sensitive. Whether or not the program planner wishes to encourage gender-specific clubs or to mix participants has also been considered. Understanding the developmental period of the participant will assist the planner who wishes to place a program within a club in selecting an appropriate club structure from existing ones or in the creation of rules and structures for a new club.

Existing club structures have been described such as the 4-H clubs, Jane Goodall's Roots and Shoots clubs, Boys and Girls Clubs of America, and the YMCA/YWCA. Examples have been provided for occupation-centered clubs within the aforementioned existing club structures. In addition, the development of two freestanding clubs, the Ice Cream Cart Club and the Jazz Club, have been briefly described. All of the examples involve collaborations and partnering with the community. The concept of "club" within developmentally appropriate contexts and rule-bound structures can provide a frame for the placement of successful occupation-centered programs for all ages.

# References

Abraham, B., Feldman, S. S., & Nash, S. C. (1978). Sex role self-concept and sex role attitudes: Enduring personality characteristics or adaptations to changing life situations? *Developmental Psychology, 14*, 393–400.

American Psychiatric Association. (2003). *Diagnostic and statistical manual of mental disorders* (5th ed.). Washington, DC: Author.

Archer, S. L. (1982). The lower age boundaries of identity development. *Child Development, 53*, 1,551–1,556.

Archer, S. L. (1992). A feminist's approach to identity research. In G. R. Adams, T. P. Gulotta, & R. Montemayor, (Eds.), *Adolescent identity formation* (Advances in Adolescent Development, Vol. 4). Newbury Park, CA: Sage.

Arendt, H. (1986). Communicative power. In S. Lukes, (Ed.), *Power* (p. 64). Oxford: Basil Blackwell.

Batsleer, J. (1996). *Working with girls and young women in community settings*. London: Arena.

Battle, J. (1981). Culture free self esteem inventory, self-esteem inventory for children and adults. Seattle, WA: Special Child Publications.

Battle, J., & Blowers, T. (1982). A longitudinal comparative study of the self-esteem of students in regular and special education classes. *Journal of Learning Disabilities, 15*, 100–102.

Beetham, D. (1991). *The legitimation of power*. London: MacMillan.

Bruininks, V. L. (1978). Actual and perceived peer status of learning disabled students in mainstream programs. *Journal of Special Education, 12*, 51–58.

Bryan, T. H., & Pearl, R. (1979). Self-concept and locus of control of learning disabled children. *Journal of Clinical Child Psychology, 8*, 223–226

Chamberlin, J. (1997). A working definition of empowerment. *Psychiatric Rehabilitation Journal, 20*(4), 43–46.

Clark, F., Azen, S., Zemke, R., Jackson, J., Carlson, M., Mandel, D., et al. (1997). Occupational therapy for independent-living older adults. *Journal of the American Medical Association, 278*(16), 1,321–1,326.

Csikszentmihalyi, M., & Larson, R. (1984). *Being adolescent*. New York: Basic Books, Harper and Row.

Erikson, E. (1968). *Identity: Youth in crisis*. New York: Norton.

Florey, L. (1998). Psychosocial dysfunction in childhood and adolescence. In M. Neistadt, & E. Crepeau, (Eds.), *Willard and Spackman's occupational therapy* (pp. 622–635). Philadelphia: Lippincott.

Florey, L. (2003). Psychosocial dysfunction in childhood and adolescence. In E. Crepeau, E. Cohn, & B. Schell, (Eds.), *Willard and Spackman's occupational therapy* (pp. 731–744). Philadelphia: Lippincott.

Florey, L., & Greene, S. (1997). Play in middle childhood: A focus on children with behavior and emotional disorders. In L. D. Parham, & L. S. Fazio, (Eds.), *Play in occupational therapy for children* (pp. 126–143). St. Louis, MO: Mosby.

Freud, S. (1935/1953). *A general introduction to psychoanalysis.* (J. Riviere, Translator). New York: Permabooks.

Gibson, C. M. (1993). Empowerment theory and practice with adolescents of color in the child welfare system. *Families in Society, 74*(7), 387–396.

Gilligan, C. (1982). *In a different voice: Psychological theory and women's development.* Cambridge, MA: Harvard University Press.

Grotevant, H. D., Cooper, C. R., & Kramer, K. (1986). Exploration as a predictor of congruence in adolescents' career choices. *Journal of Vocational Behavior, 29,* 201–215.

Grotevant, H. D., & Durrett, M. (1980). Occupational knowledge and career development in adolescence. *Journal of Vocational Behavior, 17,* 171–182.

Harter, S. (1982). The perceived competence scale for children. *Child Development, 53,* 87–97.

Harter, S. (1985). *Manual for the self-perception profile for children.* Denver, CO: University of Denver Press.

Harter, S. (1990a). Issues in the assessment of the self-concept of children and adolescents. In A. M. LaGreca, (Ed.), *Through the eyes of the child: Obtaining self-reports from children and adolescents.* Boston: Allyn and Bacon.

Harter, S. (1990b). Processes underlying adolescent self-concept formation. In R. Montemayor, G. R. Adams, & T. P. Gullotta, (Eds.), *From childhood to adolescence: A transitional period?* Newbury Park, CA: Sage.

Havighurst, R. (1972). *Developmental tasks of education* (3rd ed.). New York: David McKay.

Hooks, B. (1984). *Feminist theory: From margin to center.* Boston: South End Press.

Inhelder, B., & Piaget, J. (1958). *The growth of logical thinking from childhood to adolescence.* New York: Basic Books.

The Jane Goodall Institute for Wildlife Research, Education and Conservation. (1995). Roots and Shoots Fact Sheet. Ridgefield, Connecticut.

Keating, D. P. (1980). Thinking processes in adolescence. In J. Adelson, (Ed.), *Handbook of adolescent psychology.* New York: Wiley.

Kohlberg, L. (1984). *The psychology of moral development: The nature and validity of moral stages.* New York: Harper and Row.

Marcia, J. (1966). Development and validation of ego identity status. *Journal of Personality and Social Psychology, 3,* 551–558.

Markstrom-Adams, C. (1992). A consideration of intervening factors in adolescent identity formation. In G. R. Adams, T. P. Gullotta, & R. Montemayor, (Eds.),

*Adolescent identity formation (advances in adolescent development)* Vol. 4. Newbury Park, CA: Sage.

Markus, H. R., & Kitayama, S. (1991). Culture and the self: Implications for cognition, emotion, and motivation. *Psychological Review, 98,* 224–253.

Neville-Jan, A., Fazio, L. S., Kennedy, B., & Snyder, C. (1997). Elementary to middle school transition: Using multicultural play activities to develop life skills. In L. D. Parham, & L. S. Fazio, (Eds.), *Play in occupational therapy for children* (pp. 144–157). St. Louis, MO: Mosby.

Nowicki, S., & Strickland, B. R. (1973). A locus of control scale for children. *Journal of Consulting and Clinical Psychology, 40,* 148 – 154.

Parham, L. D., & Primeau, L. (1997). Introduction to play and occupational therapy. In L. D. Parham, & L. S. Fazio, (Eds.), *Play in Occupational Therapy for Children* (pp. 2–21). St. Louis, MO: Mosby.

Piaget, J. (1960). *The psychology of intelligence.* Patterson, NJ: Littlefield, Adams.

Siegler, R. S. (1981). Developmental sequences within and between concepts. *Monographs of the Society for Research in Child Development, 46*(2, Serial No. 189).

Sigelman, C., & Shaffer, D. (1995). *Life-span human development* (2nd ed.). Pacific Grove, CA: Brooks/Cole.

Spencer, M., & Markstrom-Adams, C. (1990). Identity processes among racial and ethnic minority children in America. *Child Development, 61,* 290–310.

"Take a Closer Look." (1998). Roots and Shoots Los Angeles: A curriculum packet to connect community, environment and wildlife. (Limited publication supported by The Los Angeles Roots and Shoots Steering Committee, The Los Angeles Zoo, and The University of Southern California Department of Occupational Science and Occupational Therapy).

The Dunbar Economic Development Corporation. (1996). *Organizational history.* Los Angeles: The Dunbar Economic Development Corporation.

Young, K. (1992, April). Work with girls and young women: Losing the purpose? *Youth Clubs, 67,* 17.

## Internet Sites

4-H: http://www.4h-usa.org

4-H Afterschool: www.4hafterschool.org

YMCA: http://www.tased.edu.au/tasonline/ymca/history1.htm

YWCA: http://www.ywca.org;
   http://www.ywca.org/mission/shelter_services_victims.html

Boys and Girls Clubs: http://www.ncnatural.com/UCYOUTH/youthweb.htm;
   http://www.bgca.org/html/numbers.html

# CHAPTER 18

# Shelter Programming for Homeless Persons with HIV/AIDS and Mental Illness: Exploring Prevocational and Vocational Skills

## Learning Objectives

1. To appreciate the complexity of programming necessary to meet the multiple needs of those homeless persons with HIV/AIDS who may be mentally ill
2. To examine the development of a sample program to meet the goals and multiple objectives of a selected group of homeless persons with HIV/AIDS and mental illness
3. To understand the contributions of task analysis to the success of an occupation-centered program designed to meet multiple objectives

## Key Terms

1. HIV/AIDS and Homelessness
2. Mental Illness and Homelessness
3. Shelter
4. Prevocational and Vocational
5. Occupational Balance
6. Task Analysis

The population introduced in the title of this chapter appears to be cumbersome in description, but it is, in fact, quite common in today's shelter and mission system to find **HIV/AIDS, mental illness**, substance abuse, and physical illness existing simultaneously in one individual who is **homeless**. This truly challenges the skills of the occupational therapy practitioner to bring to the forefront all of the academic information and experience he or she can accumulate while maintaining a focus on meaningful occupation and the self-assigned needs of the person.

Of course, successful programs can be conducted in the community for all of the aforementioned groups, individually, with entirely different objectives; however, when working in the community, it can be more beneficial to combine groups whenever possible and to remember that the presence of a diagnosis or disease entity has little bearing on your programming. Rather, it is your challenge to design meaningful programming for the individual and to remember that your intervention occurs within and is strongly influenced by the orientation of community.

You must also remember that even though a population may share the condition of homelessness, this is by no means perceived in the same way by each individual. For some it may be disabling; for others it is desirable and enabling. The condition or circumstance of homelessness represents a *community* of individuals who must be treated as such.

# The Population Characteristics of Our Program Example

Individuals living with schizophrenia make up a large portion of the population of the mentally ill who are homeless, and this was true for the program we will describe. Chronicity with acute episodes is a frequent pattern, and failure to obtain and/or maintain medications is a common occurrence (albeit a result of neglect, misinformation, fear, or lack of availability). Self-medicating behaviors through street drugs or alcohol complicate and exacerbate already unpleasant symptoms such as hallucinations and delusions. In addition, depression is a common factor and is even more likely to prompt self-medicating behaviors than perhaps the symptoms of schizophrenia. In combination with mental illness or existing alone, HIV/AIDS must also be considered.

There are approximately 30.6 million people worldwide living with HIV/AIDS, and approximately 612,078 reported cases in the United States (Centers for Disease Control and Prevention, 2005; Karon, 1996). Assuming that all cases are not recognized or reported, it is difficult to obtain an accurate estimate, and the official estimates are probably low. This population also is often homeless and may use street drugs and alcohol to mediate their symptoms. On a more optimistic note, according to 1997 statistics provided by the Los Angeles County Department of Health Services, the fatality rate in Los Angeles County has dropped from

95 percent in 1983 for advanced HIV disease to 11 percent in 1996. These statistics are encouraging for those with HIV disease and AIDS and for those who care for them.

## The Site of Our Program Example

The site/location of the "papermaking" program was within a **shelter** system consisting of seven houses, each supporting the combined mission to provide residential care and supportive housing to assist those in transition to independent living. There were from five to seven residents in each home, and all were considered to be homeless before coming into the residential system. To receive funded services in this particular system, residents were first required to be HIV positive and symptomatic. Other illness as described previously (alcoholism/substance abuse, mental illness) was secondary to the HIV/AIDS diagnosis. In addition, a small number of HIV/AIDS persons came to the system on a daily basis for food, showers, medications, and activities but remained living on the street. It should be considered that for many, remaining homeless was the desirable option.

The seven houses were located within a geographic region with similar community characteristics. All were surrounded by small, single-family homes with a few scattered apartment structures. Other residents of the community were largely Black, Hispanic, and Asian and would generally be considered low-income/poverty level. The seven residences easily could be linked through public transportation and on foot. This was an important characteristic that permitted programming to be established at one site while meeting the needs of all residents of the system.

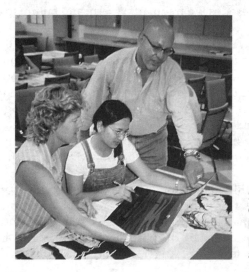

Silk-screen, paper-making, or both? Choosing the craft that will best meet the needs of members with HIV/AIDS and psychiatric disability is a task shared by all involved.

# Assessing Need and Planning
# the Paper-Making Program

Planning for the residents was not unlike other programs described in this text. The sponsoring system was engaged to provide the mission and purpose and to elicit the goals each residential advisor had for his or her residents. The goals were examined in light of the mission and purpose of the full system, and these were utilized to structure a needs assessment for the individual residents. Resources available from regional and county social services and private donations were examined.

Information received from these combined efforts stimulated the establishment of goals and objectives that were deemed appropriate to the needs of the shelter system and to the needs of the individuals who would be involved in the program. Shared goals were drafted around several central themes: (1) the establishment and strengthening of a *community* to incorporate all of the residents of the seven houses; (2) the creation of a balance of occupations demonstrated through a daily routine of independent living skills for each resident; and (3) the establishment of a venue for the testing and practice of **prevocational and vocational skills** appropriate for residents' transition to other communities of their choice.

Objectives were then drafted with each individual who wished to participate in programming, including those who wished to remain homeless. Regardless of individual interests, each participant was required to attend one *community* meeting a week conducted in each house. The meetings were intended to provide the route for self-governance and self-empowerment, which may accompany the shared responsibility of achieving positive outcomes. When the paper-making business was initiated, this meeting also became the place where group business decisions were made.

Previous to this program, the second theme of **occupational balance** and daily routine of independent living skills had had little success with residents who spent much of their time watching television, smoking, and sleeping. Some previous residents had experienced success with the third theme of prevocational and vocational exploration, but the residential managers felt that something more was needed at a more achievable foundational level since many of the residents had never worked in what might be described as a socially acceptable system (for example, some had worked as prostitutes and some as drug dealers, and some had participated in petty thievery).

Following evaluation of all of the information collected in on-site interviews, through paper/pencil assessments, and substantial library and Internet research of the population and the systems supporting the existing programs, it was time for some substantial brainstorming between the students assigned to this opportunity and the instructor. Through this process and a review of the basic tenets of occupation and occupational therapy, it was determined that all of the theme-goals of the program could be incorporated through the use of a carefully selected activity and could also meet the therapeutic objectives of individual residents through the employment of the foundation skills of **task analysis**. Further, the activity to be selected would have the potential to become a profit-producing mechanism.

In today's language of self-efficacy, empowerment, and personal advocacy, the above conclusion may seem too simplistic to some and may provide a bit of an enlightening experience for others. Whichever it is, it is important to remind ourselves to continue to cultivate our historical roots and to recognize that some of our most significant strengths reside in that soil. The mix of a well-understood and carefully selected occupation/activity, comprehensive and skillful task analysis, and the combination of clinical reasoning and a strong therapeutic self can be powerful in achieving occupation-centered outcomes, even within the most sophisticated paradigms.

# The Selection of an Activity to Meet the Program Goals

Following lengthy discussion, it was determined that the task ahead was to select an occupational activity that would (1) produce a relatively inexpensive but marketable product (2) with good or at least tolerable profit margin, and that the production of this product would be (3) broad and flexible enough to meet the shared goals and objectives of each resident while (4) offering a realistic example of the business characteristics appropriate to umbrella the development of prevocational and vocational skills.

Contiguous to the discussion was that the selected activity must be meaningful and relevant to the participants and to the potential market. Arts and crafts were considered because they can offer a certain mystique in today's mechanized and mass-produced environment. For these reasons and more, it was anticipated that they would be taken seriously by street-smart participants who likely had numerous agendas for being in the program but perhaps none of them were the ones expressed to the planners.

Some of the students had heard of similar projects with varying populations. Suggestions were made to include the packaging of dry ingredients for a favored soup recipe, selling produce and/or flowers from a community gardening venture (perhaps also packaging the seeds from an organic garden), making candles and soap, or collecting and mixing potpourri. Constructing small wooden toys and compiling books of poems, personal journal notes, or recipes were suggested as well.

All ideas were entertained with equal enthusiasm, but when these and numerous other suggestions were measured against the desired goals and objectives, the desired characteristics of the project, potential collaborations, available space, and proposed cost, paper-making—or more accurately, paper-recycling—was selected. The first step was to research paper-making and paper-recycling, select an appropriate recipe, and obtain the necessary supplies and equipment. (Resources for task analysis and paper-making are included in the recommended reference list.)

The next step involved the actual experimentation with recycled-paper production so that all members of the student group could gain some experience with the media before attempting a task analysis of the steps involved. Finally, a step-by-step list of the tasks involved in the process was completed. Following some experimentation, it was determined that small packets of blank note paper would be packaged as well as sheets of wrapping paper that would be printed with natural object impressions (such as shells and flower petals). Following further experimentation and later consultations with the residents, it was decided that pre-designed stamps would be used to print the name of the program on attached cards and raffia would be used to tie the packages. Plastic bags were the preferred product packaging, although equipment for shrink-wrapping could be a future consideration.

The most formidable task was the completion of the full task analysis of the process from the first step to the last, including preparing and maintaining supplies and equipment, actually making and drying the paper sheets, printing, packaging, obtaining retailers, marketing, and accounting. Several resources were used to assist in formatting the task analysis, and these are included in the reference list.

The next step of this first stage was to locate space and to obtain funding for start-up. Space was provided in an empty garage at one of the residential sites and was brought to functional use through donations from a local builder's supply and several residents, students, and volunteers with suitable carpentry skills. It was determined that several corporate groups were accustomed to offering assistance to charitable groups in need through volunteer days, and these were utilized as well. A small $3,000 start-up grant was received from a local philanthropic organization, which was a satisfactory sum to obtain the supplies and equipment to initiate the program. Most of these contacts were identified through early collaborations, marketing, and research.

The next phase involved a fairly lengthy evaluation period to determine the perceived and actual baseline skills of the residents and a matching of these to the steps of the activity. Following initiation, it was planned that the residential project would be able to support the work of a supervisory occupational therapist, one occupational therapy assistant, and one resident who would function as an aide. This group, along with the community of participants and volunteer retired business entrepreneurs, would determine the future direction of the project. The occupational therapy staff would provide individual evaluation and recommendations to appropriate professionals regarding the prevocational and vocational readiness of participants and would also monitor the evaluation of the program in general.

This program provides an exciting model that easily can be tailored to the needs of many populations in the community and is one that challenges us to use all of our skills as occupation-centered practitioners. Survey your community, and you will find the challenges to which this model is responsive.

# Summary

This chapter has continued to provide discussion of those persons who are homeless with mental illness and has also provided a description of the complex needs of those with HIV/AIDS who are homeless. The problems of both groups may be further complicated by the presence of self-medicating behaviors in the form of substance abuse and often physical illness. A multi-shelter program has been described that is structured around goals to establish and strengthen "community," to balance individual occupations, and to create a venue for the testing and practice of prevocational and vocational skills. The program example emphasizes the importance of task analysis to ensure that the selected activity/project matches the individual needs of the participants while meeting the goals of the program for all participants.

# References

Centers for Disease Control and Prevention (CDC). (1997). Update: Trends in AIDS incidence—United States. *Morbidity and Mortality Weekly Report, 46*(37), 861–867.

Centers for Disease Control and Prevention (CDC). (1997). *HIV/AIDS Surveillance Report, 9*(1), 1–37.

Karon, J. M. (1996). Prevalence of HIV Infection in the United States, 1984 to 1992. *Journal of the American Medical Association 276*(2): 126–131.

Los Angeles County Department of Health Services. (1997). *Advanced HIV disease surveillance summary*. Los Angeles, CA: HIV Epidemiology Program.

UNAIDS. (1997, December). *Report on the global HIV/AIDS epidemic*. New York: Author.

## Recommended Reading

Lamport, N., Coffey, M., & Hersch, G. (2001). *Activity analysis and application* (4th ed.). Thorofare, NJ: Slack.

Toale, B. (1983). The Art of Papermaking. Worcester, MA: Davis.

Watson, D. (1994). *Creative handmade paper*. Kent, Great Britain: Search Press.

Watson, D., & Wilson, S. (2003). *Task analysis: An individual and population approach*. (2nd ed.) Bethesda, MD: American Occupational Therapy Association.

# CHAPTER 19

# Programming for the Homeless Adolescent in Transitional Shelter: Film-Making for High School Credit

## Learning Objectives

1. To appreciate the conditions that prompt running away and resulting homelessness in children and adolescents
2. To understand the particular challenges experienced by children and adolescents when living on the street
3. To identify services offered to homeless children and adolescents
4. To review the example of the development of an occupation-centered program for an adolescent shelter population

## Key Terms

1. Family Shelters
2. Homeless Adolescents
3. Crisis Intervention
4. Transitional Living

Homelessness is a condition that cuts across cultures, socioeconomic considerations, and gender, as well as age and family structure. Although not nearly adequate, shelters and temporary housing are available across the country to individuals, families, and teens. In Los Angeles County there were approximately 82,096 homeless persons in 2004; of these, approximately 20–40 percent are single mothers and children. (Just the Facts, 2004). Certainly many families disintegrate under the pressures of homelessness.

A trends analysis of the constant flux in the job market and of affordable housing in this urban area and others like it does not appear optimistic for families who are presently low income or who rely on vocational skills that may become obsolete. **Family shelters** are excellent communities for occupation-centered services, for they provide access to a family system within the protected environment of the shelter.

Programming in such shelters can include life skills for adults and teens, vocational assessment, and prevocational training for adults, developmental screening and creative play opportunities for young children, and educational support services for school-aged children. Family shelters are generally nonprofit organizations with a mission to provide food, shelter, and other services to homeless families. They are often funded by city governments, foundations/corporations, and private donations. The residences may include a family bedroom, common dining room and bathrooms, a day care/play room for infants and toddlers, a tutoring/educational support room for school-aged children, and a playground. Occupation-centered services, therapeutic or formative, find a comfortable fit with this structure.

Although teens may be found as part of the homeless family, when they are alone and homeless, their problems and concerns are quite unique. The next program description will provide a view of the special concerns of **homeless adolescents**.

# The Population Characteristics of Our Program Example

Homeless youth, who are most frequently runaways, dot the United States as they make their way to various perceived *utopias* around the country. According to The U.S. Department of Health and Human Services (1991) and the National Network of Runaway and Youth Services (1995), upwards of one million youth run away from home each year (2,740 of them every day). Shelters of many kinds may be found in virtually every city, urban or rural, in an effort to stop or at least postpone this exodus from home. Although there are many popular destinations for runaways, Hollywood, California, has the dubious distinction of being the "runaway capital" of this country, with an estimated 4,000 children and adolescents surviving on the streets and in the abandoned buildings (Covenant House Fact Sheet, 1994, and Esperanza, 1997). More recent figures suggest the numbers vary from 4,800 to 10,000. (Just the Facts, 2004). Although runaway children and adolescents include all ethnicities, the Hollywood Covenant House, whose mission it is to serve runaway teens, reported that Caucasian youths accounted for nearly half of all of their contacts in recent years (Covenant House Fact Sheet, 1994; Covenant House of California; www.coventhouse.org/about_loc_la.html, 2005.).

The largest population seems to be those between the ages of 18 and 21 who are too young for adult shelters and yet too old for the shelters and systems caring for minor children. Many of them "aged out" of the foster care system at age 18, and even though they were ill-prepared for adult life, they were released to the street. According to a 1991 study by the U.S. Department of Health and Human Services, 45 percent of homeless youth in California were in foster care in the year before they took to the streets. Perhaps surprisingly, 42 percent of the homeless youth across the country were locked out by their parents, as was reported in a 1995 survey by the National Network of Runaway and Youth Services.

According to Esperanza (1997), 81 percent of Covenant House clients in Hollywood have been victims of some kind of abuse, which includes physical, sexual, and emotional abuse, neglect, and abandonment (1997). Approximately 11 percent of these children had sex before the age of 9, and 46 percent had sex before the age of 15. Other statistics that are significant in understanding this group include that 83 percent have a family history of substance abuse, and 74 percent have substance abuse problems themselves. An estimated 93 percent have an array of emotional disorders, which include depression, suicidal ideation, and psychosis. Most have not graduated from high school (92 percent) and have inadequate skills for any employment.

Wherever there are large numbers of homeless adolescents, there are those who victimize them with promises of notoriety, money, and affection. One out of three runaway children is lured into prostitution within 48 hours of leaving home, and it is estimated that nearly 30 percent of youths on the street have been paid for sex and 22 percent have traded sex for food or shelter (Covenant House of California. 2005). Unfortunately, opportunities to become victims far exceed the available shelters and services.

When we review the developmental considerations of adolescence, it is not difficult to see how vulnerable they may be to those so-called temptations that are believed to accompany the perceived freedoms, attributes, and rights of adulthood. The community of homeless adolescents, wherever it exists, is a strong one with many of the *club* characteristics noted in the previous chapters. There are perhaps more covert rules than in the adult homeless community, and adolescents are more likely to group and support each other than homeless adults. Considering that they are all likely to be either "running away from" or "running to" something and considering that many are being searched for by families, they tend to be less trusting, more furtive, and more secretive than the communities of homeless adults.

# The Site of Our Program Example

A fairly common model for programs targeting homeless youth is a frontline **crisis-intervention** outreach program of some sort. Intervention counselors, often volunteers from the police departments or churches, go to the streets where homeless youth are likely to congregate. Crisis intervention often takes the form of assisting youth who are endangered by excessive drug use or a "bad drug trip" or those who are being pursued by pimps or pornographers. Although occupational therapy intervention is not likely to find a foothold in crisis intervention, it is an opportunity to observe and to begin to understand what this community is about, which is critical for those who wish to provide programming to this group. It is also an excellent way to become familiar with the other service providers and volunteer organizations and a way to become known to them, for they are your potential allies and partners.

Beyond this front line is usually an emergency bed shelter that may also provide medical services as well as counseling. In addition, there may be a **transitional living** environment that offers support directed toward the skills necessary to live independently and to remain off the streets. Transitional living is generally reserved for those adolescents who have demonstrated the motivation, interest, and initiative to benefit from this opportunity. There are paid personnel who work in the transitional living environment who may be social workers, teachers/tutors, and occupational therapists, and there are many volunteers from the surrounding community to provide role-modeling and skill development.

## Assessing Need and Planning the Programming

The mission of the selected transitional living unit provided in this example was developed by the Catholic church when the first such shelter was established in New York in 1967. The mission statement included directives for immediate needs and for sanctuary. The mission further offered structure, trust, respect, and choice. Following several evenings with the crisis-intervention teams, reading of the mission, and discussion with personnel as well as observation of existing programming (collectively constituting the Phase I needs assessment), it was determined that occupation-centered providers could best match their body of knowledge and expertise with the aspect of programming that was directed toward life skills development. It was the interest of the director to offer small, individualized opportunities for learning. These opportunities were preconceived as modules with a similar format and structure to what is expected in formal education, which was a large part of the residents' day.

A Phase II needs assessment to be given to residents was developed according to the structure and content requested by the director and in keeping with the mission and philosophy of the facility. This assessment included life skills development modules in the areas of communication, goal setting, time and task management, and sexuality. Through this assessment, which was conducted in personal interviews, specific concerns were elicited in each of the areas first noted by the director. Most of the residents were fairly disinterested in the idea of yet "another class" and were not as helpful in this stage of program development as might be desired.

Although the occupational therapy student group conducting the needs assessment was fairly disheartened by the response, after some discussion they came to the conclusion that the respondents might be more motivated if they had a hand in selecting how the content of the modules would be disseminated or investigated. Another series of interviews gleaned an assortment of creative but often impractical (generally because of time and/or cost) ideas. It was clear though, as was mentioned in the previous chapter, that street-smart clients offered a substantial challenge for the creation of stimulating and engaging programming.

# Community "Partnering" to Provide the Program

Bringing together the larger program goals and objectives that incorporated the enhancement of communication, setting realistic and manageable life goals, managing time and tasks, and exploring developmentally appropriate and safe sexuality in an informative and captivating programming package was the challenge. The response came in the form of a series of documentary videos.

Through investigation of volunteer resources of persons and companies, it was discovered that one of the local movie studios had previously offered an internship program, along with high school credit, for the experience to residents of the transitional living unit. The occupational therapy students first prepared a proposal for the approval of the director of the shelter. Following this step, a similar proposal that outlined the program and the purpose was developed for the studio executives. Although it had different goals than the traditional internship had offered, the proposal was received positively and the studio agreed to offer the internship/high school credit format. In addition, the studio offered the services of other college film program interns to advise and assist and to be responsible for video equipment to be loaned to the program; a resulting collaboration that exceeded the initial expectations!

The film interns supplied the technical expertise and advice, and the occupational therapy students offered the structure to make sure that the content of the scripts and the process of residents' involvement met the goals of the program established from the earlier needs assessment. A time line was developed; tasks were determined, analyzed, and distributed; the product was developed; and the process was evaluated.

The goals of establishing realistic objectives—time and task management— were accomplished in the process of planning and scripting, filming, and editing. The goals of developing communication skills and learning about sexuality were accomplished through the group decision that the film would be a documentary of individual "life story" vignettes provided by each of the participants. Not only were individual goals met through this activity, but there also were numerous other positive outcomes related to prevocational and vocational exploration (for example, discovering talents for writing, directing, and acting).

The initial format for formative program evaluation was eventually discarded in favor of a qualitative analysis of the filmed vignettes for the five participants. Since numerous practice films were made, there was substantial footage available for analysis. This was conducted both by the occupational therapy students and by the participants, with shared observations of progress and identification of areas still needing improvement.

Videotaping or film-making is an excellent tool for occupation-centered interventions. If there are film students in the community, they are most likely looking for practice opportunities and generally have access to equipment. If not, then perhaps the local television station can become involved, particularly if the programming can be developed to advance the station's public relations as well as benefit participants. If no television stations are available, then consider "oral histories" and radio or audio taping as the medium.

Even if these external resources are not available, the seemingly simple process of using a camcorder can still utilize the development of a script through the telling of personal stories or story-making, and review of the film can be a powerful evaluative tool for both respondents and for students in the classroom.

This review of programming for homeless adolescents has presented some of the advantages and potential dilemmas you may find working with this community. They are perhaps the most challenging of the homeless persons for which you may wish to develop programs. They offer all of the characteristics of the homeless alongside the particular characteristics of the developmental phase of adolescence. Frequently they are abused and neglected, and they are often the most disenfranchised of all—rejected from family systems while in many ways still children.

## Summary

The problems of homeless children and adolescents, whether part of a homeless family unit or alone, are complicated by their developmental characteristics and their lack of preparation for the adult roles that may be thrust upon them (or that they are seeking). Communities of homeless children and adolescents resemble the structure of clubs discussed in previous chapters. There are often more covert rules than in adult homeless communities, and adolescents as well as younger runaway children who may be present are more likely to group together and support each other.

Children and adolescents are more difficult to engage in programs because they are often being searched for by families or are engaging in law-breaking behavior and fear being found or identified. The program described in this chapter provided an example of how homeless adolescents might be engaged in an occupation-centered program targeting the development of age-appropriate life skills. You may also wish to revisit the Denver Sanctuary Program for Homeless Teens described in Chapter 7.

# References

Covenant House Fact Sheet. (1994). Hollywood, CA: Covenant House.

Covenant House of California. 2005: www.coventhouse.org/about_loc_la.html

Esperanza, M. L. (1997). *Covenant house California: Service plan, 1996–97.* Hollywood, CA: Covenant House.

Just the Facts. (2004). Institute for the Study of Homelessness and Poverty at the Weingart Center. (August)

National Network of Runaway and Youth Services. (1995). *A report on anti-homeless laws, litigation and alternatives in 50 United States Cities.* Washington, DC: National Law Center on Homelessness and Poverty.

United States Department of Health and Human Services (HHS). (1991). *Runaway youth annual report.* Washington, DC: Author.

# CHAPTER 20

# Promotion of Health, Well-Being, and Community: An Intergenerational Program for Older Adults Living in a Senior-Care Facility

## Learning Objectives

1. To explore health promotion and wellness programming for older adults who are living in a senior-care institution
2. To become aware of the need for older adult programming that is culturally relevant and linked to the larger community
3. To examine ideas and theories that assist in our understanding of effective programming for older adults in institutional care
3. To examine intergenerational programming as a viable and effective mode for encouraging community in institutions for older adults
4. To become familiar with one site-linked example of an intergenerational/culturally relevant older adult program designed to support health, well-being, and a sense of community membership

## Key Terms

1. Health Disparities
2. Health Promotion and Well-Being
3. Cultural Traditions
4. Aging in Place/Aging in a Familiar Context
5. Self-Determination Theory (Competence, Autonomy, Relatedness)
6. Expectancy, Self-Efficacy, and Outcome Expectations
7. Kinship and Social Connectedness
8. Intergenerational Programming/Mentoring

For two decades, the U.S. Department of Health and Human Services (DHHS) has encouraged the use of health promotion and disease prevention objectives to improve the health of American people (DHHS, 1990). Since the 1970's there has been a growing social movement that encourages people of all ages to look at wellness as optimal physical, mental, and spiritual well-being. It is no surprise that the first goal of *Healthy People 2010* is to increase the quality as well as the years of healthy life. Today's older adult is more fully aware of this agenda than ever in preventing illness and disability, improving functioning, and living fully in the world. Granted, escalating health care costs may be a motivating factor across the economic continuum for many aging adults, but most want more than simple disease and illness prevention. They wish to live fully engaged in lives of choice and all hope to live independently in their homes for all, or most of their lives.

Occupational therapy practitioners endorsed the objectives of the above reports in their 2001 American Occupational Therapy Association official statement: *Occupational therapy in the promotion of health and the prevention of disease and disability* (AOTA, 2001). We know that people are living longer. Atchely (1994, p. 520) predicted that by 2050 there would be about 68.5 million Americans 65 and older. In 1990 there were about 500,000 people 85 and over living in long-term care facilities. At that rate of utilization and anticipating the aging of even the old-old population (95+) we can expect 3 million people 85 and over to need long-term care by 2050. Of course trends in long-term care will likely evolve to shift from nursing home to more independent living spaces with less standardized menus of care in the future and will likely encourage older adults to remain connected to their previous lives, but how will this occur, and who will be involved in the orchestration of this transition? Occupational therapy practitioners seem ready to move to the forefront as the programming example in this chapter might suggest. Engagement in occupations of choice that are linked to the larger community is key to successful living, and aging.

Sultz and Young (2004) describe already evolving innovations in long-term care to meet the diverse medical needs, personal desires, and lifestyle choices of older Americans. Concepts such as aging in place, life care communities and high technology home care are some of the changes that offer enriched alternatives to long-term care recipients. The future of physical aging, according to Atchely, will be influenced by the impact of biomedical research, trends in morbidity and mortality, and the impact of a general movement toward wellness (Atchely, 1994; p. 521). Other advancements, such as improved diagnosis, prevention, and treatment of diseases such as Alzheimer's and other dementias will lead to an older, more viable population of aging adults.

In the U.S., it is predicted that Hispanic and Asian populations will triple over the next half century and non-Hispanic whites will represent about one-half of the total population by 2050. (More Diversity, Slower Growth: U.S. Census Bureau, March 2004, retrieved 2/11/06). Such trends will obviously call for more bilingual programming and programs to meet various cultural demands provided by a culturally diverse health promotion work force. A culturally diverse workforce of occupational therapy practitioners adequate to meet such needs does not presently exist. As a profession, we all have some work to do to encourage academic admission and retention of ethnically diverse students or we'll likely become marginalized in this evolving culturally diverse future.

These reports and statements deal specifically with the U.S. population, but we know that aging and older adults around the world are utilizing all resources available to them to maintain a viable place on the planet. The world's population age 65 and older is growing by an unprecedented 800,000 people a month. (An Aging World: 2001. U.S. Census Bureau, 2001; retrieved 2/11/06).

Global aging will likely continue well into the 21st century with the numbers and proportions of older people continuing to rise in both developed and developing countries. According to the United States Census Bureau, the ratio of older people to total population differs widely among countries (An aging world: 2001). The U.S. was 32nd on a list ranking countries with a high proportion of people age 65 and older. Italy was the "oldest" country in 2000 with 18 percent of Italians having celebrated at least a 65th birthday. In many countries the "oldest old" (80 and above) were the fastest growing component of the population.

Certainly we know that not all of the world's older population has equal access to the social and economic factors that invite the characteristics of "aging well." Even in the US, there are wide and obvious health disparities. The Trans-NIH Work Group on Health Disparities has defined the term **health disparities** as "the difference in the incidence, prevalence, morbidity, mortality, and burden of diseases and other adverse health conditions that exist among specific population groups (NIH, 1999)." The NIH work group notes that health disparities arise from a complex combination of social and economic factors, the physical environments, cultural beliefs and values, educational level, personal behaviors, and genetic susceptibilities. Previously in this text we discussed the work of Wilcock (1998). Her concepts of occupational imbalance, occupational deprivation, and occupational alienation help us to understand health disparities from an "occupation" perspective.

Occupational therapy practitioners are well positioned to offer assistance in several of these areas of disparity that will even the odds for all persons, and, for aging adults in particular. Clearly, we have ample justification from demographics alone to devote substantial funded research efforts in community programming for older adults to encourage broader education of students in matters of older adulthood, and to establish occupation centered parameters for health promotion and wellness in our aging populations.

# Health Promotion and Well-Being

The title of this chapter uses the terms health promotion, well-being, and community. From earlier discussions in this text we know that Green and Kreuter (1991, p. 5) define **health promotion** as any planned combination of educational, political, regulatory, environmental, and organizational supports for actions and conditions of living conducive to the health of persons, groups, or communities. The World Health Organization tells us that health promotion is simply "the process of enabling people to increase control over and to improve their health" (WHO, 1986, p. iii). Complex or simplistic, by definition, occupation is central to health promotion and occupation-centered practitioners are central as well.

Scaffa (2001) describes occupation-based health promotion interventions that may be conducted at an individual level, group level, organizational level, community (societal) level, and the governmental/policy level. Some examples of each for older adults are: driving evaluation, safety checks and perhaps compensatory instruction for the "individual" older adult, and programs to encourage "groups" of older adults to remain engaged in meaningful occupation. Chapter 17 of this text provides an example of an exercise program for groups of older adults with Parkinson's disease and their significant others. Providing consultation to businesses and potential employers regarding the benefits of hiring older adults in the part-time work force, or providing information on accessibility and universal design to local building suppliers, hardware stores, and contractors, and encouraging accessible public transportation in the community are examples targeting organizations and, at the governmental/policy level, for example, we may promote policies that offer affordable, accessible health care for all older adults.

**Well-being** is defined quite simply as "the state of being healthy, happy, or prosperous" (*The American Heritage Dictionary*, 1976; p. 1454). *Mosby's Dictionary (Medical, Nursing and Allied Health)* offers a definition perhaps more appealing to occupational therapy practitioners: "achievement of a good and satisfactory existence as *defined by the individual*" (1994, p. 1664). Granted these definitions are subjective, as, of course, the phenomenon of well-being should be. If we are to place "well-being" within an appropriate context according to the *Occupational Therapy Practice Framework: Domain and Process*, it would undoubtedly be in the spiritual context but certainly informed by and interconnected with the cultural, physical, social, personal and temporal contexts (2002). For our purposes, it is a significant goal for intervention and a direct outcome of our health promotion efforts. The following program example links attention to all of these domains with the combined goals of health promotion and well-being.

# Occupation-Centered Programming for Older Adults: Lunalilo Home on the Island of Oahu, Hawaii

This particular programming example is selected to best illustrate the encouragement of individual health and well-being by linking the institutionalized older adult to the larger cultural community. The bulk of this work was accomplished by Lum, occupational therapy doctoral graduate and resident of Oahu; and it showcases a blend of traditional program planning as described in this text with an integration of **cultural tradition** and attention to the specific characteristics of the ethnic community (Fazio and Lum, in press, 2008).

## Background

Aging seniors in Hawaii are little different than many other aging populations around the world except that their population appears to be growing at a rate more than two times the national average. In 2002 there were approximately 160,601 seniors age 65 and older, showing a 28.5 percent increase over 125,005 seniors living in Hawaii in 1990 (Star Bulletin, 2002, February 19). This increase may be due, in part, to increased health agendas targeting prevention and management of diabetes and other life threatening illnesses linked to diet and genetic predisposition.

Not unlike other similar regions where many families live at or below the poverty line, there may be little planning for older adult years. The traditional mode of many generations living under one roof, or clustered housing is likely being undermined by the need and desire for the middle generations, particularly women/daughters, to work outside the household. If the older generation lives to require nursing care, there is little recourse. The Island of Oahu, although sophisticated in many respects, has not created sufficient support services for this growing contingent of the population. Certainly this is a problem, but the larger dilemma may be that if such services were available (particularly low-income senior care housing), would they meet the broader cultural needs of a population that has always relied on family and tradition for sustenance and well-being.

## Lunalilo Home

Lunalilo Home provides an example of a senior care residence and is the site of this experiment in creative programming that focuses on the cultural family traditions of the indigenous population demonstrating Hawaiian ancestry. Perhaps exotic in that this population may be confined by choice to an Island, it is not unlike many we are aware of in pocketed urban areas, small towns, and rural areas throughout the United States. The characteristics of the population and the programming may be transferred to many scenarios we encounter as practitioners and programmers.

### Key Elements Contributing to the Program Design

Following an extensive investigation and multiple interviews with residents of Lunalilo, their family members, and members of the surrounding community, the combined needs assessment supported the initial hypothesis of the programmers suggesting the readiness for a "renaissance" celebrating indigenous Hawaiian craft and tradition. Central to this awareness were the Curators and Directors of Cultural Anthropology and Artifacts, Indigenous Arts, and Indigenous Horticulture at the University of Hawaii, the Bishop Museum Library and Archives, and the Edith Kanaka'ole Foundation for the Preservation of Indigenous Traditions. In the needs assessment process, several strong partnerships were developed that, through volunteerism and funding, would support this program's goals. One does not have to investigate deeply to know that many groups have lost cultural traditions, often turning them aside in favor of efficiency and current social trends. Resurrecting such traditions by accessing older adults who remember and practice them offers purposeful engagement benefiting the community at all levels.

Central ideas or organizing elements for potential programming that were gleaned during the above assessment process and were in danger of being lost to younger generations were deemed to be these:

1. shared traditional culture: preservation of information gleaned through oral tradition/storytelling; art and craft knowledge and skills; music and dance traditions, both in archival form and to be shared with younger generations;
2. the importance of kinship, family, intergenerational systems; staying "connected" to family and community; and
3. health and wellness for aging adults (diet, activity, "meaning," efficacy, engagement, and empowerment).

### Supporting Ideologies

The above organizing elements have within their structure several supporting ideas and theories that provide scaffolding for the development of the day-to-day programming.

**Aging in Place** is a phrase found in the literature of many disciplines. Carol Siebert, in her AOTA Continuing Education module *Aging in Place: Implications for Occupational Therapy*, described the values and goals of "aging in place" (AOTA, 2002; CE5). These values and goals are offered as autonomy, engagement, community living, and a healthy active lifestyle. Generally, when one thinks of "aging in place," we think of the older adult continuing to live in their own residence in the community that has always supported their values and interests, and in the presence of family and friends. It was the intention of the Lunalilo program to respect the notion of aging in place but, for these residents, to expand this notion to **aging in a familiar context**: that of the community and the culture.

**Self-Determination Theory** (SDT) is an approach to human motivation and personality that uses traditional empirical methods while employing an organismic metatheory that highlights the importance of humans' evolved inner resources for personality development and behavioral regulation (Ryan, Kuhl, and Deci, 1997). When people are at their fullest potential they appear to be curious, vital, and self-motivated. They are agentic and inspired, striving to learn, extend themselves, and master new skills. We know, however, that these persistent, proactive, and positive tendencies of human nature are not always apparent, and perhaps not present. When thinking of older adults in institutional care, we are not likely to describe them with any of the above terms. . . . Why not? Ryan and Deci (2000) have identified three needs that, when satisfied, provide the basis for self-motivation, personality integration, optimal functioning, and, most importantly, personal well-being. These three needs are the need for competence, relatedness, and autonomy. The foundations for self-determination theory begin with the nature of motivation—whether one is internally motivated to function in the world with action and intention or externally pressured to act. Our interest in providing programming for older adults (or any population) is to encourage an environment that fosters internal motivation observed as actions with energy and direction. We have all, too often, seen older institutionalized adults forced from the bed to the chair to the lunch room, which then becomes the activity room, and then back to bed. Throughout this series of events, we seldom see any action from the person that appears to be intentional, and certainly not any that express interests or values.

Our first act as therapists and programmers is to establish an environment that encourages internal motivation and opportunities for engagement in activities of interest, skill, and value that satisfy what Ryan and Deci (2000) describe as the "need for competence" (Ryan and Deci, 2000; p. 69). In our programming example, this environment is rich with opportunities to engage in various components of cultural tradition that one is good at, is interested in, and values—a "valuing" that is shared by all members of the culture. **Competence** and **autonomy** are related in that competence is fulfilled by the experience that he or she can effectively bring about desired effects and outcomes, and autonomy involves the perception that one's activities are endorsed by or congruent with the self. **Relatedness** then pertains to feeling that one is close and connected to significant others (Reis, Sheldon, Gable, Roscoe, and Ryan (2000, p. 419). The ultimate outcome is a general sense of well-being.

**Expectancy, Self-Efficacy, and Outcome Expectations** are terms from the work of Bandura (1977a, 1977b). Related to the above concepts that support self-determination theory, expectancy is an important feature of self-efficacy. **Expectancy** is described as a value an individual places on a particular outcome. **Efficacy** expectations are related to competence and stem from previous and present skills and knowledge. Successful accomplishment enhances ones' expectation for future efforts. Key to "revisiting" old knowledge and skill sets is the evidence to support the fact that the more similar the current task to ones performed successfully in the past, the greater the efficacy expectations will be (Bandura, 1977b). This is of great significance to the programming for Lunalilo in that the skills and knowledge sets of the residents are central to the selected programming. A programmer's encouragement and ability to structure (perhaps through task analysis and adaptation) circumstances for a successful outcome are critical to the development of efficacy expectations, as well as expectations for general outcomes. Bandura (1977a) describes **outcome expectations** as the individual's belief that a given behavior will lead to specific outcomes. In our example, these outcomes may be praise, playful pleasures, a greater perceived sense of health, and a general sense of well-being. It is also the programmer who must orchestrate environmental expectations, what Bandura (1997a) describes as how events are related to each other and what one may expect from a given environment. It is often partnering with other individuals and groups in the community that establishes the supportive environment and solidifies expectations for program performance and success.

**Kinship** and the maintenance of social connectedness or relatedness (as described above) is central to the health and well-being of people regardless of age; but is perhaps most significant as adults age and may become isolated from families. Baumeister and Leary (1995) discuss relatedness as a significant component in the satisfaction of innate psychological needs. This desire for interpersonal attachments can perhaps best be satisfied in a somewhat predictable and reliable fashion through connections with family. Kendig (1986) strongly suggests that social status impacts an older person's options and abilities to form and maintain supportive bonds, whether within the boundaries of kinship or in wider circles. Over time, older adults undergo reduced social opportunities as they lose power and respect and become increasingly dissimilar from those in the mainstream of adult life; this may be described as a loss of **social connectedness**. We would question, then, the impact of institutionalization and removal from mainstream family and cultural life for our population of indigenous Hawaiian individuals as well we might for any older adult who is living within an institution. Our compelling question, as occupational therapy practitioners, is how might we establish programming that would encourage power, respect and social opportunities, rather than diminish them. How can we maintain the rights and obligations associated with kinship and assist the older adult to stay connected and related toward optimal functioning and personal well-being? According to Dowd (1980), the concept of "exchange" provides a valuable way to understand the interactions that take place within informal, as well as formal, relationships and may, in fact, form them. Older people who are institutionalized experience a retracting social world that is marked by the withdrawal of dominant younger people who may no longer receive the returns commensurate with investments but also of subordinate older people whose independence and self-esteem is compromised in each encounter. How can we offer programming that will encourage engagement rather than disengagement, activity and interrelatedness rather than isolation? Clearly, if we think of establishing an exchange system, the "commodities" must be considered of importance and valued by all levels of the social network and layers of kinship. Can we think of disappearing traditions (stories, arts, crafts, music and dance) as the valued media for exchange? Can we develop and encourage relationships between our Lunalilo residents (the ancestral/elder keepers of these traditions) and those institutions and persons in the community who hold power relationships that cross generations and who sanction and encourage the collection, documentation, and teaching of these traditions (the museums, the foundations, and the Universities)? For every craft, art, music, dance, and oral or written tradition to continue there must be a craftsman, an artist, a musician, a dancer, a storyteller, and a writer . . . teachers! They are, perhaps not always rewarded, but are appreciated and generally respected. This provides a potential path to empowerment and an important concept for a program linking art/craft knowledge and production to family and community.

**Intergenerational Mentoring Programs** offer two or more generations of persons the opportunity to experience meaningful and supportive relationships that result in social and emotional fulfillment and growth. It is my preference, whenever possible, to engage at least three generations in programming of this type: the elders (in our programming example, the direct recipients of services); the middle (sons and daughters, perhaps siblings); and children through adolescence/young adulthood. These generations encompass not only family members but also friends and neighbors and often strangers in the initial encounter. The task then is to link generations in what becomes a shared microcosm of "community," with resulting effort toward shared goals of solidarity, integral responsibility, and better life quality for all involved.

The origins of intergenerational programming may be in the foster grandparent programs established by the federal government in the 1960's (Newman, Ward, Smith, Wilson, and McCrea, 1997). Over time, these earlier programs have evolved into three main models: youth serving older adults; older adults serving youth; and young and old united in serving the community (Hawkins, McGuire, Backman, 1999). Shared engagement in occupation is the common characteristic of all these programs, and most often the benefits are mutual. It's sometimes hard to know if the "giver" or the "recipient" of a gift enjoys the process more.

Newman, Ward, Smith, Wilson, and McCrea (1997) suggests that the original concept of intergenerational programming may have developed through recognition of the bond that occurs in a family, across generations. Transfer of knowledge, values, and experience benefits both adults and children. In a less obvious exchange, adults gain a sense of enhanced purpose, well-being, and life satisfaction (Newman, Ward, Smith, Wilson, McCrea, 1997; p. 4).

The term **mentoring** is used to describe a supportive relationship between a more experienced person and, usually, a younger, less experienced person. A mentoring relationship involves mutual caring, commitment, and trust (Taylor and Dryfoos, 1998/1999; p. 44). Such programs often involve a youth population considered to be "at risk." Although still emerging, intergenerational programs have been field tested widely and have generally been found to be effective (Kaplan, 2001; Lewis, 2002). For at-risk youth in particular, such programs offered by older adults with perhaps similar life experience can present a life perspective that is "rooted in survival" and can provide a continuity between past, present, and future generally not available to children and young adults (Taylor and Dryfoos, 1998/1999; p. 44).

For most older adults, the benefits of involvement in such programs are the combined results of the opportunity to remain useful, vital, and, most importantly, to make a positive difference in the life of a child/adolescent and in the community (Kaplan, 2001). Of interest for older adult programming in institutional care, Lewis (2002) observed that older adults in a nursing care facility who previously would not participate in activities came out of their rooms when (the) children

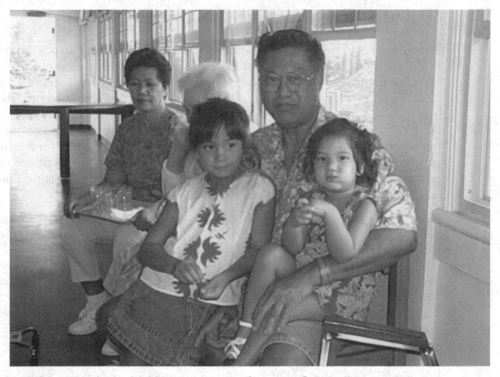

Grandparent and grandchildren enjoying an afternoon of storytelling.

arrived. Of importance is that these older adults continued to be involved in the life of the facility even when children were not present. This suggests that there are concomitant changes in feelings of efficacy and relatedness not necessarily requiring the continued presence of the children (or mentees). It is this kind of lasting engagement in meaningful occupations, after the completion of programming, which we wish to encourage for all of our program recipients.

For children and older adults a common intergenerational model may involve an adult senior day care center, nursing care facility, and/or long-term care facility and an organization that provides after-school or day-care programming for children from lower-income families (the YMCA is such an organization). These children may or may not be "at risk;" however, programming goals generally are to support community wellness through the promotion of healthy aging and prevention of further illness or disability for the older adult, and optimal development for the children.

In many cities across the country, adult facilities and organizations offering programming for children are coupled in ethnic, culturally circumscribed communities. Programs that utilize the mutual sharing of cultural (and perhaps religious) traditions, holidays, rituals, writings, stories, costumes, toys, etc. are particularly engaging for both groups and may be more akin to the foster grandparent programs in goals and purpose. The Lunalilo Home example is such a program but is more global in intergenerational scope and purpose than the typical foster grandparent programs.

## Art, Craft, Music, Dance and Oral Traditions . . . Why?

To someone of shared native Hawaiian ancestry, it may appear an obvious answer; these traditions are so linked to the expression of life that one cannot realistically separate them. It is not a unique phenomenon that all generations of an indigenous Hawaiian family engage in ceremonies and rituals involving dance and music. It is, perhaps, less likely for arts, crafts and story telling, but nevertheless the traditions are there in the making of the flower Lei and the music and dance instruments. One can also argue that the perhaps romantic desire for a return to a simpler life through resurrection of art, craft, and surrounding traditions can be a powerful motivator, as well as the more practical notion of protecting one's heritage by protecting the objects and rituals associated with it.

# The Goals to Structure Programming and Outcomes

The programming goals for the Lunalilo residents were generated following the comprehensive needs assessment in a focus group format with the residents, families, and potential partners all engaging in participatory leadership. The resulting goals are powerful, subjective statements of what would be achieved. They are appropriately charismatic, in an effort to attract positive attention to the program. Objectives are attached to all of the goals to provide a map to achievement of the larger goals. Considering all of the above information, organizing ideas, and literature, the following goals were established for the Lunalilo Home project:

1. To empower kupuna (grandparent) living in the Lunalilo Home and residents of the adjacent communities to embrace and celebrate their cultural identities through intergenerational, community-centered programming;
2. To foster and encourage opportunities for engagement in meaningful occupations that promote and enhance health, well-being, and the perceived quality of life for the individual and the community while preserving indigenous/native Hawaiian culture;
3. To perpetuate the knowledge of indigenous/native Hawaiian ancestors through the integration of activities that are imbedded with symbolic and spiritual meaning; and
4. To build an awareness of occupational choices that facilitate, integrate and motivate individuals to engage in respected roles appreciated and honored by the family and the community.

# The Programming

The programming was developed in phases that were symbolic of the spiritual context within which the native cultural arts evolved. The first phase was the *community garden*. It is fitting that the various arts, crafts, music, and dance traditions be traced backwards to the plant materials which are so closely associated with them. Multiple generations of adults and children from families and the surrounding community, working alongside kupuna restoring and preparing the land, selecting native plants that would become musical instruments, dance skirts, fabric dyes, sculpted forms and holiday foods, planting, and cultivating—*the Native Hawaiian Community* Garden was the place to begin.

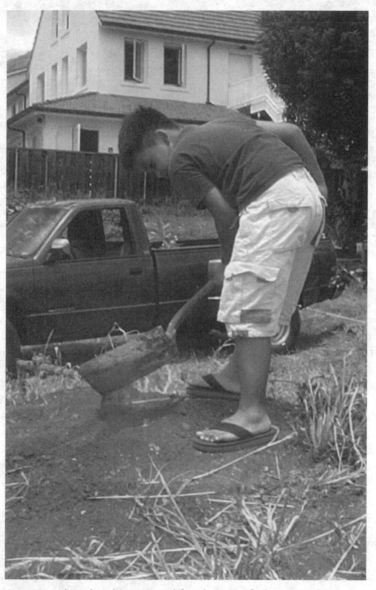

Great grandson breaking ground for planting of a banana palm.

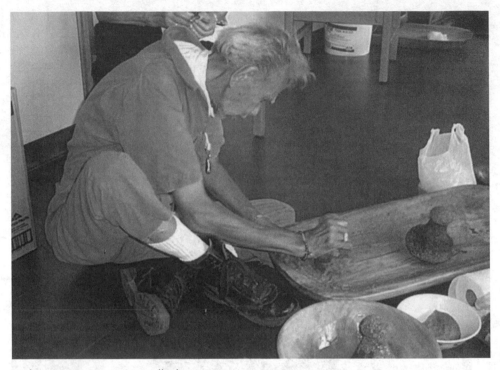

Making poi as it was originally done.

Overall, the program was designed to encourage the residents of Lunalilo Home to explore occupational choices intended to promote and improve health, well-being, and their perceived quality of life while engaging with their families and those of the surrounding communities in the enjoyment and celebration of traditional Hawaiian culture. These activities ran the gamut from how to plant and tend a banana palm to the weaving of a grass skirt, the construction of a ukulele, the making of poi, and to the storytelling dance traditions. These activities formed cultural bridges to validate the knowledge and skills of residents in the cultural/social traditions of indigenous/native Hawaii by offering them the opportunities to share this knowledge and skills with their children and grandchildren and other multi-generational residents of the community. The cultural legacy of what it is to be "native Hawaiian" will be protected and preserved through the personal empowerment of every individual involved in the experience, both young and old.

Additional phases of programming have included the fabrication of craft implements and materials, dance implements, and musical instruments followed by the actual production of art, craft, dance traditions, and music. Songs and oral traditions are being collected in the development of archival material for an anticipated on-site museum. Recently, an adult day-care program was added to the facility and has contributed to the ongoing programming. Further planned production

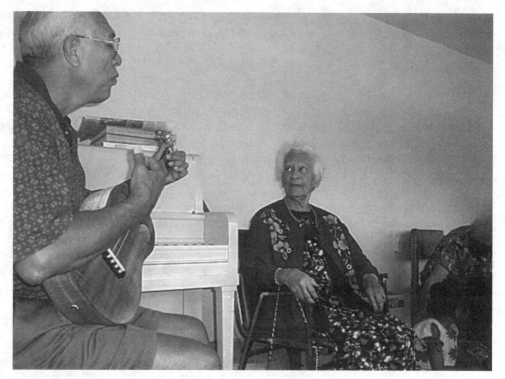

Playing the ukulele.

and demonstrations will include flower and seed lei making, lauhala weaving (mats, hats, etc.), 'meke (gourd bowls and containers), woodworking and carving, fishing tools, and featherworking. Classes and demonstrations will always be cross-generational.

# Program Outcomes

Present outcomes are subjectively demonstrated in connectedness to community resulting in maintenance of emotional, social, and physical health and modified independent living *within* a residential facility. Regular interviews are conducted with residents and they are encouraged to maintain journals of daily activity with indications of perceived well-being daily and weekly. The *Self-Determination Scale* (Sheldon, Ryan, and Reis, 1996) may be useful in providing measures of competence and autonomy as compared to the journal entries. As the work progresses we could evaluate the level of engagement against objective measures of health and well-being, lowered blood pressures, reduction in pain, and reduction of symptomology associated with depression and perhaps dementia. The use of both subjective and objective measures strengthen the program outcomes.

# Summary

Adults are living longer and, generally, better than in years past. They are more knowledgeable about exercise, nutrition, stress, and general conditions of wellness. Most hope to enjoy their older adult years at home and in good health. Many may be able to do so with advances in technology and information; however, there will always be those who will live out their lives in institutions designed for senior care. Occupational therapy practitioners are in an excellent position to assist older adults toward continued lives of competence, autonomy, and general well-being, regardless of where they live. This chapter has offered some examples of the considerations that are necessary to provide creative and relevant programming that will assist residents of a senior care facility to engage in meaningful activity that will promote health, well-being, and membership in the larger community. You can easily translate some or all of these ideas to senior-care programming where you live and work.

# References

Ackermann, K., Chow, K., Hongo, M., & Levine-Dickman, A. (2005). *Intergenerational Bridges: Finding a sense of well-being through shared meaningful activities*. Unpublished proposal, Los Angeles, CA: USC-OT.

American Occupational Therapy Association (2002). *Occupational Therapy Practice Framework: Domain and Process*. Bethesda, MD: AOTA.

American Occupational Therapy Association. (2001). *Occupational therapy in the promotion of health and the prevention of disease and disability*. Bethesda, MD: AOTA.

(The) American Heritage Dictionary of the English Language. Morris, Wm. (Ed.). (1976) Boston: Houghton Mifflin.

Atchley, R. (1994). *Social forces and aging: An introduction to social gerontology*. Belmont, CA: Wadsworth.

Bandura, A. (1977a). *Social learning theory*. Upper Saddle River, NJ: Prentice-Hall.

Bandura, A. (1977b). Self-efficacy: Toward a unifying theory of behavioral change. *Psychological Review, 84*, 191–215.

Baumeister, R., & Leary, M.R. (1995). The need to belong: Desire for interpersonal attachments as a fundamental human motivation. *Psychological Bulletin 117*, 497–529.

Dowd, J. J. (1980). *Stratification Among the Aged*. Monterey, CA: Brooks/Cole.

Fazio, L., & Lum, K. (2008 in press). Empowering older adults through the intergenerational sharing of native Hawaiian cultural traditions. In M. Scaffa, M. Reitz, & M. Pizzi, (Eds.), *Occupational Therapy in the Promotion of Health and Wellness*. Philadelphia: FA Davis.

Green, L., & Kreuter, M. (1991). *Health promotion planning: An educational and environmental approach*. Mountain View, CA: Mayfield.

Hawkins, M. O., McGuire, F. A., & Backman, K. F. (Eds.). (1999) *Preparing participants for intergenerational interaction: Training for success*. New York: Haworth Press.

Star Bulletin, H. (2002, February 19). Group seeks ways to address growing needs of isle seniors. Honolulu, Hawaii.

Kaplan, M. (2001). Intergenerational programs: Some what's and why's of intergenerational programming. Retrieved Feb. 2006 from Penn State, College of Agricultural Sciences Web Site: http://intergenerational.cas.psu.edu/Docs/whatswhys.pdf.

Kendig, H. (1986). Perspectives on ageing and families. In H. Kendig, (Ed.). *Ageing and Families*. Sydney, Australia: Allen and Unwin.

Lewis, L. (2002, August). Intergenerational programs that really work. Retrieved Feb. 2006 from American Medical Director's Association: http://www.amda.com/caring/August 2002/intergenerational.htm.

Mandel, D., Jackson, J., Zemke, R., Nelson, L., & Clark, F. (1999). *Lifestyle Redesign: Implementing the Well Elderly Program*. Bethesda: American Occupational Therapy Association.

Mosby's Medical, Nursing, and Allied Health Dictionary. (4th ed., 1994) St. Louis: Mosby.

National Institute of Health. (1999). Trans-NIH work group on health disparities. Retrieved 2006 from: http://www.nider.nih.gov/Research/Health Disparities/Trans Work Group.htm.

Newman, S., Ward, C. R., Smith, T. B., Wilson, J. O., & McCrea, J. M. (1997). *Intergenerational Programs: Past, present and future*. Washington, DC: Taylor and Francis.

Reis, H. T., Sheldon, K. M., Gable, S. L., Roscoe, J., & Ryan, R. M. (2000). Daily well-being: The role of autonomy, competence, and relatedness. *Personality and Social Psychology Bulletin 26*(4), 419–435.

Ryan, R., & Deci, E. (2000). Self-determination theory and the facilitation of intrinsic motivation, social development, and well-being. *American Psychologist 55*(1), 68–78.

Ryan, R. M., Kuhl, J., & Deci, E.L. (1997). Nature and autonomy: Organizational view of social and neurobiological aspects of self-regulation in behavior and development. *Development and Psychopathology 9*, 701–728.

Scaffa, M. (2001). *Occupational Therapy in Community-Based Settings*. Philadelphia: Davis.

Sheldon, K. M., Ryan, R. M., & Reis, H. (1996). What makes for a good day? Competence and Autonomy in the day and in the person. *Personality and Social Psychology Bulletin 22*, 1270–1279.

Siebert, C. (2002). Aging in place: Implications for occupational therapy. *O.T. Practice.* (May 5, 2003; CE 1–17). Bethesda, MD: American Occupational Therapy Association.

Sultz, H. & Young, K. (2004). *Health Care USA: Understanding its' organization and delivery.* Sudbury, MA: Jones and Bartlett.

Taylor, A. S., & Dryfoos, J. G. (1998/1999). Creating a safe passage: Elder mentors and vulnerable youths. *Generations* 22(4), 43–48.

United States Census Bureau. (2004). More diversity, slower growth. (retrieved 2/11/06) http://www.census.gov.

United States Census Bureau. (2001). An aging world. Washington, DC: author. http://www.census.gov

United States Department of Health and Human Services. (1998). Healthy people 2010: Objectives: draft for public comment. Washington, DC: author.

United States Department of Health and Human Services. (1990). Healthy people 2000: National health promotion and disease prevention objective. Washington, DC: author.

Wilcock, A. (1998). *An occupational perspective of health.* Thorofare, NJ: Slack.

World Health Organization (1986). The Ottawa charter for health promotion. *Health Promotion*, I, iii–v.

# Index

*Note:* Page numbers followed by *f* denotes figures.